Techniques in Bedside Hemodynamic Monitoring

Techniques in Bedside Hemodynamic Monitoring

ELAINE KIESS DAILY RN, BS

Consultant in Clinical Cardiovascular Research and Education
Madison, Wisconsin

JOHN SPEER SCHROEDER MD

Professor of Medicine (Cardiology)
Cardiology Division, Department of Medicine
Stanford University School of Medicine
Stanford, California

FIFTH EDITION

with 275 illustrations

M Mosby

St. Louis Baltimore Berlin Boston Carlsbad Chicago London Madrid
Naples New York Philadelphia Sydney Tokyo Toronto

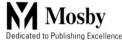
Mosby
Dedicated to Publishing Excellence

Editor: Timothy M. Griswold
Developmental Editor: Jolynn Gower
Project Manager: Patricia Tannian
Senior Production Editor: Betty Hazelwood
Senior Book Designer: Gail Morey Hudson
Cover Designer: Teresa Breckwoldt
Manufacturing Supervisor: Betty Richmond

FIFTH EDITION

Printed in the United States of America
Composition by Graphic World, Inc.
Printing/binding by Maple-Vail Book Mfg Group

Mosby–Year Book, Inc.
11830 Westline Industrial Drive
St. Louis, Missouri 63146

Library of Congress Cataloging in Publication Data

Daily, Elaine Kiess.
    Techniques in bedside hemodynamic monitoring / Elaine Kiess Daily,
John Speer Schroeder. — 5th ed.
        p.   cm.
    Includes bibliographical references and index.
    ISBN 0-8016-7260-0
    1. Hemodynamic monitoring.   2. Hemodynamics.   I. Schroeder, John
Speer.   II. Title.
    [DNLM: 1. Monitoring, Physiologic—methods.   2. Hemodynamics.   WG
106 D133t   1994]
    RC670.5.H45D35   1994
    616.1'0754—dc20
    DNLM/DLC
    for Library of Congress   93-46952
                                                                                      CIP

94 95 96 97 98   /   9 8 7 6 5 4 3 2 1

Contributors

PAT O. DAILY, MD

Director
Cardiac Surgery
Sharp Memorial Hospital
San Diego, California

MARY FRAN HAZINSKI, RN, MSN

Pediatric Critical Care Clinical Specialist
Vanderbilt University Medical Center
Nashville, Tennessee

RONALD PEARL, MD

Associate Director
Intensive Care Unit and Stanford Medical Transport Program
Stanford Medical Center
Stanford, California

To
AUBURN

Preface

The abilities and the responsibilities of members of the critical care team have expanded substantially over the past few years. The advances made in hemodynamic monitoring within the past two decades relate not only to technologic changes, but also to our increased knowledge of pathophysiologic mechanisms, as well as the more aggressive medical management of the critically ill patient.

Technologic advances in hemodynamic monitoring have provided the clinician with the ability to rapidly determine and monitor numerous cardiopulmonary and tissue oxygenation parameters at the bedside. However, these advances must be accompanied by a clear understanding of the physiologic and technologic principles of hemodynamic monitoring to make hemodynamic monitoring safe, appropriate, and helpful.

Several studies have identified deficiencies in critical care physicians' and nurses' knowledge of important aspects of hemodynamic monitoring—particularly in the correct identification and accurate measurement of the pulmonary artery wedge (PAW) pressure waveform.[1,2,3] The average accuracy in the correct identification of a PAW waveform by critical care physicians was 57% in Komadina's study and 53% in Iberti's study.[1,2] A recent survey of critical care nurses revealed very similar knowledge deficiencies, with only 58% correctly identifying a PAW waveform.[3] Overall knowledge of hemodynamic monitoring was somewhat lower among critical care nurses (48.5%) compared with that of physicians (67%).[2,3]

Because the PAW pressure represents one of the basic components of hemodynamic monitoring, correct identification of this waveform is essential to safe hemodynamic monitoring. Decisions regarding therapeutic interventions are based on the assumed accuracy of the hemodynamic data obtained. In addition, serious complications associated with spontaneous catheter wedging can be avoided only if the waveform can be identified and corrective measures undertaken rapidly. Clearly, the onus of this responsibility falls to the critical care nurse who is vigilantly monitoring the patient.

---

[1] Komadina KH, Schenk DA, LaVeau P, Duncan CA, Chambers SL: Interobserver variability in the interpretation of pulmonary artery catheter pressure tracings, *Chest* 100:1647-1654, 1991.

[2] Iberti TJ, Fischer EP, Leibowitz AB, et al. and the Pulmonary Artery Catheter Study Group: A multicenter study of physicians' knowledge of the pulmonary artery catheter, *JAMA* 264:2928-2932, 1990.

[3] Iberti TJ, Daily EK, Leibowitz AB, et al. and the Pulmonary Artery Catheter Study Group: Critical care nurses' knowledge of the pulmonary artery catheter, *Crit Care Med* (in press).

The purpose of the revised, fifth edition of this book continues to be the presentation of the principles and techniques of hemodynamic monitoring in a simple, practical way that will ensure its utility to all health care personnel involved in hemodynamic monitoring. Its goal is to expand the knowledge base of the critical care practitioner such that hemodynamic monitoring of the critically ill patient becomes helpful—not detrimental.

We have updated and expanded the technical aspects of this book by including a discussion of the principles and methods of continuous cardiac output monitoring, as well as right ventricular volumetric measurements. More waveforms have been included to enhance correct waveform identification and interpretation. However, the reader is referred to our companion book *Hemodynamic Waveforms: Exercises in Interpretation and Analysis* to obtain greater practice and skill in waveform identification.

Recommendations regarding specific technical aspects of hemodynamic monitoring have been included and/or updated when scientific evidence is available to support them. This represents a major change from the first edition of this book, in which little or no data were available to support certain practices, and allows the ability to standardize techniques to promote accuracy, as well as efficiency.

It is our hope that this book will continue to be used and referred to frequently to help the novice, as well as the experienced critical care practitioner, to minimize all potential risks of hemodynamic monitoring while maximizing its potential benefits.

Elaine Kiess Daily
John Speer Schroeder

Acknowledgments

We are grateful to many of our colleagues who have shared their expertise, as well as unique or interesting waveform samples — some of which are depicted in this book. In particular, we thank the critical care nurses at the University of Wisconsin Hospital, Madison, and at Stanford University Medical Center, Laura Toledo of San Diego, Sue Engelbaugh of Madison, Wisconsin, and Dr. Michael Jastremski of New York for providing a variety of interesting and educational waveform samples and a case study.

Contents

Appendixes

Chapter 1

The Heart as a Pump

The function of the heart is to pump blood returning from other parts of the body to the lungs and into the aorta. This process delivers oxygenated blood and nutrients to peripheral tissues via the vascular system and removes metabolic waste products. Bedside hemodynamic monitoring permits minute-to-minute surveillance of the cardiovascular system and provides the physiologic data to guide therapy. This chapter reviews basic principles of cardiac physiology and anatomy as they pertain to hemodynamic monitoring.

FUNCTIONAL ULTRASTRUCTURE OF THE MYOCARDIAL CELL

The myocardial cell, or myocardial fiber, is the basic unit of the ventricular myocardium (Fig. 1-1). Composed of multiple linearly arranged myocardial fibrils and a cell nucleus, it is separated from other myocardial fibers by intercalated disks. These intercalated disks are true cell boundaries but have very low electrical impedance, so that electrical impulses can travel rapidly throughout the myocardium. The myocardial fibril, or myofibril, is composed of *sarcomeres,* the basic functional unit of the myocardium. These sarcomeres are composed of contractile proteins called *myofilaments,* specifically *myosin filaments* and *actin filaments.* Mitochondria are distributed in the myocardial cell between myofibrils and, by the process of oxidative phosphorylation, are the major source of energy for cell function. The last major component of the myocardial cell is the *sarcoplasmic reticulum,* which surrounds the cell. The sarcoplasmic reticulum is a complex network that interconnects between myofibrils, so that it is adjacent to the surfaces of individual sarcomeres. Not only is it in direct relationship to the sarcomere, but it also is in continuity with the extracellular space and serves as the transport mechanism for ionic movement and ionic control of contraction. Individual myocardial fibers are also surrounded by cell surface membranes, the *sarcolemma.*

The sarcomere is the contractile unit of the heart and is similar to the contractile unit of skeletal muscle. The thicker myofilaments of the sarcomere are the myosin filaments and are limited to the A band of the sarcomere. The thinner actin filaments begin at the Z band and interdigitate with the myosin filaments (see Fig. 1-1, C). The relationship between the actin and myosin filaments depends on the sarcomere length, which is determined by the amount of stretch of the myocardial fibers. There is maximal contact between the actin and myosin filaments when the sarcomere is 2.2

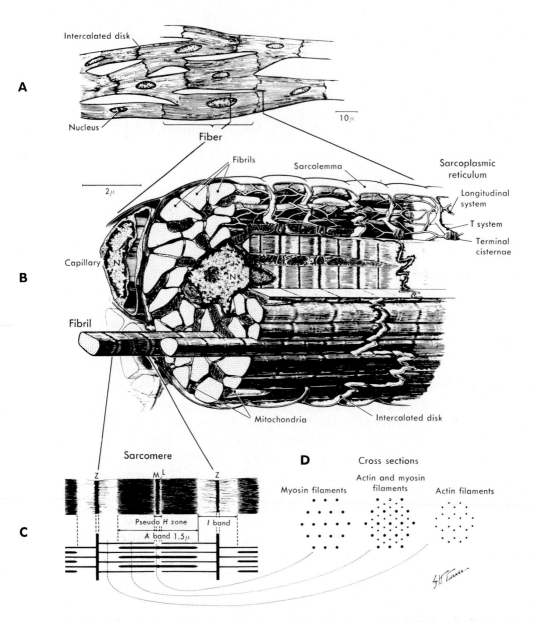

Fig. 1-1. Microscopic structure of heart muscle. **A,** Myocardium as seen under the light microscope. Branching of fibers is evident; each fiber contains a centrally located nucleus. **B,** Myocardial cell or fiber reconstructed from electron micrographs; the arrangements of the multiple parallel fibrils composing the cell and of the serially connected sarcomeres composing the fibrils are apparent (*N,* nucleus). **C,** Arrangement of myofilaments making up an individual sarcomere from a myofibril with thick (myosin) filaments 1.5 μ in length, forming the A band, and thin (actin) filaments 1.0 μ in length, extending from the Z band through the I band into the A band, ending at the edges of the H zone. (An H zone exists in the central area of the A band, where thin filaments are absent; overlapping of thick and thin filaments is seen only in the A band.) **D,** Cross sections of the sarcomere indicating the specific lattice arrangements of the myofilaments. In the center of the sarcomere *(left)* only thick filaments arranged in a hexagon are seen; in the distal portions of the A band *(center)* both thick and thin filaments are found (each thick filament is surrounded by six thin filaments); in the I band *(right)* only thin filaments are present.

From Braunwald E et al: *N Engl J Med* 277(15):794-800, 1967. Reprinted by permission from the *New England Journal of Medicine.*

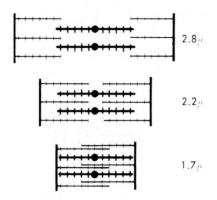

Fig. 1-2. As the sarcomere is shortened or lengthened from 2.2 μ, actin-myosin interactions are fewer and less contractile force is generated.

μ in length. If the sarcomere is shorter or longer than 2.2 μ, force development decreases (Fig. 1-2). When the sarcomere is stretched to approximately 3.6 μ, tension development no longer exists, because there is no contact between the actin and myosin filaments. In contrast, when the sarcomere is shorter than 2.0 μ before contraction, tension development is less, since the filaments bypass one another and overlap. As the volume and radius of the ventricle increase in response to either increased diastolic filling pressure or volume, the myocardial fibers lengthen, reflecting an increase in sarcomere length.

Huxley and others explained the shortening of the sarcomere by the sliding filament or ratcheting mechanism. It is believed that when the sarcomere is activated electrically, interaction between the actin and myosin filaments takes place, so that the filaments actually slide or ratchet by each other, shortening the sarcomere. This contractile process requires adenosine triphosphate (ATP) and proper concentrations of calcium, magnesium, and other ions. The sarcoplasmic reticulum plays a critical role in initiation, control, and reversal of reactions between the actin and myosin filaments. This basic function of the sarcomere serves as the basis for length-tension curves and for the Frank-Starling law. Studies by Braunwald, Ross, and Sonnenblick on the relationship of the sarcomere to cardiac performance have been reviewed.

To explain relaxation of the sarcomere, Hill proposed a model involving a series elastic element that is stretched during contraction and results in return of the original sarcomere length during relaxation (Fig. 1-3). This model also considers viscous elements to explain changes in the sarcomere's rapidity of relaxation when it returns to its original length. More recently, Sonnenblick and associates have proposed other models to explain certain characteristics of the isolated heart muscle. The elastic element is probably not a separate anatomic entity in the sarcomere; rather, it serves primarily as a model to explain characteristics of relaxation and resting tension.

In summary, the basic functional unit of contraction is the sarcomere, which is composed of myofilaments—contractile proteins that interdigitate and slide by one another during contraction, shortening the sarcomere. Physiologic and pharmacologic agents used to change contraction operate to affect this interaction.

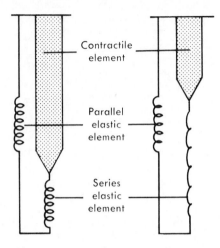

Fig. 1-3. Hill model for muscle contraction-relaxation. As the contractile element contracts, the series elastic element is stretched. When the contractile element relaxes, the series elastic element returns the contractile element to its resting length. The parallel elastic element is primarily responsible for resting tension and viscosity (resistance to sudden stretch).

FUNCTIONAL GROSS ANATOMY OF THE CARDIOVASCULAR SYSTEM

It is beyond the purpose of this book to describe the basic anatomy of the heart and vascular system. The following is a review of several aspects of the functional anatomy of the cardiovascular system that are pertinent to the understanding of hemodynamic changes in the critically ill patient.

Cardiac Innervation

Autonomic innervation to the heart is extensive. Sympathetic nerve fibers are found throughout the atria and the ventricles, including the sinoatrial (SA) and atrioventricular (AV) nodes. Parasympathetic fibers are found primarily in the atria and SA and AV nodes but extend into the ventricles as well. The autonomic nervous system has a significant influence on regulation of impulse formation and on conduction of the excitation impulse. It also influences contractility of both the atria and the ventricles.

Sympathetic innervation arises in the upper thoracic spinal cord and reaches the heart via cervical ganglia, giving rise to the cardiac nerves. These nerves form the cardiac plexus, which surrounds the root of the aorta and has fibers extending to the SA and AV nodes and to the right and left coronary arteries.

Parasympathetic innervation originates in the medulla oblongata and goes to the heart via the vagus nerve, joining sympathetic fibers in the cardiac plexus. Stimulation of the vagus nerve produces cardiac slowing and inhibits AV conduction. Because there are few parasympathetic nerve fibers in the ventricular myocardium, the vagus nerve has little effect on contractility except by its indirect effect on heart rate.

Sensory pain fibers are present in the pericardium, connective tissue adventitia, and myocardium and pass via sympathetic plexuses through thoracic dorsal ganglia.

The impulses then ascend via the ventral spinal thalamic tract, terminating in the posteroventral nucleus of the thalamus. These fibers may be important for reflex responses of the heart to ischemia and injury.

Regulation of the Peripheral Vascular System

Peripheral blood flow is controlled by local autoregulation and the nervous system. The exact function of autoregulation is poorly understood but may depend on several mechanisms:

1. Local metabolic tissue demands. Blood flow is regulated to meet the oxygen requirements of the tissues. With decreased flow, metabolic byproducts increase causing vasodilation and increased blood flow.
2. Intraluminal stretch and pressure. Autonomic constriction of smooth muscle of the vessel wall occurs in response to increased intraluminal stretch and pressure. With decreased stretch and pressure, the vessel relaxes and dilates.
3. Turgor. Increased luminal pressure causes increased fluid in surrounding local tissue (turgor), which compresses small, thin-walled vessels and reduces blood flow.

Nervous system control is accomplished primarily by sympathetic effects on peripheral vessels from a vasomotor center in the medulla oblongata. This sympathetic activity affects mainly the arterioles, capillaries, and venules. The vasomotor center operates in conjunction with a vagal parasympathetic center, which affects cardiac performance and some capacitance vessels. The vasomotor center is influenced by many autonomic, reflex, and supratentorial factors, including barore-ceptors, chemoreceptors, the hypothalamus, and the cerebral cortex.

Baroreceptors are pressure and stretch receptors that are located in the carotid sinus and aortic arch. As arterial blood pressure rises, these receptors sense the pressure rise and respond with an increased rate of firing signals, which inhibit the vasomotor center, with a resultant fall in vessel tone and pressure. Reflex vagal-induced bradycardia contributes to this response. In arterial hypotension the reverse effect occurs, and increased vasoconstriction causes the blood pressure to rise.

Chemoreceptors in the carotid sinus and elsewhere regulate respiration by responding to changes in Pa_{CO_2} and Pa_{O_2}. These changes also influence the vasomotor center.

The *hypothalamus* affects the vasomotor center principally in response to temperature-regulating mechanisms, resulting in changes in peripheral circulation.

The *cerebral cortex* influence on the vasomotor center can be noted during excitement (blushing may occur) or emotionally induced syncope.

The end result of these varying metabolic and neurally mediated influences generally is termed *peripheral resistance*. Because inappropriate increases in periph-eral resistance can adversely affect cardiac output and tissue perfusion, this calculation provides a major means of monitoring the circulatory status of the seriously ill cardiac patient. Clinically, the systemic pressure gradient is divided by the cardiac output (CO) to estimate resistance and then is multiplied by 80 to yield $dynes/sec/cm^{-5}$.

$$\text{Peripheral resistance} = \frac{\text{Mean arterial pressure} - \text{Central venous pressure}}{\text{CO (L/min)}} \times 80$$

Because it is possible to accomplish rapid reductions in peripheral resistance with pharmacologic agents (such as nitroprusside), which improve cardiac output at little "expense" to the myocardial oxygen requirements, this measurement is an essential one in critical care cardiology.

Pulmonary Circulation

The pulmonary arterial vessels differ markedly from the systemic vessels; they have thinner walls, less medial muscle, and a resistance to flow that is approximately 6 times less than that of the systemic vessels. For example, in patients with left-to-right shunts there can be a threefold to fourfold increase in flow before any significant rise in pressure or resistance occurs. The pressure in the systemic capillaries is 25 to 35 mm Hg; the pressure in the pulmonary capillaries is 7 to 10 mm Hg. Thus there is relatively little interstitial fluid in the lung at these pressures, and pulmonary edema does not occur until a pulmonary capillary pressure of 25 to 30 mm Hg is reached.

Coronary Circulation

The right and left anterior descending and circumflex coronary arteries are epicardial arteries that run along the surface of the heart and act as passive conduits, each carrying approximately 100 ml of blood per minute. This blood flow is distributed by perforating dividing branches that terminate in arterioles, which account for the majority of autoregulation. A dense capillary network supplies the working myocardium with 6 to 8 ml of oxygen/100 g/min — approximately 20 times the oxygen utilization of skeletal muscle. At rest, only about one third of the capillaries are perfused. In response to increased myocardial oxygen demands, oxygen utilization increases threefold to sixfold, coronary vasodilation occurs, and capillaries open to allow additional perfusion of the myocardium. This dramatic ability to alter coronary blood flow in the normal heart is referred to as *autoregulation* and responds to changes in myocardial tension. Autoregulation usually is maintained at coronary perfusion pressures of 60 to 80 mm Hg. Coronary perfusion pressures less than 40 mm Hg generally result in little or no flow or myocardial perfusion.

Coronary blood flow is a phasic process that is affected by the degree of vasoconstriction or vasodilation of the epicardial as well as the resistance vessels. In addition, flow is markedly reduced during systole when myocardial tension development tends to collapse the coronary arteries and veins. Therefore the majority (as much as 85%) of coronary flow to the myocardium — at least to the left ventricle — occurs during diastole. As heart rate increases, the diastolic period shortens and adversely affects coronary flow, with as much as 50% of the coronary flow occurring during systole at high heart rates.

Atherosclerotic lesions adversely affect coronary flow once approximately 75% of the coronary lumen becomes occluded with plaque. Multiple lesions in a vessel result in further pressure gradients, which are difficult to estimate but which, almost certainly, result in ischemia downstream when myocardial oxygen demands rise. Recently it has been demonstrated that areas of atherosclerotic plaquing tend to be *hyperreactive* to vasoactive influences and do not respond appropriately to autoregulatory demands. For example, localized *vasoconstriction* in a plaque has been demonstrated during exercise in patients with occlusive coronary artery disease and exertional angina. This suggests that not only mechanical obstruction, but dynamic obstruction can contribute to exertional angina. The use of anti-ischemia drugs, which vasodilate, may be especially beneficial in such patients.

Local autoregulation of a coronary vessel likely reflects metabolic changes, as well as possible myogenic alterations. One proposed autoregulatory agent is adenosine, which is a metabolic product of ATP released during muscle contraction. The amount of adenosine released is related to the degree of work (and demand). Adenosine diffuses into the vascular wall and causes local vasodilation. Local control is also affected by endothelium derived relaxant factor (EDRF), which is believed to be nitric oxide (NO), a potent vasodilator. Multiple other local substances, such as prostaglandin/prostacycline, catecholamine, and serotonin, likely further influence the vascular tone at any given moment.

CARDIAC CYCLE

The sequence of events occurring during the cardiac cycle is best divided into systole and diastole, as described by Wiggers' classic diagram (Fig. 1-4). *Isovolumic contraction* is the first phase of systole and results in mitral and tricuspid valve closure, which produces the first heart sound. With a continuing rise in ventricular pressure the aortic and pulmonic valves open and blood is ejected from the ventricles. As the volume of ejecting blood falls, the pressure decreases until the aortic and pulmonic valves close, producing the second sound. *Isovolumic relaxation* then follows as the pressure continues to fall in the ventricles until it is lower than the pressure in the atria. At this time there is *rapid ventricular filling,* which is initiated by the opening of the mitral and tricuspid valves. If the mitral valve is stenotic, there may be an opening snap at this point. As blood rushes into the ventricles, the ventricular walls suddenly expand; if there is decreased compliance because of disease or hypertrophy, an S_3 sound, or gallop, may occur. As diastolic filling continues, ventricular diastolic pressure rises until atrial systole occurs, which causes further ejection of blood from the atria into the ventricles. This rapid filling can produce an S_4 sound if there is resistance to filling or if atrial systole is vigorous.

Abnormalities in impulse conduction patterns may result in one ventricle contracting and relaxing before the other, causing abnormalities in the relationship between the first and second sounds. Abnormalities in flow across valves, either during diastole or systole, result in murmurs caused by turbulence of blood flow. These murmurs and sounds are described more completely in Chapter 2.

CONTROL OF CARDIAC PERFORMANCE

Homeostatic mechanisms regulating cardiac output involve not only factors controlling performance of the pump, but also factors affecting the peripheral vascular system and resistance. Normally, the heart can vary its cardiac output up to 5 or 6 times the resting level, depending on the age and physical condition of the person. Some aspects of the regulatory mechanism vary continuously; for example, sinus dysrhythmia during the respiratory cycle is a result of continuous change in the balance between parasympathetic and sympathetic tone on the sinus

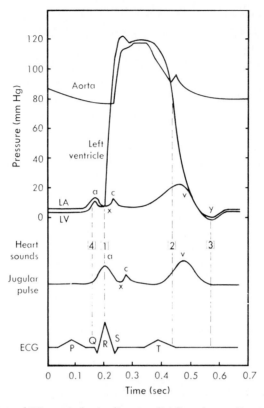

Fig. 1-4. Modification of Wiggers' classic diagram dividing the cardiac cycle into systole and diastole. Simultaneous ECG, jugular pulse, heart sounds, and left-sided pressure events are diagramed. Right atrial (RA) and right ventricular (RV) pressure tracings are omitted for the sake of simplicity. The *a* wave of the left atrial (LA) pressure follows electrical atrial systole (the P wave) and may produce an S_4 heart sound. As ventricular systole occurs, the mitral valve closes, causing part of the first heart sound and producing a *c* wave in the atrial pressure tracing. As isovolumic contraction continues, pressure rises in the left ventricle until it exceeds the aortic pressure and opens the aortic valve. In late systole a *v* wave in the left atrium and jugular venous tracing reflects bulging of the atrioventricular (AV) valve into the atrium. As the left ventricular (LV) pressure falls, the aortic pressure exceeds it, closing the aortic valve and producing part of the second heart sound. The LV pressure continues to fall until the LA pressure exceeds it, opening the mitral valve. As blood rushes into the left ventricle from the left atrium, an S_3 sound may occur. Note the delay in transmission of pressure waves to the jugular pulse in comparison with LA or ECG timing.

Modified from Hurst JW, Logue RB, editors: *The heart,* New York, 1974, McGraw-Hill.

node. Other regulatory mechanisms vary little until challenged by disease or a demand for increased cardiac output. This section briefly describes regulatory mechanisms affecting the hemodynamic performance of the heart as they relate to cardiovascular monitoring.

There are two basic methods by which the heart regulates cardiac output in response to stress or disease. Because cardiac output equals heart rate times stroke volume, the heart may respond by altering either of these factors to maintain or increase the output.

Changes in Heart Rate

Because of the rapidity of its response, a change in heart rate is the most effective method of changing cardiac output. An increase in heart rate can double or triple the cardiac output, particularly in a healthy person, who could develop a heart rate of 170 or 180 beats per minute (bpm). In the patient with cardiac disease, however, a heart rate over 120 bpm may have deleterious effects because of the resultant increased myocardial oxygen demand and the decreased time for diastolic coronary blood flow. Rapid or instantaneous changes in heart rate are effected by the autonomic nervous system via its influence on the SA pacemaker. In addition, the heart rate can increase in response to circulating catecholamines, as can be seen in the denervated heart during exercise. When the heart rate increases, a slight increase in ventricular contractility occurs (Bowditch's law).

Decreases in heart rate to approximately 50 bpm may not decrease cardiac output, because diastolic filling time is increased, which increases stroke volume. However, below this rate cardiac performance may be affected, particularly in the diseased heart.

Changes in Stroke Volume

The stroke volume of an intact ventricle is influenced by three factors: (1) ventricular end-diastolic volume (preload), (2) ventricular afterload, and (3) contractility. Although these three factors operate simultaneously to determine the stroke volume, they are discussed separately as they relate to the hemodynamic performance of the heart.

Ventricular end-diastolic volume (preload)

Because the end-diastolic volume profoundly influences the myocardial fiber length and ultimately the sarcomere length (as discussed earlier), it also has a great influence on myocardial performance. The Frank-Starling law describes the principle for this factor and was based on work by Wiggers and Straub, who concluded that the mechanical energies set free when the sarcomere moves from a relaxed to a contracted state depend on the area of chemically interactive surfaces between the actin and myosin filaments; therefore these energies depend on the length of the muscle fibers. Because a change in myocardial fiber length affects sarcomere shortening and stroke volume, the Frank-Starling law accounts for minute-to-minute changes in stroke volume of both the right and the left ventricles. In response to disease, rises in end-diastolic pressure and volume also provide a compensatory increase in stroke volume because of the increase in the myocardial fiber length of the remaining functioning myocardial cells. However, the diseased and markedly dilated heart actually can have a decreased stroke volume because of areas of fibrosis and slippage of myocardial fibers past one another.

Fig. 1-5 shows the relationship between left ventricular (LV) end-diastolic fiber length and stroke work or volume. As fiber length increases, stroke work increases until the sarcomere is stretched past the optimal length of 2.2 μ, at which point there is maximal contact between actin and myosin filaments. A change in the relationship between end-diastolic fiber length and stroke volume therefore reflects a change in contractility.

In the normally functioning heart the end-diastolic volume is determined by four major factors: (1) diastolic filling pressure, (2) total blood volume, (3) distribution of

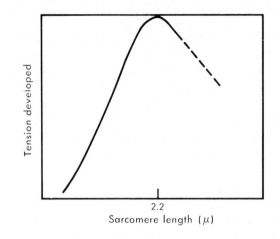

Fig. 1-5. Ultrastructural basis for the Frank-Starling curve showing that peak tension development occurs at a sarcomere length of 2.2 μ; whether a downslope of the curve after peak tension exists is questionable.

blood volume, and (4) atrial systole. The major determinants of *diastolic filling pressure* are central venous return, blood volume, and pressure generated in the atria. In general, an increase in diastolic filling pressure results in increased myocardial stretch and, by the Frank-Starling law, increased shortening. If the *total blood volume* is depleted, as during hemorrhage, diastolic-filling pressures may fall and affect stroke volume. The *distribution of blood volume* is of critical importance, because it affects central venous return to the right side of the heart. Such factors as body position, intrathoracic pressure, intrapericardial pressure (as in cardiac tamponade), and venous tone will affect blood return from the body to the right side of the heart and will thus affect stroke volume. *Atrial systole* results in an increase in atrial pressure and increased diastolic filling of the left ventricle at the end of diastole just before ventricular systole. This mechanism is particularly important for increasing end-diastolic volume in the patient with decreased ventricular compliance, such as that seen with LV hypertrophy. These patients may have a disastrous fall in stroke volume and cardiac output when atrial fibrillation occurs because of the loss of atrial systole.

Ventricular afterload

The ventricular stroke volume is critically determined by the extent of myocardial fiber shortening during systole. The primary factor that determines the extent of shortening, in addition to the fiber's initial length, is the *afterload* or resistance to flow from the ventricle. Thus as the LV outflow pressure increases because of hypertension or other factors (such as aortic stenosis), stroke volume may gradually decrease because of increased resistance to systolic ejection of blood from the ventricle. Conversely, as resistance falls (during exercise, sepsis, or therapeutically induced afterload reduction), stroke volume increases at the same level of myocardial contractility. The concept of decreasing afterload or resistance to flow during systole is important and can be applied pharmacologically or mechanically to treat the failing ventricle.

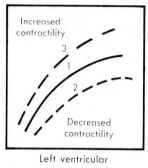

Fig. 1-6. Relationship between left ventricular (LV) end-diastolic fiber length (sarcomere length) and LV work. Curve 1 represents normal function; curve 2 shows depressed function (negative inotropy or contractility); and curve 3 shows increased function (positive inotropy or contractility) at the same fiber length.

Contractility

The level or degree of ventricular performance at any given end-diastolic volume and afterload depends on the contractile state of the ventricle. Multiple influences can modify the simple relationship between ventricular end-diastolic volume and performance (Fig. 1-6). Each of these influences may shift the ventricular performance to a different curve or change the relationship between end-diastolic volume and performance or stroke volume.

Sympathetic influence is one of the most important regulatory factors for myocardial contractility. Rapid changes may be initiated via the sympathetic nervous system or more slowly via catecholamines circulating from the adrenal medulla and other sympathetic ganglia outside the heart. The heart rate has a slight effect on contractility (Bowditch's law), as discussed, but changes in rhythm can have a marked effect on the relationship between end-diastolic volume and performance.

Metabolic abnormalities (e.g., hypoxemia, hypercapnia, or metabolic acidosis) decrease myocardial contractility regardless of the cause. Loss of myocardial viability can decrease performance of the remaining normal myocardium because of changes in ventricular diameter and wall stress.

Finally, pharmacologic agents that can alter the contractile state of the ventricle can be administered. Positive inotropic agents include epinephrine, digitalis, isoproterenol, dopamine, dobutamine, amrinone, and milrinone. There are also multiple agents that can decrease the contractile state of the ventricle. These agents include antidysrhythmic agents, such as procainamide, and drugs that cause beta-receptor blockade, such as propranolol.

Other factors, such as the ionic state and abnormalities in metabolism, may influence the intrinsic contractile state of the ventricle, but these factors are poorly understood at this time.

DETERMINANTS OF MYOCARDIAL OXYGEN CONSUMPTION

As an aerobically pumping organ, the heart requires a continuous supply of oxygen to develop sufficient energy to maintain its pumping function. The primary determinants of the amount of oxygen needed or consumed by the myocardium ($M\dot{V}O_2$) are wall tension, contractility, and heart rate.

Factors that cannot be influenced as much by pharmacologic or mechanical means are (1) the basal resting metabolism of the myocardium, (2) the external work performed by the heart, and (3) the energy required for activation-relaxation of the ventricle. This section concerns only those factors that can be easily altered during hemodynamic monitoring.

Myocardial Tension

It is now recognized that wall tension is a major factor in determining myocardial oxygen demands. The myocardial tension of the ventricle is a direct function of the intraventricular pressure (systolic pressure) and the ventricle's radius and is inversely related to wall thickness. This is expressed by the LaPlace Law:

$$T = \frac{Pr}{2h}$$

where: T = Wall tension
P = Intraventricular pressure
r = Radius of the ventricle
h = Thickness of the ventricle

From this formula, it is clear that wall tension, and therefore myocardial oxygen consumption ($M\dot{V}O_2$), increases with increases in heart size and intraventricular pressure, but decreases with hypertrophy.

Monitoring of systolic arterial blood pressure and heart rate (rate pressure product) provides a global reflection of myocardial oxygen demands.

Contractile State

A direct relationship exists between an increase in the contractile state and myocardial oxygen demands. Changes in the contractile state must be differentiated from other effects of changes in the heart rate and preload or afterload.

Heart Rate

A direct relationship exists between heart rate and myocardial oxygen demands, primarily because of the increase in the number of times tension is being exerted per minute. This relationship is a major factor in determining oxygen consumption and is important in the treatment of the patient with myocardial ischemia, particularly since the increased heart rate also decreases the diastolic period and therefore myocardial oxygen delivery.

Summary

In summary, stroke volume may be affected by factors influencing total blood volume and central venous return, resistance to forward systolic ejection of the blood in the ventricle, and the contractile state of the myocardium, which responds to multiple factors, including autonomic tone, disease, and drug intervention.

The coronary circulation can respond to wide changes in demand for myocardial perfusion and oxygenation. Autoregulation is a complex neural and hormonal process, which can be affected adversely by the atherosclerotic process. The relationships between these factors during myocardial insult, such as infarction, are discussed in subsequent chapters. Their physiologic relationships must be kept in mind during hemodynamic monitoring of the critically ill patient with cardiovascular disease.

REFERENCES

Benzig G III et al: Evaluation of left ventricular performance: circumferential fiber shortening and tension, *Circ* 49:925-932, 1974.

Berne RM, Knabb RM, Ely SW, Rubio R: Adenosine in the local regulation of blood flow: a brief overview, *Fed Proc* 42:3136-3142, 1983.

Braunwald E: Regulation of the circulation, *N Engl J Med* 290:1124-1129, 1974.

Braunwald E, Ross J, Jr, Sonnenblick EH: Mechanisms of contraction of the normal and failing heart, *N Engl J Med* 277:795-800, 1967.

Feigl EO: Coronary physiology, *Physiol Rev* 63:1-205, 1983.

Guyton AC: Regulation of cardiac output, *N Engl J Med* 277:805-812, 1967.

Hill AV: Heat of shortening and dynamic constants of muscle, *Proc R Soc Lond Biol* 126:136-195, 1938.

Honig CR: *Modern cardiovascular physiology,* ed 2, Boston, 1988, Little, Brown.

Huxley HE: Structural arrangements and contraction mechanism in striated muscle, *Proc R Soc Lond Biol* 160:442, 1964.

Huxley HE: The mechanism of muscular contraction, *Sci Am* 213:18-27, 1965.

Olsson RA, Bunger R: Metabolic control of coronary blood flow, *Progr Cardiovasc Dis* 19:369-387, 1984.

Sarnoff S: Myocardial contractility as described by ventricular function curves: observations on Starling's law of the heart, *Physiol Rev* 35:107, 1955.

Sarnoff S et al: Homeometric autoregulation in the heart, *Cir Res* 8:1077-1091, 1960.

Schlart RC: Normal physiology of the cardiovascular system. In Hurst JW, Schlart RC, editors: *The heart,* New York, 1990, McGraw-Hill.

Sonnenblick EH: Myocardial ultrastructure in the normal and failing heart, *Hosp Pract* 5:35-43, April 1970.

Sonnenblick EH, Shelton CL: Myocardial energetics: basic principles and clinical implications, *N Engl J Med* 285:668-675, 1971.

Starling EH: The Linacre lecture on the law of the heart, given at Cambridge, 1915, London, 1918, Longman Group, Ltd.

Strobeck JE, Krueger J, Sonnenblick EH: Load and time considerations in the force-length relation of cardiac muscle, *Fed Proc* 39:175-182, 1980.

Strobeck JE, Sonnenblick EH: Myocardial and ventricular function, *Cardiovasc Rev Rep* 4:568-581, 1983.

Wiggers CJ: Some factors controlling the shape of the pressure curve in the right ventricle, *Am J Physiol* 33:382, 1914.

Chapter 2

Monitoring Signs and Symptoms

The patient's history and physical examination are critical components in monitoring minute-to-minute and day-to-day cardiovascular status. The use of invasive and noninvasive monitoring procedures augments and complements rather than replaces these basic techniques. This chapter reviews the techniques of history-taking and physical examination that are applicable to cardiovascular monitoring.

HISTORY AND ANALYSIS OF SYMPTOMS

The patient's complaint, whether it is the severe chest pain of an acute myocardial infarction or transient dizziness during an episode of ventricular tachycardia, is frequently the precipitating factor in initiating medical care. Symptoms can reflect spontaneous changes in cardiovascular status or response to therapy. For example, a patient may complain of progressive dyspnea before any x-ray or auscultatory findings of pulmonary edema are actually detected. Another patient may develop uneasiness or a sense of doom before a major catastrophic event. However, because symptoms may be common to many problems or diseases, a careful analysis of each symptom is necessary to relate its importance to the current illness.

Depending on both the severity of the illness and the patient's individual personality, an open-ended question may provide helpful information. More frequently, however, the person caring for the patient will need to direct the patient's answers through skilled questioning based on the questioner's knowledge of the problem and disease process, triggering responses about certain aspects of the illness. The following is a procedure for clarifying the characteristics of symptoms:

Location: Define the location and origin of the pain, discomfort, or unusual sensation. Radiation to other areas is particularly important.

Severity: Attempt to quantitate the extent and severity of the symptoms in relation to the patient's attitudes and pain or complaint threshold.

Character: Determine the descriptive quality of the symptoms. Is the pain sharp, dull, or burning?

Associated symptoms: Determine whether other sensations accompany the primary symptom. For example, aching in the left arm associated with transient epigastric pressure is much more suggestive of angina than of gastrointestinal problems.

Timing: Determine the duration of the symptoms in comparison with previous episodes. Does the pain last for a longer or shorter time?

Factors altering the symptoms: Determine what factors affect the symptoms. What initiated the symptoms? Do they occur during activity, rest, or sleep? What relieves or partially relieves them? What aggravates them?

These descriptions of a patient's symptoms may allow one to assess progression of disease or development of a new problem or provide a guide for requesting further diagnostic information.

PHYSICAL EXAMINATION
General Inspection

General inspection of the patient may sometimes be overlooked during intensive invasive hemodynamic monitoring. Its importance cannot be overemphasized, because the inspection may provide important information concerning the cardio-vascular status of the patient.

Does the patient appear to be the stated age? Physical appearance may be a better indication of the physiologic status of the patient than is the chronologic age.

Does the patient appear to be in distress? The patient complaining of dyspnea while lying comfortably in bed may have a low complaint threshold. On the other hand, the denying patient may have obvious tachypnea and respiratory distress yet not complain about it.

Does the patient respond appropriately to your questioning and care? Lack of cooperation may reflect a changing mental status caused by either physiologic or psychologic factors.

Is the patient cyanotic or pale? Careful, continued observation for cyanosis may provide the first clue to a diagnosis of decreased peripheral perfusion or pulmonary embolus.

The restless, anxious patient who cannot get comfortable or who is constantly tossing and turning may reflect a deteriorating cardiovascular status. Not only is the distress disconcerting, but the resulting anxiety and movements may demand increased cardiac output and cause further deterioration of the patient's cardiovascular condition.

Mental Status

A changing mental status in the critically ill patient with cardiovascular disease may indicate the development of a postoperative psychosis or a decrease in cardiac output. Depending on the patient's status, the examination might include evaluation of the following mental abilities:

1. Appropriateness of responses
2. Orientation to time, place, and person
3. Memory for recent and past events
4. Retentive ability, such as the ability to repeat five random numbers from memory

Ability to do calculations, such as serially subtracting 7 from 100
Understanding of the meaning of proverbs

Venous Pulses

Examination of the neck veins is one of the easiest components of the cardiovascular examination and may yield important information regarding a patient's cardiovascular status. Fig. 2-1 shows the distended external jugular vein, which is easiest to examine because it is superficial to the sternocleidomastoid muscles. When distended, the external jugular vein accurately reflects the venous pressure of the right atrium, although apparent lack of distention may be caused by obesity or fibrosis of the vein. At times the external jugular vein can be so distended that it does not pulsate and is actually not noticed until the patient assumes a semiupright or upright position. The anterior jugular vein is of a smaller caliber but usually can be seen when distended. The internal jugular vein is more difficult to examine because of its position below the sternocleidomastoid muscles and next to the carotid artery.

If the venous pressure is normal or near normal, the patient's head and trunk can be elevated just slightly above the horizontal plane. The patient's head should be rotated away from the examiner's side of the bed and the external jugular vein examined for distention. A bedside lamp arranged to shine tangentially across the area being inspected may help to detect a slightly distended vein. If there is no distention, the examiner's finger should be placed horizontally across the base of the suspected location of the external jugular vein (Fig. 2-2). If the external jugular vein fills during

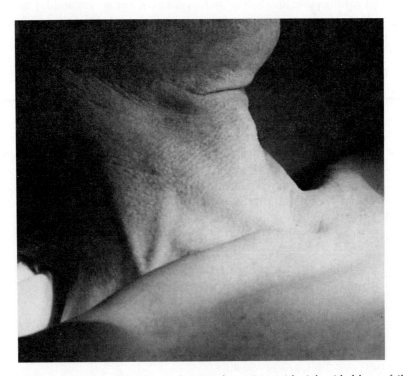

Fig. 2-1. Distended external jugular neck vein of a patient with right-sided heart failure.

pressure application and collapses when pressure is released, the examiner can be sure that the venous pressure is low. The patient's head can then be lowered further to determine the actual venous pressure. Conversely, if the venous pressure is very high, the external jugular veins may be markedly distended without visible pulsation when the patient is in a flat or only slightly upright position. The patient's head should be raised until visible pulsations can be seen in the external jugular vein. A patient with cardiac tamponade, constrictive pericarditis, or severe right heart failure may have a venous pressure higher than 30 cm H_2O, resulting in distended neck veins above the level of the upper neck when the patient is in an upright or standing position. In these patients the veins may be distended even in the temporal area or the forehead.

Venous Pressure

The right-sided venous pressure reflects the right atrial (RA) pressure and right ventricular (RV) end-diastolic pressure. This venous pressure can be measured directly by a central venous catheter or estimated by examination of the neck veins. Although the central venous pressure (CVP) has been shown to have a poor correlation with the pulmonary arterial wedge (PAW) or left atrial (LA) pressure (which reflects left ventricular diastolic filling pressure), the trend of changes in the CVP during monitoring of the seriously ill patient can provide important information concerning the patient's hemodynamic and volume status.

Noninvasive assessment of the venous pressure is particularly important when there are contraindications to invasive measurement or when there is difficulty using

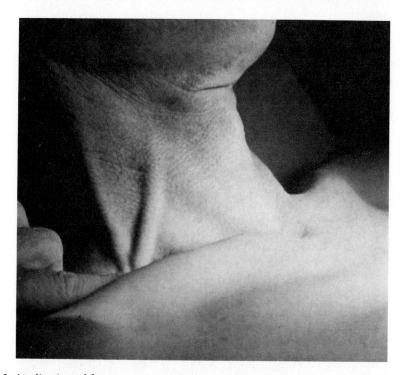

Fig. 2-2. Application of finger pressure at the base of the external jugular vein, causing venous distention. When the finger pressure is released, the venous pressure falls and can be estimated.

or inserting the central venous catheter. In these situations estimation of the pressure from examination of the neck veins may be invaluable in deciding whether pressure measurements are correct or whether the central venous catheter requires replacement.

Method of measurement

An accurate noninvasive measurement of the CVP (RA pressure) is contingent on the following criteria: (1) there is no obstruction to venous flow from the neck veins to the right atrium; and (2) one can approximate the location of the right atrium in the chest. If these criteria are met, CVP can be estimated accurately by the following procedure (Fig. 2-3):

1. Raise the patient's head to a semiupright position. If the patient is in severe RV failure, raise the patient's head to an upright position.
2. Examine the neck for pulsating and distended internal or external jugular veins. If the patient is able to cooperate, have the patient breathe in; look for a fall in the amount of venous distention.
   a. If the neck vein is completely distended, increase the elevation of the patient's head or have the patient stand beside the bed.
   b. If there is no venous distention, lower the patient's head until you can see filling of the vein.
3. Estimate the level at the top of the fluid column within the vein.
4. Estimate the location of the middle of the right atrium.
5. Using a centimeter rule, measure the *vertical* distance between the two locations.

Sources of error. The following are sources of error in the noninvasive measurements of CVP:

1. Inability to visualize the vein in a short, fat neck or in one without a visible external jugular vein.

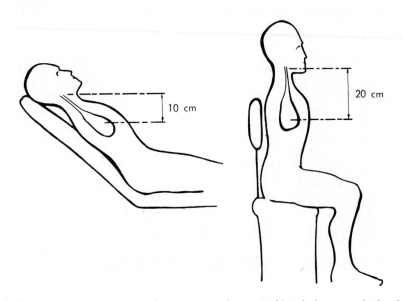

10 cm

20 cm

Fig. 2-3. Estimate of venous pressure by measuring the *vertical* height between the level of the right side of the heart and the meniscus of the distended neck veins.

2. Inability to see the neck veins because of marked distention when the patient is in a supine or semiupright position. (This error is a common one in patients who have constrictive pericarditis or cardiac tamponade and extremely high venous pressures.)
3. Inability to estimate the top of the fluid column because the patient's head cannot be raised.
4. Confusion in identification of venous versus arterial pulsations. (Venous pulsations are easily obliterated by pressure on the neck at the level of the clavicle.)
5. Hypovolemia causing poor distention of neck veins in a supine position.
6. Neck surgery or previous procedures on the neck veins causing local venous distention, which does not reflect true central venous pressure.

Clinical application

CASE 1

A 49-year-old man was admitted to the coronary care unit with an extensive anterior myocardial infarction. Except for frequent premature ventricular contractions that were suppressed by lidocaine hydrochloride, he appeared to be doing well on hospital day 1. Routine CVP ranged from 2 to 6 cm H_2O. On hospital day 3 his CVP steadily rose to as high as 17 cm H_2O. This rise in CVP was accompanied by a slight rise in heart rate, but there was no change in respiratory rate or blood pressure. Blood had been difficult to withdraw from the inserted catheter, although the IV infused fairly well.

Examination of his neck veins revealed no venous distention, and it was suspected that the readings were inaccurate. A new catheter was inserted by Seldinger's technique, and a CVP of 3 cm H_2O was confirmed. This simple examination of the neck veins prevented inappropriate treatment based on artifactual, high venous pressures.

CASE 2

A 35-year-old woman with severe RV and LV failure caused by an idiopathic cardiomyopathy was admitted to the hospital because of increasing dyspnea. Examination revealed severe dyspnea and marked venous distention. With bed rest, oxygen therapy, and repeated IV injections of furosemide, she had an excellent diuresis and showed marked improvement. On hospital day 5 she complained of fatigue and had a resting heart rate of 100 beats/minute. Despite continued treatment, she became worse and developed a narrowed pulse pressure and hypotension. The use of IV diuretics effected no improvement. It was then noted that her neck veins were barely distended, even in a supine position. A diagnosis of iatrogenic hypovolemia resulting from excessive diuresis was made. Diuretics were discontinued, and salt was restricted; 500 ml of 0.2% NaCl with 5% dextrose in water was administered, resulting in striking improvement.

Venous waves

Venous neck pulsations of the patient with normal sinus rhythm reflect the same waves seen in RA pressure tracings (Fig. 2-4). The *a* wave is produced by atrial contraction and in timing just precedes the arterial pulsation that can be timed by simultaneous palpation of the other side of the neck. The *a* wave precedes the first heart sound if the heart is simultaneously auscultated. When atrial fibrillation is present, atrial contraction does not occur and no *a* wave will be visible.

The second wave seen in the neck is the *c* wave, which is small in amplitude and frequently not seen. This wave reflects the closing of the tricuspid valve at the beginning of ventricular systole.

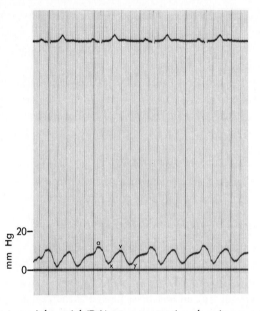

Fig. 2-4. Central venous or right atrial (RA) pressure tracing showing *a* and *v* waves with *x* and *y* descents. No *c* wave is seen in this pressure tracing.

The third wave is the *v* wave, which reflects changes of pressure in the right atrium as the AV valve bulges into the right atrium during ventricular systole. The descent of the *a* wave is termed the *x descent,* and the descent of the *v* wave is termed the *y descent.*

Venous wave abnormalities. Elevations of right-sided pressures, for any reason, result in increased RA and venous pressure; likewise, abnormalities of the tricuspid valve (either stenosis or insufficiency) result in abnormalities in venous pulsation.

Rhythm disturbances also may result in abnormalities of venous waves. For example, AV dissociation results in a lack of synchronization between atrial and ventricular systole, and atrial contraction may take place at a time when ventricular systole is occurring. This atrial contraction against a closed tricuspid valve results in giant *a* waves (called *cannon waves*) in the right atrium and neck veins. Similar abnormalities can be seen in complete heart block and ventricular pacing.

Patients with mitral stenosis and pulmonary hypertension, pulmonic valvular stenosis, and tricuspid stenosis have abnormally high *a* waves.

An exaggerated *v* wave is seen with tricuspid insufficiency, whether it results from RV hypertension and dilation of the annulus or from valvular disease.

Severe constrictive pericarditis, or cardiac tamponade, can cause a marked elevation of the neck veins that may be overlooked during superficial examination. This distention of the neck veins is one of the most valuable diagnostic clues to this life-threatening problem. In constrictive pericarditis and tamponade, both the *a* and *v* waves are prominent and have rapid *x* and *y* descents. In chronic constrictive pericarditis, Kussmaul's sign occurs with a rise, instead of a fall, in the venous pressure during inspiration.

Arterial Pulses

Examination of arterial pulsations provides monitoring of the patient's heart rate and information regarding the stroke volume. During the initial examination, it is important to palpate all major pulses, that is, the carotid, radial, brachial, femoral, popliteal, dorsalis pedis, and posterior tibial pulses. Although not all of these pulses need to be monitored continuously, regular observation of their presence or absence and their character is helpful for making an accurate assessment of changes in the critically ill patient.

Simultaneous assessment of both the brachial and radial pulses is an efficient and useful method of assessing both pulsations. In younger patients or patients with well-developed biceps, the brachial artery may be hidden beneath the belly of the biceps muscle, requiring heavier pressure or some manipulation of the arm for accurate assessment. Elderly patients with arterial tortuosity may have lateral displacement of the artery. Various elbow flexion positions may be necessary to properly palpate the brachial arterial pulses in these patients.

During the initial examination or periodic reevaluation, taking the patient's hand can be extremely valuable — not only for palpation of the radial pulse, but also for an overall assessment of the patient's mental and physical status. The patient's response to this action may provide clues about his or her mental status. A desperate grasp of the examiner's hand may indicate anxiety or fear that the patient may not be able to express verbally. A sweaty, moist hand may indicate anxiety or a diffuse, hypersympathetic state. A cool, limp hand may indicate a low cardiac output in a patient with cardiovascular disease. Examination of the nail beds for color and arterial pulsation can provide information about the arterial system. Finally, palpation of the radial pulse not only measures the heart rate but also determines the character of the pulse, which may indicate a changing stroke volume. In addition to providing information, taking the patient's hand provides a physical contact that gives the patient important psychologic support.

This section discusses common cardiovascular abnormalities that affect arterial pulsations.

Absent or weak pulsations

Determining the presence or absence of arterial pulses during the initial examination and thereafter is vital in monitoring the critically ill patient with cardiac disease. Diffuse atherosclerosis may result in absence of the dorsalis pedis or posterior tibial pulse before the patient is admitted to the hospital. It is helpful to document this absence to differentiate it from a new catastrophic event, such as an arterial embolus. After a cardiac procedure involving catheterization of femoral or brachial arteries, monitoring of distal pulses is critical for the early detection of local thrombosis or distal embolization, either of which might require urgent thrombectomy or Fogarty catheterization. Finally, the sudden disappearance of a pulse may be indicative of a systemic embolus. The source of this embolus may be a thrombus in the left ventricle from an artificial valve, from the left atrium (particularly in atrial fibrillation or mitral valvular disease), or more rarely from a myxomatous tumor in the left atrium. Arterial embolization is usually accompanied by pain and frequently by pallor of the extremity distal to the embolus. Temperature may differ between the two extremities. Arterial pulsations may be weak because of low stroke volume or abnormalities of the arterial vessel. Patients who have had previous coronary arteriography by the Sones technique may have a diminished or absent brachial artery pulse. Information concerning a previous arteriogram can be obtained through the history; an arteriotomy scar also may be present in the antecubital area. Some disease states, such as dissecting aortic aneurysms, may result in cessation of arterial pulsation and should be considered an emergency. Patients with diffuse atherosclerosis may have diminished or absent femoral pulses and absent distal pulses in the legs. Although this disease process is bilateral, one pulse may well be stronger than the other. Similar abnormalities may occur in the carotid vessels in elderly patients. In these situations palpation of the carotid arteries should be performed carefully to prevent complete occlusion of flow for any period of time.

Auscultation of the artery

Bruits may be heard over arteries (particularly the femoral and carotid arteries) with diminished pulsation caused by occlusive atherosclerotic disease. Auscultation of the carotid arteries is performed while the patient is suspending respiration, so that bruits can be differentiated from inspiratory or expiratory noises. Abdominal bruits also may be heard but do not hold the same significance, since approximately 25% of young normal people have a systolic bruit during auscultation of the abdomen.

Rapid upstroke of the arterial pulse

The upstroke of the arterial pulse normally becomes more rapid, the more peripherally it is palpated. A quick uptake of the arterial pulse can be ascertained by the experienced examiner. This quick upstroke may indicate nothing more than an anxious patient, but it may also reflect cardiac disease. A rapid upstroke of the pulse accompanied by a rapid fall (that is, a spiking arterial pulse) may reflect mitral insufficiency with a rapid initial ejection from the ventricle followed by regurgitation into the left atrium and early closure of the aortic valve. Aortic insufficiency, when not accompanied by significant stenosis, also will be reflected by a rapid upstroke of the arterial pulse and a widened pulse pressure of as much as 100 mm Hg. One can clinically see this markedly widened pulse pressure by placing a light under the patient's finger pad and observing the pulsating nail beds while applying slight pressure to the nail. Other diseases that may result in a rapid upstroke of the pulse are systemic diseases, such as thyrotoxicosis and anemia, and arteriovenous shunts with high cardiac output and rapid distal runoff. The pulse of an elderly patient may have a seemingly rapid upstroke because of generalized arteriosclerosis and rigidity of the arterial system. Another disease resulting in a prominent early pulse is hypertrophic obstructive cardiomyopathy or hypertrophic subaortic stenosis; in this case the arterial pulse has a rapid, early peak and there is either a bifid pulse (double-peaked) or absence of the second half of the systolic pulse because of LV outflow obstruction during late systole.

Slow upstroke of the arterial pulse

A slow upstroke of the arterial pulse is associated with aortic stenosis, in which a prolonged ejection time and late appearance of the peak systolic pressure occur. Although the character of the pulse may allow differentiation between mild and severe aortic stenosis, changes in compliance of the arterial system (particularly in the elderly patient) may make this estimation difficult. A slow upstroke of the pulse also may be the result of severe congestive heart failure and a small stroke volume.

Pulsus paradoxus

During inspiration the systolic arterial pressure may fall as much as 10 mm Hg. This normal decline is caused by decreased LV stroke volume and transmission of the negative intrathoracic pressure to the great vessels during systole. A decrease in systolic pressure greater than 10 mm Hg during inspiration is called *pulsus paradoxus* and reflects either severe cardiac decompensation or, classically, cardiac tamponade. Pulsus paradoxus also occurs in about 50% of patients with constrictive pericarditis, as well as in patients with obstructive airway disease. Kussmaul first described this condition as paradoxical as the disappearance of the peripheral pulse occurred in the face of obvious apical pulsations.

The character and variations of the pulse during inspiration should be noted during palpation of the pulse. In the patient with a critically severe cardiac tamponade, the pulse may nearly disappear during inspiration and reappear during expiration. This condition is an exaggerated pulsus paradoxus that can be easily detected with a stethoscope and blood pressure cuff.

Pulsus alternans

Pulsus alternans is an alternation of peak systolic pressure and usually reflects severe LV failure. If the finding is exaggerated, the examiner may detect the variation during palpation of the pulse. These alternating stronger and weaker pulsations of the distal pulse can be confirmed by a blood pressure cuff or intraarterial monitoring.

Dysrhythmias

Abnormalities in cardiac rhythm result in abnormalities of pulsation. For example, atrial fibrillation may result in shorter R-R intervals that prevent adequate time for diastolic filling of the ventricle. When this situation occurs, even though mechanical systole occurs, insufficient volume or pressure is generated by the ventricle to open the aortic valve and produce a pulse. For this reason the peripheral pulse may be an inaccurate determinant of the true ventricular rate in atrial fibrillation. The occurrence of premature ventricular contractions (PVCs) or ventricular bigeminy may result in palpation of only the normal sinus beats. In these instances correlation of the peripheral pulse with the ECG monitor will prevent a misdiagnosis or an inaccurate measurement of the cardiac rate.

The Lungs

Examination of the lungs and respiratory status provides information regarding pulmonary problems that may be aggravating or causing serious cardiovascular difficulties. A daily chest x-ray examination cannot substitute for frequent evaluation of the respiratory rate and character, the character of breath sounds during auscultation, and the presence or absence of rales. This section briefly discusses the techniques of percussion and auscultation of the chest as they relate to monitoring the critically ill patient with cardiovascular disease.

Percussion

Percussion of the anterior chest consists of defining areas of cardiac dullness and areas of dullness from the liver and possibly the spleen. Percussion of the posterior chest is performed with the patient in a sitting position, which is not always feasible in the critically ill patient. When it is possible, the patient should be relaxed and leaning forward slightly. It is best to begin percussion at the top of the chest and proceed downward, comparing the sounds produced on each side of the chest and from top to bottom. Examination is hampered by obesity, wasting of the upper chest, asthma, distention of the bowel or stomach by gas, and incorrect positioning of the patient. Examination by percussion requires practice and skill. Because the amount of resonance obtained at any point depends on the strength of the stroke delivered, minor variations in technique can cause considerable differences in the percussion note produced.

Percussion sounds are divided into normal vesicular resonance, hyperresonance, dull or flat sounds, and tympanic resonance. Normal vesicular resonance is a low-pitched, vibrant sound that occurs over healthy, air-containing lungs. Overinflation of the lungs results in a louder and more vibrant note referred to as *hyperresonance*. Areas not containing air produce a dull or flat sound that is short, higher pitched, and without a vibrant quality. Tympanic sounds occur over hollow organs distended with air. These sounds are high pitched and similar to the sound produced by the kettledrum. Percussion to define areas of fluid in the lung is performed with the patient in an upright position. Fluid-filled areas are characterized by a dull sound occurring abnormally high above the usual diaphragmatic area or unequally from one side of the chest to the other.

Auscultation

Auscultation of the lungs is easily performed and should be a component of each cardiovascular examination. Before auscultation is begun, the patient should be observed carefully to characterize the respirations. Are they labored or quiet? Are they regular or irregular? Does the patient make audible noise during respiration that will be heard during auscultation? Characterizing these features of the patient's respiration will prevent initial confusion during examination.

Examination of the lungs traditionally is performed with the diaphragm component of the binaural stethoscope because it detects higher-pitched sounds. The earpieces should be applied properly to exclude extraneous room noise, and the diaphragm of the stethoscope should be placed firmly on the patient's chest. Skillful use of the stethoscope requires knowledge of what to listen for and what to ignore and the ability to concentrate on various components of the respiratory cycle while listening for particular sounds. A quiet room is preferred but is usually not possible when the critically ill patient is examined. A great deal of information can be obtained in a less than perfect environment. Care must be taken to disregard noise from movement of the diaphragm on the skin. This noise can be avoided by maintaining firm, light pressure of the diaphragm against the skin. In very thin patients the bell component of the stethoscope may be needed for listening between the ribs.

Normal breath sounds

The three types of sounds heard during examination of the normal lungs are vesicular, tracheal, and bronchovesicular. Experience gained from the examination of many normal people is needed so that minor deviations from normal can be detected and applied to the care of the critically ill patient. Vesicular breath sounds are heard best during inspiration and have a breathy quality. Tracheal breath sounds occur more frequently during expiration and have a tubular, harsher quality. Bronchovesicular breath sounds are a mixture of tracheal and vesicular elements and are heard best over the central areas of the chest overlying the large bronchi.

Abnormal breath sounds

Diminished vesicular breath sounds relate either to a change in the flow of air to the alveoli or to abnormalities of the pleural cavity, such as the presence of fluid, air, or scar tissue. Restriction of air movement, either because of chest wall disease or bronchial disease such as asthma, can markedly decrease vesicular breath sounds. Tubular or bronchial breath sounds are heard in diseases in which there is excessive transmission of sound from the bronchi to the chest, as in consolidation caused by pneumonia. Asthmatic breath sounds are characterized by a markedly prolonged expiratory phase with wheezing or groaning sounds and a short inspiratory phase with minimal vesicular breath sounds.

Rales are the sounds produced when air passes through bronchi that contain fluid of any kind. Rales vary greatly from patient to patient, depending on the cause and extent of the underlying cardiac or pulmonary disease. It is best to have the patient cough before auscultation so that the lungs are cleared of any minimal hypostatic fluids. Moist rales can be coarse and gurgling (rhonchi) and occur when excessive secretion that the patient cannot cough up is in the trachea and large bronchi. Rhonchi usually occur in critically ill patients or patients with decreased mental status. Medium crepitant rales are small and bubbling and occur over areas of pneumonia or pulmonary congestion. Fine rales sometimes are described as crackling and occur in conditions in which pulmonary venous congestion is present. Dry rales are caused by a small amount of thickened exudate in the bronchioles and occasionally are heard in patients with chronic bronchial disease. These rales are almost always associated with bronchial breath sounds or asthmatic sounds.

Pleural friction rubs

Sound of a friction rub may be heard during the respiratory cycle, particularly during inspiration. The rubbing sound seems very superficial, as though it were right under the diaphragm of the stethoscope. Pleural rubs are variously described as grating, rubbing, or creaking and may have even a leathery characteristic. They frequently alter with a change in the patient's position or state of inspiration. A friction rub may be important to identify because it can be caused by an underlying pulmonary infection or infarcted area.

The Heart
Inspection and palpation of the anterior chest

Diagnostic information can be obtained from brief but careful inspection and palpation of the anterior chest during monitoring of the critically ill patient with cardiac disease. This section describes briefly the technique and some of the more common abnormalities found in specific areas of the precordium. Abnormalities detected during inspection or palpation must be correlated with the cardiac cycle and auscultation. This examination is carried out in the aortic area, the pulmonic area, the lower left sternal border, and the apical area.

Aortic area. Although abnormal pulsations in the aortic area may be produced by marked dilation of the ascending aorta, its position near the sternum usually prevents any visible pulsation. During palpation, a vibratory thrill may be felt in the patient with aortic stenosis and is associated with a loud systolic murmur. The aortic valve closure occasionally can be palpated in the patient with severe hypertension.

Pulmonic area. Abnormalities of pulsation in the pulmonic area are rare except in the patient with marked dilation of the pulmonary artery because of either pulmonary hypertension or pulmonary ectasia. During palpation, a thrill may be felt in the patient with pulmonic stenosis. A loud pulmonic second sound may be palpated in severe pulmonary hypertension, and a pulmonic systolic tap may be palpated in patients with a dilated pulmonary artery.

Lower left sternal border. Palpation in the lower left sternal border area may reveal a palpable thrill in patients with a ventricular septal defect. Abnormalities of pulsation in this area most commonly are found in conditions associated with RV hypertrophy, such as pulmonary hypertension (with or without severe mitral stenosis). When RV hypertrophy is present, the sternum can be felt to move anteriorly during systole; this movement is referred to as a *substernal heave.*

Apical area. The LV apical impulse can be identified and actually pinpointed within a 1 cm area. It is normally located in the fifth intercostal space in the midclavicular line. Displacement of the point of maximal impulse (PMI) lateral to the midclavicular line is indicative of cardiac enlargement. Not only is the location of the PMI important, but its character may reflect LV contractility. A poorly palpable apical impulse may indicate poor LV contraction and stroke volume if the apex is near the chest wall. However, a very muscular chest or emphysema will obscure this finding. A systolic thrill may be palpated in this area because of mitral insufficiency from any cause. Occasionally a very loud, rumbling diastolic murmur can be palpated. A forceful or sustained apical impulse generally reflects LV hypertrophy associated with aortic stenosis or arterial hypertension. In patients with mitral insufficiency or rapid peripheral runoff (as in AV fistula), a rapid damping of the apical impulse during systole may be palpated.

Events occurring in the left ventricle during diastolic filling also can be appreciated. Palpation of an early diastolic gallop, associated with outward movement of the left ventricle during early filling, usually reflects LV failure. An early diastolic gallop may be palpated also in patients with a hyperadrenergic state and large cardiac outputs. Rarely, during late diastole, a systolic gallop or "atrial kick" may be palpated. In patients with mitral valvular disease, palpation of an opening snap in early diastole occasionally can be appreciated, but this snap is much easier to hear than to palpate.

Epigastric area. Visible or palpable pulsations of the aorta in the epigastric area are normal findings. Many people also are slightly tender in this area. For these reasons palpation in the epigastric area generally does not yield further information about cardiac events, although aneurysmal dilation of the abdominal aorta may be detected.

Auscultation

Although cardiac auscultation traditionally is thought of as a diagnostic tool, components of this part of the cardiac examination may be used to assess the current cardiovascular status of the heart and to monitor hemodynamic changes. Ideally, auscultation of the heart should be carried out in a quiet room with a cooperative patient. The stethoscope should be equipped with both a diaphragm and a bell. In general, the diaphragm is used for high- frequency sounds, such as aortic or mitral insufficiency murmurs, and the bell for low-frequency sounds, particularly diastolic gallops and the rumbling murmur of mitral stenosis. It is important to place the bell on the skin with just enough pressure to seal out extraneous noise. With further pressure on the bell, the skin itself becomes a diaphragm and accentuates any high-frequency sounds.

Auscultation of the heart involves selectively listening for each component of the cardiac cycle separately, that is, the first sound, the second sound, the period of systole, and the period of diastole. This listening should be done systematically in at least four cardiac areas: the aortic area, the pulmonic area, the lower left sternal border, and the apical regions of the precordium (Fig. 2-5). These areas do not correspond exactly to their anatomic location but to the area in which the particular valve sounds are best heard. Although each examiner develops a personal system, optimal auscultation usually is begun at the aortic area to determine cardiac cycle time and to identify the first and second heart sounds. Once these sounds are firmly identified, the listener may then move to other areas of the precordium, mentally noting murmurs and changes in heart sounds.

The character of heart sounds should be noted carefully, and specific attention should be directed to differences in intensity and constancy. Each heart sound is identified and characterized separately. The presence of extra heart sounds should then be identified, particularly in midsystole and in early and late diastole. Once they are noted, more exact timing can be ascertained in relation to the first and second heart sounds. Whenever difficulty develops in the timing of the sounds, the examiner

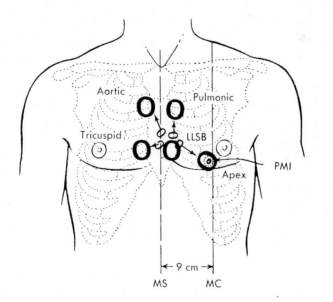

Fig. 2-5. Primary areas of cardiac auscultation. These areas correspond to the locations where sounds and murmurs are best heard rather than to an anatomic valve location. *MS,* Midsternum; *MC,* midclavicle; *PMI,* point of maximal impulse; *LLSB,* lower left sternal border.

may wish to return to the aortic area to confirm the first and second sounds, since these sounds indicate systole and diastole and can be used as a timing reference. When possible, the patient should assume other positions, including sitting upright or even standing, so that changes in heart sounds and murmurs that otherwise might not be heard may be detected.

Heart sounds

The *first heart sound* (S_1) is produced by closure of the mitral and tricuspid valves (Fig. 2-6). These AV valves open at the initiation of diastole and allow filling of the ventricles. The valves float partially closed during ventricular filling and then reopen during atrial systole. At the onset of ventricular systole, the pressures in the two ventricles quickly exceed the pressures in the atria and result in forceful closure of both valves. This closure results in vibrations that are transmitted through tissues of the body and are heard through a stethoscope as the first heart sound. Changes in conduction time and blood volume can cause alterations in the timing of valve closure, resulting in a separate sound for closure of each valve. This process is termed *splitting of the first sound*.

Conditions that accentuate the first heart sound are hyperthyroidism, anemia, tachycardia, and mitral stenosis.

The *second heart sound* (S_2) is associated with closure of the aortic and pulmonic valves and represents the onset of ventricular diastole (Fig. 2-6). Closure of the aortic valve usually precedes closure of the pulmonic valve. The aortic component of the

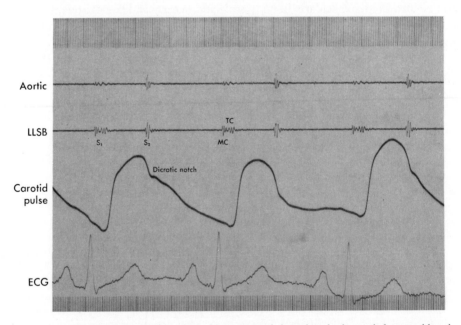

Fig. 2-6. Phonocardiogram showing normal heart sounds heard at the lower left sternal border *(LLSB)* and aortic area. Split first sound (S_1) is composed of mitral valve closure *(MC)* and tricuspid valve closure *(TC)*. Dicrotic notch in the carotid artery tracing indicates aortic valve closure.

second heart sound may be accentuated in systemic hypertension and diminished or absent in aortic stenosis, where there is restricted movement of the valve. The pulmonic component will be accentuated in pulmonary hypertension from any cause.

Splitting of the second sound normally occurs during inspiration as increased blood flow to the right side of the heart prolongs RV systole and delays pulmonic valve closure. An atrial septal defect results in wide splitting of the second sound, which varies little with respiration because of the balancing of the central venous return between the right and left atria through the atrial septal defect.

Paradoxical splitting of the second sound (pulmonic valve closure preceding aortic valve closure) occurs with (1) left bundle branch block caused by delay of LV systole and (2) severe aortic stenosis caused by prolonged LV ejection time and restricted movement of the aortic valve.

The *third heart sound* (S_3) occurs at the end of rapid diastolic ventricular filling and probably results from vibrations of the ventricular wall and by tensing of the papillary muscles. It may originate in either the right or the left ventricle and is heard best at the apex with the bell of the stethoscope. The presence of a third heart sound may be normal in adolescents, in patients with ventricular dilation from any cause, and in patients with decreased ventricular compliance (Fig. 2-7).

The *fourth heart sound* (S_4) occurs during atrial systole and is produced by the forceful movement of blood from the left atrium into the ventricle near the end of diastole. Usually it is not heard in normal patients, although it may be recorded by a phonocardiograph. This sound also is heard at the apex in patients with decreased LV compliance, which may occur with coronary artery disease, LV hypertrophy, and cardiac failure.

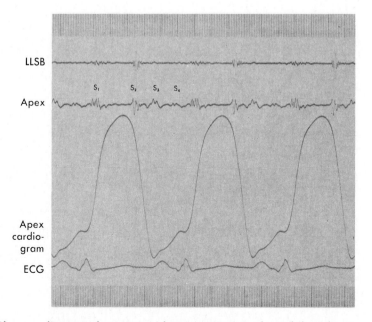

Fig. 2-7. Phonocardiogram of a patient with severe congestive heart failure showing an S_3 and S_4 gallop. Apex cardiogram records systolic outward bulging of the ventricle during systole.

Systolic sounds

Ejection clicks may occur when a partially stenotic aortic or pulmonic valve opens at the initiation of ventricular systole. Ejection clicks may result from sudden expansion of the pulmonary or aortic wall at the initiation of systole and are heard frequently in midsystole and late systole. The best-known syndrome is the midsystolic click that initiates a late systolic murmur of mitral insufficiency caused by prolapse of the mitral valve.

Diastolic sounds

Opening snaps can be heard when a stenotic mitral or tricuspid valve is forced open at the start of diastole. The sound has a snapping quality and is heard best at the left sternal border, where it may be confused with the widely split second sound. Early diastolic sounds without an opening snap may occur in pericardial disease because of sudden distention of the thickened pericardium during diastole.

Gallop rhythms

Gallop rhythms (Fig. 2-8) occur when the third or fourth heart sounds become pathologically accentuated. The summation of the third and fourth sounds during tachycardia is called a *summation gallop* and usually represents severe cardiac decompensation.

Heart murmurs

Heart murmurs are produced by turbulent blood flow through stenotic or abnormal valves or vessels, resulting in audible vibrations that can be heard with a stethoscope. Blood flow is laminar, and valve movement normally occurs in such a

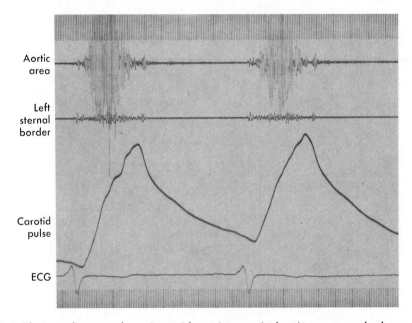

Fig. 2-8. Phonocardiogram of a patient with aortic stenosis showing a crescendo-decrescendo systolic murmur. Slow-rising carotid pulse also suggests aortic stenosis.

way as to provide unimpeded flow. When stenosis or insufficiency of a valve occurs, blood flow becomes turbulent, producing audible vibrations.

When all cardiac sounds have been identified and their timing ascertained, the presence of murmurs or other heart sounds can be identified. When a murmur is heard, it should be characterized in relation to the cardiac cycle and changes in intensity (holosystolic or crescendo-decrescendo murmurs).

Systolic murmurs

Systolic murmurs generally can be categorized as either ejection or regurgitant murmurs. Ejection murmurs result from aortic or pulmonic stenosis or increased flow through a normal valve and have a crescendo-decrescendo character (Fig. 2-8). The systolic ejection murmur of aortic stenosis is heard best at the aortic area and radiates to the suprasternal notch and carotid artery and to the apex. Regurgitant systolic murmurs begin immediately after the first sound and extend through the entire systolic period. They are termed *holosystolic,* which means they last through all of systole. Holosystolic murmurs occur with mitral insufficiency, tricuspid insufficiency, ventricular septal defects, or other AV communications.

At times it may be difficult to differentiate between ejection and regurgitant systolic murmurs. A number of maneuvers can be performed to cause alterations in the character and intensity of the murmur, and these alterations may help the examiner to identify the correct valve and the cause of the murmur. Table 2-1 outlines some commonly used methods to characterize systolic murmurs.

The occurrence of a new systolic murmur can be an extremely important development during monitoring of the critically ill patient. It may indicate papillary muscle dysfunction resulting in mitral insufficiency, or it may indicate the development of a ventricular septal defect caused by perforation of an infarcted ventricular septum.

Diastolic murmurs

As the pressure in the relaxing ventricles falls to a level below the pressure in the atria, the AV valves open and diastolic filling is initiated. If either the mitral or tricuspid valve is stenotic, low-pitched, rumbling murmurs occur as the result of the turbulence of the blood flow through these valves. In typical mitral stenosis the diastolic murmur is initiated by the opening snap of the stenotic valve. Placing the patient in the left lateral position brings the apex of the heart nearer to the chest wall and optimizes detection of a mitral diastolic rumble.

Table 2-1. Effect of maneuvers on systolic murmurs

Maneuver	Ejection murmur	Mitral regurgitation	Tricuspid regurgitation	Ventricular septal defect	Hypertrophic subaortic stenosis
Inspiration	—*	—	↑	—	—
Straining	↓	↓	↓	—	↓
Valsalva's release	↑	↑	↑	—	↓
Postextrasystolic beat	↑	↓ or —	—	—	↑
Amyl nitrite	↑	↓	↑ or ↓		↑

*—, No change; ↓, murmur decreases; ↑, murmur increases.

The other major diastolic murmurs occur in relation to insufficient aortic or pulmonic valves that produce a soft, high-frequency murmur. Diastolic murmurs may be listened for initially at the base of the heart or in the aortic and pulmonic areas. These murmurs are soft and of very high frequency when they are caused by aortic insufficiency or pulmonic insufficiency. Rather than being caused by organic valvular disease, pulmonic insufficiency usually is caused by severe pulmonary hypertension and results from dilation of the pulmonary artery and valve ring. Aortic insufficiency may be caused by aortic valvular disease or dilation of the ascending aorta and valvular ring from systemic hypertension. The appearance of a new murmur of aortic insufficiency in a patient with a suspected aneurysm or dissection of the descending aorta is an important physical sign of further proximal dissection that may be life threatening.

Continuous murmurs and sounds

Continuous murmurs are unusual but may be encountered with patent ductus arteriosus; these murmurs have a systolic and diastolic accentuation. Occasionally a continuous murmur can be heard over an arteriovenous fistula anywhere in the body.

Venous hums

Venous hums are benign murmurs that may be heard in the neck and confused with organic murmurs. Differentiation is made by the application of slight pressure to the neck to stop the venous flow, resulting in complete disappearance of the hum.

Extracardiac sounds

Pericardial rubs. Pericardial disease (particularly pericarditis) may result in both systolic and diastolic sounds. These sounds are scratching and high pitched and vary considerably during the respiratory cycle. The development of a pericardial rub is an important sign to monitor because it may reveal the cause of chest pain in the patient with diffuse ST elevation on an ECG. Its presence also may be a contraindication for anticoagulation therapy.

Mediastinal crunches. Mediastinal crunches occur when there is air in the mediastinum; they are produced by movements of the heart in the mediastinum against these small air pockets. The sounds are random or occur during ventricular systole. They may be associated with crepitation in the neck caused by subcutaneous air collection. These sounds may be heard after cardiac surgery; however, they can be an ominous sign in an accident victim, since they can be caused by rupture of the trachea or tracheobronchial tree.

The Abdomen

Examination of the abdomen during continuous monitoring provides some information about the cardiovascular status of the critically ill patient. An enlarged, tender liver in the right upper quadrant of the abdomen may signify elevated right-sided pressures and, if pulsatile, indicates serious tricuspid insufficiency. Because this situation is usually a long-standing one, it does not reflect a changing cardiovascular status.

Recurring abdominal pain may be caused by ischemia of the bowel as a result of a low cardiac output. This diagnosis is extremely difficult to ascertain; however, when excruciating abdominal pain accompanied by a rigid abdomen occurs in the patient with a low cardiac output, ischemia of the bowel must be considered. Differential diagnosis includes a peripheral embolus to one of the mesenteric arteries or to the kidneys.

Extremities

Examination of the hand and wrist is discussed in the section on arterial pulses. Pedal edema in the ambulatory patient with cardiac disease usually reflects right heart failure with retention of salt and water. However, in the bedridden patient, this fluid moves to the most dependent part of the body and should be looked for in the sacral and gluteal areas.

Peripheral cyanosis is evident when the arterial oxygen saturation falls below 75% as a result of an increase (>5 g) in the amount of unsaturated hemoglobin. Although its presence indicates severe hypoxia, its absence does not indicate the converse. The cause of this hypoxia may be pulmonary or cardiac:

Pulmonary	**Cardiac**
Emphysema	Congenital heart disease with right-to-left shunt
Atelectasis	Low cardiac output
Pulmonary edema	
Pulmonary shunts	
Pulmonary emboli	

The occurrence of cyanosis in the patient with cardiac disease is usually an ominous sign and requires prompt treatment. Recognition of this sign may be impaired by poor room lighting, anemia, or the patient's skin pigmentation. An arterial blood gas analysis is needed for a differential diagnosis.

REFERENCES

Constant J: *Essentials of bedside cardiology for students and housestaff,* Boston, 1989, Little, Brown.

Fowler NO: *Examination of the heart. Part II: Inspection and palpation of venous and arterial pulses,* New York, 1972, American Heart Association.

Hardman V, Butterworth J: Auscultation of the heart. I and II, *Mod Concepts Cardiovasc Dis* 30:645-649, 651-656, 1961.

Luisada AA, MacCanon DM, Kumar S, Feigen LP: Changing views on the mechanism of the first and second heart sounds, *Am Heart J* 88:503-514, 1974.

Tilkian AG, Conover MB: *Understanding heart sounds and murmurs,* ed 3, Philadelphia, 1993, WB Saunders.

Chapter 3

Principles and Hazards of Monitoring Equipment

In 1903 William Einthoven introduced the string galvanometer, which served as the basis for the ECG. Since then, electronic instrumentation has become an integral part of medicine. Biomedical instrumentation provides the tools for physiologic measurements in both the research laboratory and the clinical setting. Although some forms of biomedical instruments are unique to the medical field, most are applications of widely used methods for physical measurements, and an understanding of the basic principles of physiologic measurements is needed for cardiovascular monitoring with biomedical equipment to be both safe and effective.

Before discussing the components of hemodynamic monitoring equipment, let us look briefly at the characteristics of intravascular pressures measured through fluid-filled catheters. These consist of the following (Fig. 3-1):

1. The *residual,* or *static, pressure* inside the fluid-filled vessel
2. The *dynamic pressure,* which is caused by the imparted kinetic energy of the moving fluid (This component is encountered in arterial pressures when the catheter tip directly faces the flow of fluid.)
3. The *hydrostatic pressure head,* which results from the difference in height between the ends of the fluid-filled tube (that is, the catheter tip and the air-reference port of the transducer)

In hemodynamic monitoring the most desired measurement is the residual, or static, pressure within the vessel or chamber. To do this, it is necessary to eliminate both the dynamic and hydrostatic pressure components. As mentioned, dynamic pressures are encountered only in high or frequent flow rates or when the catheter tip points into the flow. This additional component is difficult to eliminate completely but can be reduced by changing the direction of the catheter tip or, more practically, by applying a damping device. It is the third pressure component, the hydrostatic

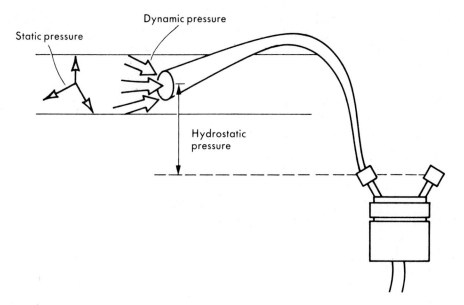

Fig. 3-1. Three components of hemodynamic pressures: static pressure within the vessel; dynamic pressure that is the imparted kinetic energy of the moving fluid; and hydrostatic pressure of a fluid-filled column.

pressure, that most consistently impacts the accuracy of pressure measurements obtained through fluid-filled systems.

Although the directions just mentioned are applicable to catheters located centrally, at the level of the heart, confusion often exists regarding appropriate "leveling" with peripheral arterial catheters. Placement of the air-reference port at the level of the tip of the arterial catheter eliminates the effect of hydrostatic pressure within the fluid-filled column and provides an accurate measurement of the static pressure within the peripheral artery. However, many clinicians, interested in a closer approximation of the aortic root pressure (as a reflection of coronary perfusion pressure), place both the catheter tip (that is, the patient's arm) *and* the air-reference port at the right atrium level, thereby eliminating the effects of hydrostatic pressure between the air-reference and the catheter tip and between the catheter tip and the aorta. This method, however, does not eliminate the normal amplification of arterial pressure that occurs distally from the aorta.

PRESSURE-RECORDING DEVICES
Principle

All biomedical recording instruments have three basic components: (1) a transducer or device to detect the physiologic event; (2) an amplifier to increase the magnitude of the signal from the transducer; and (3) a recorder, meter, or oscilloscope to display the resultant signal (Fig. 3-2).

Pressure measurement requires the transformation of a biophysical event into an electric signal that can be displayed, recorded on paper or magnetic tape, and quantified. This transformation is done with a transducer, which converts one type of energy or signal into another. Physiologic events can be transduced, but appropriate transducer selection is needed for results to be successful (Table 3-1).

Transducers

Transduction involves the sensing of a particular biophysical event and its conversion to a usable electric signal. Transducers can sense changes in flow, color, temperature, concentration, pressure, displacement, light intensity, frequency, and sound, and other physiologic changes. Transducers are classified according to the type of energy to which they are sensitive and the method of energy coupling used. The pressure transducer most commonly used in biomedical instrumentation is a mechanical, or displacement, transducer, so called because it consists of a mechanical element that is displaced as a result of changes in pressure. Although there are many types of transducers employing different physical principles to measure displacement, the strain gauge transducer is the most widely used.

External disposable pressure transducers most commonly are used in the clinical setting to measure blood pressure through a fluid column (fluid-filled catheter). Disposable pressure transducers consist of a silicon pressure-sensor chip that has a thin, etched diaphragm with a single, transverse voltage, strain gauge, piezoresistive element. Temperature compensation is done directly on the chip. The chip is mounted on an electrically isolated carrier and backplate assembly with a bonded flow-through dome (Fig. 3-3). Disposable transducers provide accuracy and sensitivity comparable to reusable transducers and eliminate the need for sterilization between patients. The transducer has two openings, each with Luer-Lok fittings. An

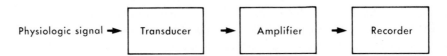

Physiologic signal → Transducer → Amplifier → Recorder

Fig. 3-2. Three basic components of a biomedical recording instrument.

Table 3-1. Characteristics of cardiovascular parameters

Parameter	Range/unit	Frequency response (cps or Hz)	Type of transducer
ECG	10 μV to 5 mV	0.05 to 85	Skin electrodes
Blood pressure	0 to 300 mm Hg	0 to 60	Strain gauge Pressure gauge
Cardiac output	2 to 15 L/min	0 to 60	Oximeter (dye) or thermistor
Temperature	25° to 40° C	Variable	Thermistor
Heart rate	45 to 180 beats/ min	0.75 to 3	From ECG or pulse
Phonocardiogram	—	2 to 2000	Microphone
Echocardiogram	—	20,000	Piezoelectric

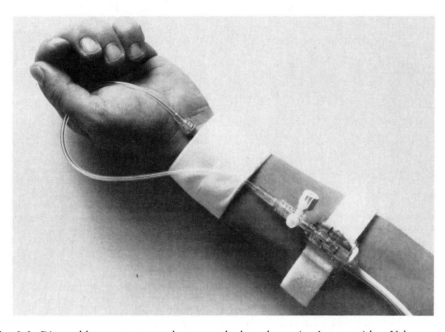

Fig. 3-3. Disposable pressure transducer attached to the patient's arm with a Velcro strap.
Courtesy Gould, Inc, Oxnard, Calif.

opening at one end allows the connection of fluid-filled tubing to the transducer; the other opening may be used for zero reference to atmospheric pressure and/or for flushing of the transducer, or to connect to the second port of the catheter. A clear plastic dome over the transducer allows detection of air bubbles or blood in the fluid, either of which can distort the pressure measurements.

Because the pressure is being measured through a fluid-filled column, any difference between the catheter tip and the air-fluid interface (the reference port) will result in an incorrect pressure. The pressure exerted by the weight of the fluid within the catheter and connecting tubing is termed *hydrostatic pressure* and is proportional to the height of the fluid column. If the tip of the catheter within the patient is higher than the level of the air-reference port, the pressure reading will be erroneously high because of the contribution of hydrostatic pressure. Conversely, if the air-reference port is placed above the level of the catheter tip, the pressure reading will be erroneously low (Fig. 3-4). To negate the effects of the hydrostatic pressure of the fluid, it is essential that both open "ends" of the system be at the same level (Fig. 3-5). In this instance, the two "ends" consist of (1) the tip of the catheter and (2) the air-fluid junction (the air-reference stopcock). Although the exact level of the catheter tip is not known, it generally is considered to be in the midchest position. To discern the patient's midchest position, measure the distance from the posterior chest to the anterior chest and place a midway mark on the patient's lateral chest wall at this location. Another method uses the phlebostatic axis at the junction of the fourth intercostal space and an imagined midaxillary line. Because no exact external anatomic site can identify the actual level of the catheter tip, any of the methods can be used to approximate its position. The air-reference port should then be set level with the patient's midchest level. Opening the air-reference port and zeroing the system

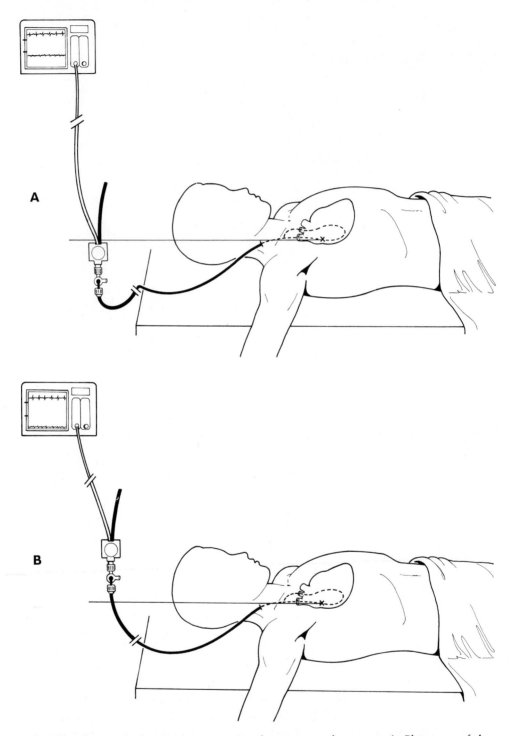

Fig. 3-4. Illustration showing improper air-reference port placements. **A,** Placement of the air-reference port *below* the catheter tip level will result in an erroneously high pressure. **B,** Placement of the air-reference port *above* the catheter tip level will result in an erroneously low pressure.

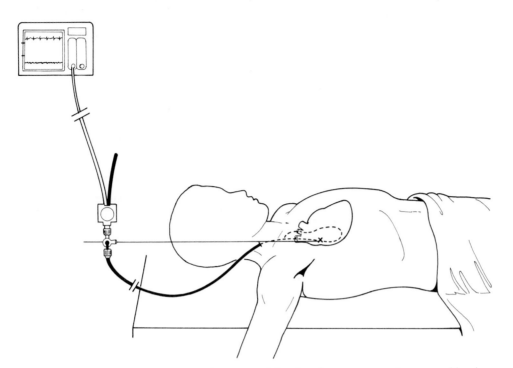

Fig. 3-5. Illustration showing proper placement of the air-reference port at the assumed level of the patient's right atrium, which corresponds closely to the patient's midchest.

at this level eliminate any hydrostatic pressure differences that exist elsewhere within the fluid-filled system. The position of either the transducer (to a certain extent) or the patient does not affect the pressure readings as long as the following criteria are met:

1. The air-reference port is level with the patient's midchest when in the supine position or level with the patient's midsternum when in the lateral position (Fig. 3-6).
2. The air-fluid reference port is opened to air and the system re-zeroed after *any* change in the position of *either* the transducer, the air-reference port, or the patient.

Although most transducers used today can accommodate the offset that exists when the transducer and the air-reference port are at different levels, the limitations of this difference have not been studied with the newer transducers. Consequently, although the transducer need not be at the same level as the air-reference port, it probably should be within approximately 6 inches of that level. This occurs with the common practice of using the stopcock located near the transducer as the air-reference port.

The electrical signal from the transducer is transmitted by the cable to an amplifier. The amplifier modifies this electrical signal by increasing voltage and filtering it for display on an oscilloscope or suitable recording device.

Strain gauge transducers are sensitive to temperature changes (typically 0.1 mm Hg/1° C) and require occasional checking of the zero-pressure baseline for drift. The room in which they are used should be kept at a fairly constant temperature.

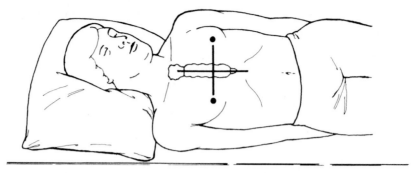

Fig. 3-6. Illustration depicting reference points for placement of the air-reference port when the patient is in a lateral position. Alternatively, air-reference placement may be done at the level of the left sternal border and the nipple line.

Solutions flushed through the transducers also can cause a temperature change and baseline drift.

Transducers also can be placed at the tip of a catheter and introduced directly into the vascular system. These transducer-tipped catheters have the advantage of not being dependent on a fluid-filled column for transmitting the pressure events at the catheter tip to the transducer. This feature eliminates problems with delay of pressure change transmittance and, more important, errors in pressure transmission caused by inherent characteristics of the diameter and compliance of the catheter. It also avoids artifacts in the pressure caused by movements of the catheter, as well as those errors involved in estimating correct placement of the air-reference port.

Amplifiers

Biomedical parameters are difficult to measure because of the relatively low energy levels generated within the body and the similarity of signals from organ to organ (for example, heart and skeletal muscle); this similarity makes discrimination of a particular signal difficult. Not only does the transducer have a certain frequency response and sensitivity to detect a particular signal accurately, but the signal generated by the transducer usually requires processing (for example, impedance matching or filtering of noise) and amplification.

Most modern transducers produce only about 6 mV above their "zero level" output when reproducing the systolic arterial pressure, whereas most monitor displays require several *volts* of signal for operation. Consequently, an amplifier is necessary to boost the size of the signal by approximately a factor of 1000 before it can be displayed.

Amplifiers can be straightforward electronic devices that simply amplify the signal from the transducer, or they can be highly complex devices that process, filter, and amplify the signal for display on an oscilloscope recorder. The signal also can be fed into a computer for further digital processing and analysis.

Amplifiers for cardiovascular measurements are designed to meet specific requirements. They must be easy to use with clearly labeled controls, and they should filter out other physiologic signals and undesired environmental noise detected by the

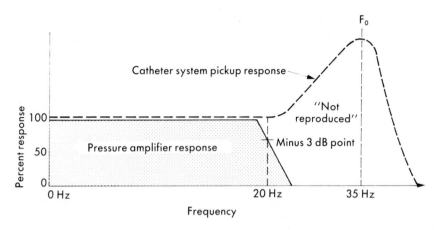

Fig. 3-7. Pressure amplifier response curve and fluid-filled catheter (plumbing) system response curve. Note the accuracy of the amplifier's response (100%) up to an upper limit cutoff frequency of approximately 20 Hz. Although the plumbing system can add distortion to the signal, if its characteristic resonant frequency is above the upper limit cutoff frequency (approximately 25 Hz), it will not be processed by the amplifier.

transducer (Fig. 3-7). The amplifier's ability to increase signal level and its faithfulness in reproducing signals from input to output should not add significant distortion (termed *linear response*). Calibration, stability, and temperature drift should minimally affect the signal. Good electronic design can accommodate all of these requirements and result in an extremely sensitive and precise diagnostic instrument.

Display devices

Physiologic pressures can be displayed on oscilloscopes and digital readout devices or on permanent recording devices using graphic recordings. The modified electrical output from the amplifier can be meaningful only when it is converted into readable form in a display or recording device. Because a display device has an upper and lower frequency limit, it is essential for faithful reproduction that the display's frequency response range match that of the input signal.

The *oscilloscope* is a display device that provides a visual image of voltage changes as a function of time. The basic component of an oscilloscope is a cathode-ray vacuum tube that produces an electron beam focused on a screen. The electron beam is visible because the interior of the screen is painted with phosphorescent chemicals that transiently emit visible light when excited by the electron beam. The brightness and persistence of the light depend on the type of phosphorescent chemical used. The horizontal sweep of the beam indicates the amount of time required for the signal to go from left to right and can be adjusted on most oscilloscopes. The vertical deflection of the beam reflects voltage changes from the amplifier and transducer. Plotting can be adjusted for optimal display of the voltage change, termed *sensitivity*, which is determined by *calibration*, the insertion of a signal of known quantity with adjustment of the amplifier and readout device to reproduce this known change accurately. Oscilloscopes can display one or more signals simultaneously. Some oscilloscopes allow the signal to remain on the scope until it is erased by a new sweep of signals.

This nonfade display allows more time for study of the waveform during monitoring of patients. Some oscilloscopes have stop-motion, or freeze ability, which permits prolonged display of a selected waveform.

Digital readout devices provide numeric values of pressure changes during specific times of the cardiac cycle. Selection of systolic, diastolic, or mean pressure values is available on most digital display devices.

To obtain a permanent record of a physiologic signal and to accurately measure pressures at end-expiration, a paper-recording device with a galvanometer often is used. The galvanometer's motion is proportional to the amount of current flowing through a wire. This flow of current generates a magnetic field, causing movement of the suspended mirror on optical recorders or movement of a writing pen on direct-writing recorders. The *direct-writing recorder* uses a stylus to record the pressure tracing on moving paper. The stylus is driven by an attached galvanometer coil. These direct-writing recorders are termed *strip chart recorders* and are used for the measurement of low-frequency parameters. Recording of high-frequency events requires an *optical recorder,* which uses a suspended mirror on the galvanometer coil to direct a light beam across moving photographic or light-sensitive paper. Ultraviolet, light-sensitive recording paper allows immediate development for review of recordings. Some recording systems use a pressurized system that squirts ink through a nozzle located in the center of the galvanometer coil and onto recording paper. This system has a very-high-frequency response and provides an immediate permanent recording of events.

Zero reference

The weight of air or the atmospheric pressure also must be eliminated from pressure measurements dependent on altitude and environmental factors (usually about 760 mm Hg at standard temperature and pressure at sea level). This is accomplished by opening the transducer to air and adjusting the display system to read zero. In this way all pressure contributions from the atmosphere are negated, and only pressure values that exist within the heart chamber or vessel will be measured.

As discussed, hydrostatic pressure differences are eliminated by leveling the air-reference port with the patient's midchest and opening the reference port to room air and adjusting the system to zero.

Calibration

Accurate quantitation of recorded pressure measurements requires precise calibration of both the transducer and its associated amplifying electrical components. Most monitor systems have a built-in electrical calibration that yields a known pressure value. This calibration should be checked before hemodynamic monitoring is initiated. To avoid electronic drift, the instruments should be allowed to warm up for approximately 15 minutes. The steps for checking the electrical calibration of the monitoring system are as follows:

1. Depress the "cal" button on the monitor system.
2. After the readout stabilizes, adjust the control knob to obtain the appropriate readout value (e.g., 200 mm Hg).
3. Release the "cal" button, and make sure the reading returns to zero.

This procedure checks the electrical calibration of the system; it does not check the calibration of the transducer. Although all disposable transducers are precalibrated and coded by the manufacturer and are considered to be accurate at the time of use, it is important to remember that transducers are sensitive instruments and easily can be damaged. The calibration of a transducer easily can be checked by following these steps:

1. Attach a 3- or 4-foot long extension tubing to the side port of an in-line stopcock.
2. Turn the stopcock open between the infusion bag and the attached extension tubing and completely fill the tubing with fluid.
3. Vertically hold or mount the filled extension tubing (Fig. 3-8).

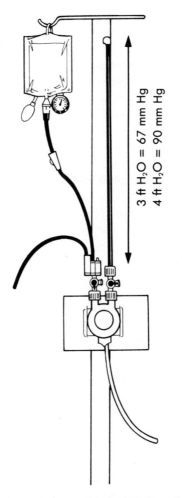

3 ft H₂O = 67 mm Hg
4 ft H₂O = 90 mm Hg

Fig. 3-8. Calibration of a pressure transducer with fluid. A 3- or 4-foot long fluid-filled tubing is extended vertically above the transducer. Pressure monitoring of the patient is discontinued temporarily, the vertical tubing is filled with fluid, and the appropriate values are observed on the monitor. This tubing can remain attached to the IV pole for additional calibration checks if necessary. As with all tubing, it should be changed every 24 to 48 hours.

4. Turn the stopcock open between the fluid-filled extension tubing and the transducer.
5. Check the digital readout on the monitor. A 3-foot fluid-filled tubing should exert a pressure of 67 (± 1) mm Hg; a 4-foot fluid-filled tubing should exert a pressure of 90 (± 1) mm Hg.

If the digital readout corresponds to the applied pressure, both the monitor and transducer are functioning correctly and may be used reliably for hemodynamic monitoring. If discrepancies occur greater than those within the specifications listed, the transducer is out of calibration and should be replaced.

Another method of calibration uses a mercury manometer to apply a known pressure directly to the transducer. However, because this method offers the possibility of introducing a large amount of air into the patient, its use is recommended only if transducer calibration check is performed before patient connection or if the system temporarily is disconnected from the patient.

Plumbing System

Transmission of a pressure signal from the patient to a transducer occurs through fluid-filled tubing. However, inherent properties of the fluid-filled system can distort the true pressure signal. The characteristics of a fluid-filled system that affect pressure wave accuracy during transmission are the resonant (or natural) frequency and the damping coefficient. Because of the inertia of the fluid in the system, pressure changes within the fluid column may differ in both amplitude and time from the action within the vessel. Thus pressure waves can be distorted before reaching the transducer. (This applies more to arterial pressures, which vary continuously, than to venous pressures, which are more static.) Because the transducer faithfully will reproduce the pressure it senses (no matter what the degree of distortion), inaccurate pressure readings can be obtained. Several factors can create pressure distortion in the plumbing system. These include the following:
1. Catheter and tubing length
2. Catheter and tubing stiffness
3. Catheter and tubing diameter
4. Air bubbles or blood clots
5. Stopcocks

Resonant frequency

The responsiveness of a plumbing system (including catheter, tubing, and stopcocks) depends on the *resonant frequency* of the system (see Fig. 3-7). This refers to how rapidly the system oscillates. This resonance is quite separate from the frequency of the pressure wave itself and is determined by the size, shape, and material of the plumbing system.

The frequency of the physiologic signal corresponds to the frequence of the patient's heart rate. At a heart rate of 60 beats per minute (bpm), the frequency of the physiologic signal is 1 per second, or 1 hertz (Hz); at a heart rate of 120 bpm, the signal frequency is 2 per second, or 2 Hz. It generally is believed that the important components of the arterial pressure wave, the most complex physiologic signal, can be reproduced at approximately 10 times the basic signal frequency, or 20 Hz, at heart rates up to 120 bpm. Thus in the critical care setting in which most patients are tachycardic, maintaining the system's *natural frequency* greater than 20 Hz is essential. If the pressure wave being transmitted has a frequency that is the same as, or near, the system's resonant frequency, the system will tend to vibrate or resonate (analogous to a bell after being struck). This produces an overshoot of the systolic pressures (accentuation), lowered diastolic pressures (attenuation), and often the appearance of numerous small oscillations in the waveform (Fig. 3-9). This error can be avoided by constructing a plumbing system whose natural, or resonant, frequency (fn) is as far away from the frequency of the physiologic signal as possible (see Fig. 3-7). Such construction includes the following:

1. **Keeping catheter and tubing length to a minimum (never longer than 3 to 4 feet).** Increased tubing length reduces the system's resonant frequency to a point at, or near, the frequency of the pressure signal. As mentioned, this results in accentuation and resonating of the signal.
2. **Using stiff, noncompliant tubing.** Soft, compliant catheters and tubing are

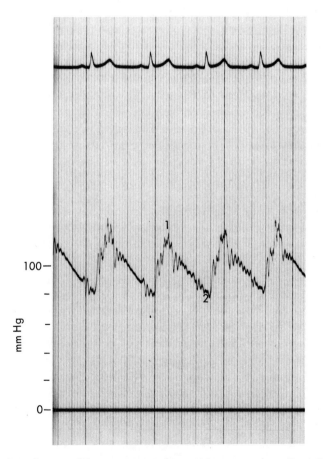

Fig. 3-9. Distortion of an arterial pressure waveform with numerous small oscillations caused by decreased resonant frequency of the plumbing system.

From Daily EK, Schroeder JS: *Hemodynamic waveforms: exercises in identification and analysis,* St Louis, 1983, Mosby–Year Book.

compressible by the transmitted pressure wave. This compression absorbs some of the pressure's energy and results in distortion and reduced amplitude of the pressure waveform (attenuation).

3. **Using large-diameter catheters (7 Fr or larger in adults; as large as possible in infants and children).** Small catheters increase the frictional resistance to movement. To overcome this, some energy from the pressure wave is lost. This generally results in reduced amplitude of the frequency components of the pressure signal. However, in the clinical setting it is necessary to strike a balance between using the smallest catheter possible to minimize the risks of thrombosis and using the largest catheter possible for faithful transmission of the physiologic signal.

4. **Eliminating all air bubbles from the system and preventing blood clot formation.** Air bubbles and blood clots are compressible. As with soft tubing, this compression of the bubble(s) by the transmitted pressure wave causes loss of the pressure wave's energy. The more energy that is lost or absorbed, the greater the amplitude reduction and distortion of the waveform. The extent of wave distortion is directly proportional to the size of the air bubble. This distortion also can occur with the formation of even small clots in the catheter tip or the stopcocks. The judicious use of anticoagulants and a continuous low-volume infusion can reduce the likelihood of clot formation.

5. **Reducing the number of stopcocks within the system.** Elimination of unnecessary stopcocks reduces the number of possible places for air bubbles or blood clots to lodge. In addition, the changes in system diameter that occur at each stopcock site alter the system's resonant frequency and can distort the signal. Basically, the system should be kept as simple and streamlined as possible.

Damping coefficient

In addition to having low natural or resonant frequencies, most catheter, tubing, and plumbing systems are *underdamped,* possessing low damping coefficients. The damping coefficient describes how quickly an oscillating system can come to rest or stop oscillating. The damping coefficient and the natural frequency of the system have a mutual effect on the system's dynamic response.

Visual inspection of the displayed waveform sometimes reveals the dynamic qualities of the monitoring system. Underdamping often is associated with amplified pressure changes ("ringing" or "fling"), or a narrow, high, very peaked systolic pressure followed by a second, less peaked, systolic curve (Fig. 3-10). An over-damped system often produces a waveform possessing a slow upstroke and a very rounded appearance. Frequently, however, alterations in the pressure signal, as a result of a low resonant frequency of the plumbing system or incorrect damping (either over or under), are less obvious, and incorrect pressures may be used as a basis for inappropriate therapeutic interventions.

Fortunately, both the system's natural frequency and damping coefficient can be measured quite easily at the bedside with the use of the in-line fast-flush device. Brief activation of the fast-flush provides a high pressure (300 mm Hg), which produces a square wave, which is followed by one or two oscillations that quickly revert to the patient's pressure wave.

Actual measurement of components of the oscillations following the square wave

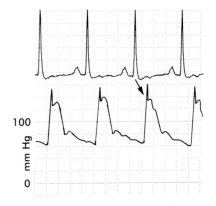

Fig. 3-10. Arterial pressure waveform with overshoot or "ringing" *(arrow)* of approximately 25 mm Hg.

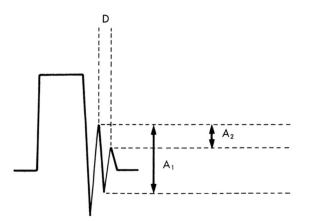

Fig. 3-11. Schematic illustration of a square wave (fast-flush) response to demonstrate measurement of the *natural frequency* (fn) and *damping coefficient* (ζ). The natural frequency is calculated by dividing the measured distance (d) between two consecutive peaks following the square wave into the speed at which the paper was run (usually 25 or 50 mm/sec). The damping coefficient can be estimated by calculating the ratio between the amplitude of two consecutive peaks (A2/A1) and then plotting that ratio on the graphic equation in Fig. 3-12, or on the scale in Fig. 3-17 to determine the corresponding damping coefficient.

can be used to determine both the natural frequency and the damping coefficient of the system. The *resonant* or *natural frequency* can be determined by measuring the distance between consecutive peaks of two oscillations after the square wave. This measurement then is divided *into* the speed of the paper recording (e.g., 25 mm/sec) to estimate the natural or resonant frequency of the system (Fig. 3-11).

The *damping coefficient* can be determined by measuring the amplitude, or height, of two consecutive peaks following the square wave. The smaller number then is divided by the larger (Fig. 3-11). This ratio then can be converted to the estimated damping coefficient by a complex formula or, more easily, with use of a graphic solution as shown in Fig. 3-12.

On a more practical basis, the dynamic response can be assessed visually at the

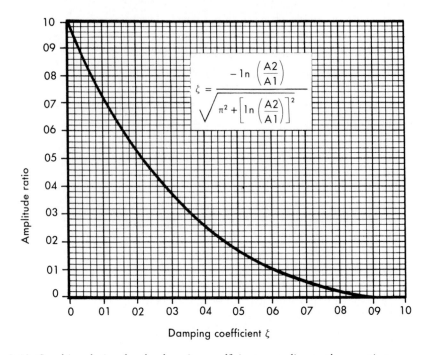

Fig. 3-12. Graphic solution for the damping coefficient according to the equation:

$$\text{Damping coefficient} = \frac{-\ln\left(\frac{A2}{A1}\right)}{\sqrt{\pi^2 + \left[\ln\left(\frac{A2}{A1}\right)\right]^2}}$$

where: A1 = Amplitude of 1st peak
       A2 = Amplitude of 2nd peak
       ln = Natural logarithm

From Gardner RM: *Anesthesiology* 54:227-236, 1981.

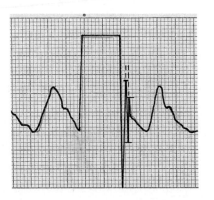

Fig. 3-13. Square wave test with undershoot followed by a small overshoot. The calculated measurements reveal an adequate dynamic response with a natural frequency (fn) of 31 Hz (25 ÷ 0.8) and a damping coefficient of 0.1 (12 ÷ 16.5 = 0.72 ratio).

bedside by simply observing the response to the fast-flush. In an optimally responsive system, the square wave should be followed by an undershoot spike, which is followed by a small overshoot before returning to the patient's waveform (Fig. 3-13). The appearance of numerous oscillations after the square wave is associated with an underdamped system, whereas the absence of any overshoot is seen in overdamped systems (Figs. 3-14 and 3-15). Ideally, the distance between two successive peaks should be 1 box or less if the paper is run at a speed of 25 mm/sec. This corresponds to a fn of 25 Hz, or more, at which level the damping coefficient is irrelevant. However, if the distance between two successive peaks is 1.5 to 2 boxes (at 25 mm per second paper speed), the amplitude ratio of the two spikes should be less than or equal to 0.3 (i.e., the second spike should be one-third, or less, the height of the first spike) (Fig. 3-16). This corresponds to a damping coefficient of 0.3 to 0.7, which is

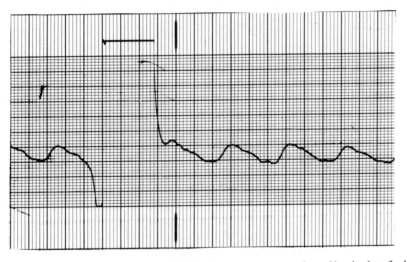

Fig. 3-14. Excessively damped arterial waveform by appearance confirmed by the fast-flush test, which has no downward spike and slowly returns to the waveform signal.

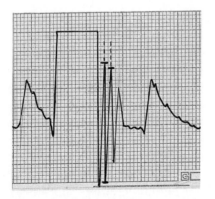

Fig. 3-15. Square wave test of this arterial waveform reveals a calculated natural frequency (fn) of 13 Hz (25 ÷ 2) and a damping coefficient <0.1 (30 ÷ 31.5 = 0.95 ratio). This is an unacceptably underdamped system, and efforts should be made to, first of all, increase the fn and then, if still necessary, increase the damping coefficient.

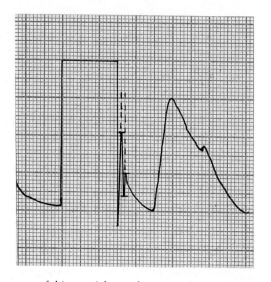

Fig. 3-16. Square wave test of this arterial waveform reveals a calculated natural frequency (fn) of 25 Hz (25 ÷ 1) and a damping coefficient of 0.35 (5.8 ÷ 17 = 0.34 ratio). This is an optimally damped system, which should provide accurate intraarterial pressure data. Even without doing the calculations, the adequacy of this system's dynamic response can be deduced from the fact that the peaks are no more than 1 mm apart and that the second peak is less than one-third the height of the first peak.

necessary to accurately reproduce the waveform components when the fn is low. When the distance between two peaks is greater than or equal to 2.5 boxes (again, at 25 mm/sec paper speed), the fn is less than 10 Hz and at this level it does not make any difference what the amplitude ratio is, because no amount of damping will satisfactorily improve the response. This basic analysis allows quick assessment of the system's dynamic response. Several repetitive square wave tests should be evaluated to adequately assess the system's dynamic response.

Fig. 3-17 plots the relationships between the natural frequency and the damping coefficient, as well as the acceptable ranges in which distortion of the pressure waveform is prevented. The best dynamic responses are obtained with a high natural frequency (20 Hz or higher) and optimum damping (i.e., with a damping coefficient between 0.6 and 0.75). As depicted in Fig. 3-15, the lower the natural frequency (particularly at or below 20 Hz), the higher the required damping coefficient (up to an approximated damping coefficient of 1.0).

Because optimum damping is difficult to achieve, all efforts should be made to increase the system's natural frequency by following the five steps previously outlined. The higher the system's natural frequency, the greater the latitude with the damping coefficient. With a natural frequency greater than 20 Hz, the damping coefficient may range from 0.2 to 1.0 and still faithfully reproduce the pressure wave. However, if the natural frequency of the plumbing system cannot be increased by minimizing the length of the tubing between the patient and the transducer, eliminating stopcocks, or meticulously removing any air bubbles, attempts should be made to increase the damping coefficient. (Even very tiny air bubbles can significantly lower the natural frequency to 10 Hz or less, resulting in gross overestimation of the actual pressure.)

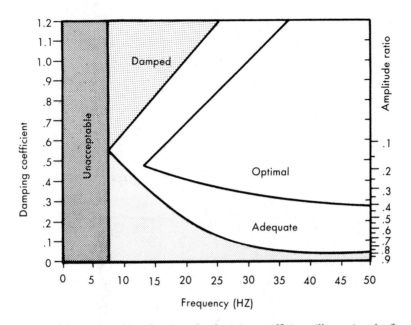

Fig. 3-17. Natural frequency plotted against the damping coefficient, illustrating the five areas into which catheter-tubing-transducer systems fall. Systems in the optimal area will reproduce even the most demanding (fast heart rate and rapid systolic upstroke) arterial or pulmonary artery waveforms without distortion. Systems within the adequate area will reproduce most typical patient waveforms with little or no distortion. All other areas will cause serious and clinically important waveform distortion. Note the scale on the right can be used to estimate the damping coefficient from the amplitude ratio determined during fast flushing.

From Gardner RM, Hollingsworth KW: *Crit Care Med* 14:651-658, 1986.

The damping coefficient can be altered mechanically with the addition of commercial damping devices. These damping devices are attached to the plumbing system and permit adjustment of resistance to increase the damping coefficient without changing the natural frequency.

If the systolic and diastolic pressures are considered important parameters to measure, the resonant frequency and damping coefficient of the system should be checked regularly to ensure accuracy. (The mean arterial pressure [MAP] is less likely to be affected by amplitude distortion.) The dynamic response of the monitoring system should be checked on a regular basis (at least once a shift) and any time the system has been opened to permit introduction of air or blood accumulation at some point within the system. The best way to avoid overshoot, peaking, or ringing in a recording system is to ensure that the natural frequency is far out into the high-frequency range—that is, far above those of the physiologic signal frequency.

This problem becomes accentuated when the frequency of the physiologic signal (the patient's heart rate) becomes high. Ringing and overshoot distort and overestimate the arterial pressure of patients who are tachycardic, producing an even greater need to achieve optimum dynamic response, with a natural frequency greater than 20 Hz.

REFERENCES

Abrams JH et al: Use of a needle valve resistor to improve invasive blood pressure monitoring, *Crit Care Med* 12:978-982, 1984.

American Association of Medical Instrumentation: ANSI standard: safe current limits for electromedical apparatus, 1982, AAMI.

Boutros A, Albert S: Effect of the dynamic response of transducer tubing system on accuracy of direct pressure measurement in patients, *Crit Care Med* 11:124-127, 1983.

Chandraratna PAN: Determination of zero-reference level for left atrial pressure by echocardiography, *Am Heart J* 89:159-162, 1975.

Donovan KD: Invasive monitoring and support of the circulation, *Clin Anesth* 3:909-953, 1985.

Falsetti HL et al: Analysis and correction of pressure wave distortion in fluid-filled catheter systems, *Circ XLIX*:165-173, 1974.

Gardner R: Direct blood pressure measurement-dynamic response requirements, *Anesthesiology* 54:227-236, 1981.

Gardner RM, Hollingsworth KW: Optimizing the electrocardiogram and pressure monitoring, *Crit Care Med* 14:651-658, 1986.

Geddes LA: *The direct and indirect measurement of blood pressure,* Chicago, 1970, Mosby–Year Book.

Gibbs NC, Gardner RM: Dynamics of invasive pressure monitoring systems: clinical and laboratory evaluation, *Heart Lung* 17:43-51, 1988.

Hunziker P: Accuracy and dynamic response of disposable pressure transducer-tubing systems, *Can J Anaesth* 34:400-414, 1987.

Jock CL, Hyman WA: Pressure wave fidelity in catheter introducers, *Cathet Cardiovasc Diagn* 27:57-65, 1992.

Kleinman B: Understanding natural frequency and damping and how they relate to the measurement of blood pressure, *J Clin Monit* 5:137-147, 1988.

Kleinman B et al: The fast flush test measures the dynamic response of the entire blood pressure monitoring system, *Anesthesiology* 77:1215-1220, 1992.

Landin Z, Trautman E, Teplick R: Contribution of measurement system artifacts to systolic spikes, *Med Instr* 17:110-112, 1983.

Morton BC: Basic equipment requirements for hemodynamic monitoring, *Can Med Assoc J* 121:879-892, 1979.

Shapiro GG, Krovetz LJ: Damped and undamped frequency responses of underdamped catheter manometer systems, *Am Heart J* 80:226-236, 1970.

Shinozaki T, Deane RS, Mazuzan JE: The dynamic responses of liquid-filled catheter systems for direct measurements of blood pressure, *Anesthesiology* 53:498-504, 1980.

Tojik RAN: Measurement of intracardiac pressure, *Herz* 11:283-290, 1986.

Yanof HM: *Biomedical electronics,* Philadelphia, 1972, FA Davis.

Chapter 4

Vascular Access

Access into either the venous or arterial system can be done via the percutaneous or surgical cutdown approach. Both techniques should be performed under aseptic conditions (except in emergency situations), with adequate administration of local anesthesia. The procedure should be explained to the patient (and family, if appropriate) and informed consent obtained.

VENOUS ACCESS
Access Sites

Access to the venous system for insertion of a central venous pressure (CVP) or pulmonary artery (PA) catheter can be obtained via peripheral arm veins (basilic, cephalic, median, cubital, or axillary), peripheral leg veins (femoral, saphenous), the peripheral neck vein (external jugular), the central neck vein (internal jugular), and the central chest vein (subclavian). Selection of a particular site depends on the patient's needs, individual anatomic considerations, and the operator's experience. In an emergency situation the first choice is any site that is available for rapid cannulation with the least amount of risk. Successful cannulation has been shown to closely correlate with the amount of operator experience. Table 4-1 lists some of the advantages and disadvantages for each venous insertion site.

Skin Preparation

Infection may be prevented by proper preparation of the skin surface before catheter insertion via percutaneous or venous cutdown routes. The site should be shaved, and an iodine preparation such as povidone-iodine complex (Betadine) should be applied for 1 minute and allowed to dry. A solution of 70% alcohol should then be applied and allowed to dry, and sterile drapes with a small opening should be placed around the area. Sterile gown and gloves should be worn, and sterile techniques should be maintained throughout the procedure.

Catheter Preparation

For insertion of a CVP, the length of catheter insertion required for proper positioning of the tip in the superior vena cava (SVC), just above the right atrial (RA) junction, should be estimated. This can be done by holding the packaged or protected catheter over the patient from the proposed insertion site to the sternal notch.

Before its insertion, the outside of the catheter should be wiped with sterile

Table 4-1. Advantages and disadvantages of venous insertion sites

Site	Advantages	Disadvantages
Internal jugular vein	Less risk of pleural puncture and pneumothorax Easier insertion with constant landmarks If hematoma occurs, it is visible and usually can be compressed Malposition of central venous catheter rare with direct path to right side of heart from right internal jugular vein Best approach for emergency transvenous pacing during chest and abdominal surgery (most accessible direct route to right side of heart)	Difficult to cannulate in hypovolemic patients "Blind" puncture Restriction of patient's neck mobility Increased risk of catheter movement or kinking with head movements Trendelenburg position for catheter insertion may not be possible for some patients Risk of carotid artery puncture
Subclavian vein	Remains open even in profound circulatory collapse Catheter fixation more secure Less restricting for patient Direct route to right side of heart	Pleural space easily entered "Blind" puncture Risk of subclavian artery puncture Difficult to apply compression if subclavian artery inadvertently punctured Higher incidence of catheter malposition
Femoral vein	Easy to cannulate Fewer major complications Accessible during cardiopulmonary resuscitation (CPR), but may not be best route	Possible increased risk of infection "Blind" puncture Less mobility for patient Risk of femoral artery puncture Malposition of central venous catheter unless fluoroscopy used
External jugular vein	Fewer major complications "Nonblind" puncture Accessible during operation	Increased difficulty negotiating catheter for central venous placement Increased risk of central venous catheter malposition Vein not always visible
Basilic and median cubital veins	Easy to cannulate when visible or palpable Safe Preferred route during CPR	Vein not always visible or palpable Difficult to cannulate in hypovolemic patients High rate of malposition if fluoroscopy not used for central catheter placement Not optimal for rapid fluid infusion or emergency transvenous pacing
Cephalic vein	Same as for basilic and median cubital veins	Same as for basilic and median cubital veins Sharp angle at shoulder may preclude entry into central vein without use of a guide-wire

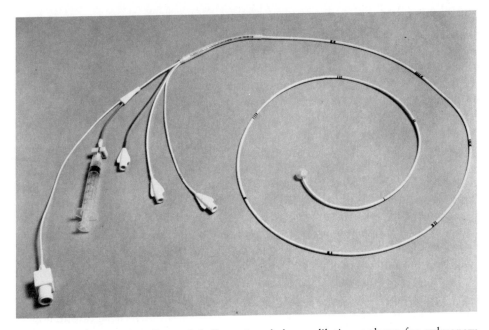

Fig. 4-1. Swan-Ganz flow-directed, balloon-tipped thermodilution catheter for pulmonary artery (PA) and right atrial (RA) pressure monitoring and cardiac output measurement. Syringe is used for inflating the balloon with air.

Courtesy American Edwards Laboratories, Santa Ana, Calif.

solution and all open lumens thoroughly flushed. The balloon of the flotation catheter should be inflated with the recommended volume of air (written on the shaft of the catheter) and immersed in sterile water to check for possible leaks as indicated by the presence of small bubbles in the water.

If a thermodilution catheter is used, the thermistor wires should be checked before insertion by adjoining the cardiac output (CO) cable to the appropriate thermistor hub of the catheter (Fig. 4-1). The CO computer will flash "Faulty cath" if the thermistor wires are damaged. In this case, a new PA catheter should be used.

If an Svo_2 catheter is being inserted, calibration of the fiberoptics should be performed by inserting the catheter tip into the provided calibration receptable according to the manufacturer's directions. This is performed under sterile conditions.

The distal lumen of the pulmonary artery catheter should be connected to a transducer via fluid-filled tubing so hemodynamic waveforms can be monitored during insertion and advancement of the catheter.

Percutaneous Catheterization

In 1953 Dr. Sven-Ivar Seldinger, a Stockholm radiologist, described the procedure for percutaneous arterial insertion of a catheter using a guidewire. This simple but revolutionary technique has stood the test of time and now is the preferred method of catheter insertion into either an artery or a vein.

Percutaneous insertion of central venous catheters has become widely accepted, not only because of speed of placement, but also because of the reduced risk of infection. In addition, percutaneous venous catheterization often preserves the integrity of the vessel, thus permitting future access.

The basic tools of the Seldinger technique of catheterization consist of an introducing needle, a guidewire, and a catheter. Although any type of needle could be used for the Seldinger technique, thin-walled needles are preferred, because the lumen can accommodate a guidewire without substantially increasing the outside diameter. Consequently, today virtually all percutaneous puncture needles have thin walls.

Fig. 4-2 illustrates the basic steps involved in percutaneous catheterization.

Procedure

Internal jugular vein. Catheterization of the internal jugular vein in the adult was first described by Hemosura in 1966. Since that time the internal jugular vein has been commonly used for percutaneous insertion of central venous, PA, and pacing catheters because its anatomic location provides a straight path to the right side of the heart, its landmarks are more definite and constant, and the complication rate is lower than with the subclavian approach.

ANATOMY. The internal jugular vein emerges from the base of the skull to enter the carotid sheath, which also contains the carotid artery and the vagus nerve. Initially, the internal jugular vein is posterior and lateral to the more superficial carotid artery. However, near the terminal portion of the vein, above its juncture with the subclavian vein, the internal jugular vein becomes lateral and slightly anterior to the carotid artery.

The lower portion of the internal jugular vein lies within the triangle formed by the sternal and clavicular heads of the sternocleidomastoid muscle (Fig. 4-3). It is within this triangle that the internal jugular vein is best cannulated. Behind the sternal end of the clavicle, the internal jugular vein unites with the subclavian vein to form the innominate vein.

EQUIPMENT. The basic percutaneous equipment tray is required, as well as the catheter of choice (central venous, PA, or pacing).

PATIENT PREPARATION. The patient should first be prepared as described on p. 53. Additional specific patient preparation consists of the following:

1. If the patient is obese or muscular with a short neck, place a small pillow or rolled towel under the shoulders to extend the neck.
2. Locate the carotid artery by palpation.
3. Identify the internal jugular vein and mark it if necessary.
4. Turn the patient's head to the contralateral side.
5. Place the patient in a 15- to 25-degree Trendelenburg position to distend the veins and prevent air embolism.

PROCEDURE. The literature describes at least 13 different variations of two basic approaches to percutaneous internal jugular vein cannulation. A high entry can be approached via a posterior (or lateral) route, an anterior (or medial) route, or a central route. Likewise, a low internal jugular puncture can be approached from a lateral or central route. Although either the right or left internal jugular vein can be cannulated, most physicians prefer the right internal jugular vein because it is larger, it forms a straight line to the superior vena cava and right atrium, the dome of the right lung and pleura lies lower than on the left side, and the large thoracic duct is not endangered. However, when right internal jugular vein cannulation fails and there is no hematoma, successful cannulation usually can be carried out on the left side.

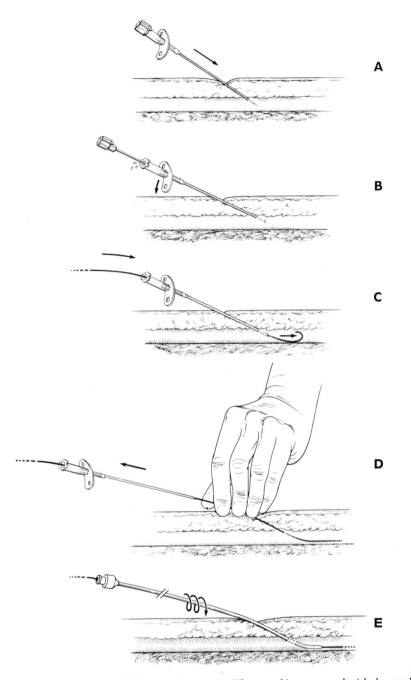

Fig. 4-2. Basic procedure for the Seldinger technique. **A,** The vessel is punctured with the needle at a 30- to 40-degree angle. **B,** The stylet is removed, and free blood flow is observed; the angle of the needle is then reduced. **C,** The flexible tip of the guidewire is passed through the needle into the vessel. **D,** The needle is removed over the wire while firm pressure is applied at the site. **E,** The tip of the catheter or sheath is passed over the wire and advanced into the vessel with a rotating motion.

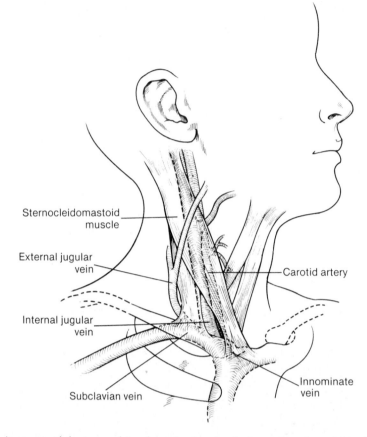

Sternocleidomastoid
muscle

External jugular
vein

Carotid artery

Internal jugular
vein

Innominate
vein

Subclavian vein

Fig. 4-3. Anatomy of the internal jugular vein showing its lower location within the triangle formed by the sternocleidomastoid muscle and the clavicle.

Discussion here will be limited to cannulation of the internal jugular vein via the central approach described by Daily et al.

1. Identify the internal jugular vein by drawing a triangle from marks placed on the medial aspect of the clavicle, the medial aspect of the sternal head, and the lateral aspect of the clavicular head of the sternocleidomastoid muscle (Fig. 4-4). The center of the triangle is directly over the center of the internal jugular vein. (Having the awake patient lift his or her head slightly off the bed makes this triangle more visible and palpable.)

2. With a #11 blade, make a small (2 to 3 mm) stab wound at the insertion site (or do this after guidewire insertion).

3. Administer a local anesthetic and locate the internal jugular vein via a small (22- or 25-gauge) needle 3 to 4 cm above the medial aspect of the clavicle and 1 to 2 cm within the lateral border of the sternocleidomastoid muscle.

4. Attach a 3- or 5-ml syringe containing 2 or 3 ml of sterile saline or 1% lidocaine to the 18-gauge vascular needle. (The smaller syringe is easier to handle.)

5. Align the needle with the syringe (see Fig. 4-4) parallel to the medial border of the clavicular head of the sternocleidomastoid muscle. Direct the needle caudally at a 30-degree angle to the frontal plane directly over the internal jugular vein

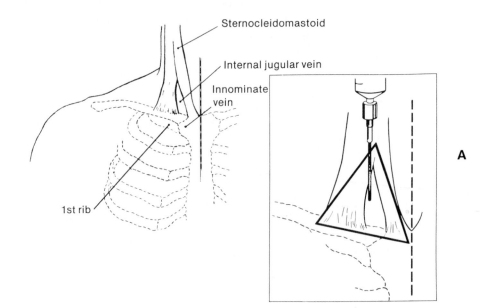

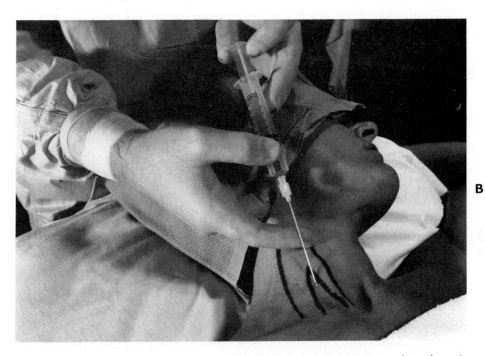

Fig. 4-4. Relationship of external anatomic landmarks to underlying internal jugular vein. **A,** Triangle drawn over clavicle and sternal and clavicular portions of sternocleidomastoid muscle is centered over internal jugular vein (inset). **B,** Alignment of the needle in the central portion of the triangle formed by the sternal and clavicular sections of the sternocleidomastoid muscle.

A from Daily PO, Griepp RB, Shumway NE: *Arch Surg* 101:534-536, 1970. Copyright 1970, American Medical Association.

and aiming toward the ipsilateral nipple. (If the needle is positioned with its bevel side directed medially, the bevel aids in directing the guidewire medially into the central circulation.)

6. Puncture the skin and advance the needle while maintaining a slight negative pressure in the syringe until free flow of blood is obtained.

7. If the internal jugular vein is not entered initially, withdraw the needle while maintaining suction with the syringe and then redirect it 5 to 10 degrees more laterally. If the vein still has not been entered, direct the needle more in line with the sagittal plane. Do not direct the needle medially across the sagittal plane lest the carotid artery be punctured. If possible, have the patient perform the Valsalva maneuver to distend the vein and improve the chance of successful cannulation.

8. After you observe free flow of venous blood into the syringe, instruct the patient to hold his or her breath or hum. During this time, quickly remove the syringe from the needle, place a thumb over the needle hub, and insert the soft, flexible tip of the appropriate guidewire through the needle approximately 10 to 15 cm. Remove the needle and wipe the guidewire with a sterile, moist gauze pad. Instruct the patient to resume normal breathing.

9. Insert the catheter introducer set over the guidewire until 10 to 15 cm of wire extends beyond the hub of the sheath. Advance the dilator and sheath through the skin and subcutaneous tissue into the vein. If the introducer has a side arm, this should be closed to the patient.

10. Remove the dilator and the guidewire together from the sheath.

11. Aspirate and flush the sheath side arm with saline and temporarily close the stopcock toward the patient or connect it to a heparin IV infusion.

12. Insert the catheter of choice through the sheath and position it in the heart.

13. Aspirate and flush the catheter and sheath side arm and connect them to a heparinized IV infusion or pressure tubing.

14. Suture the sheath and catheter to the skin.

15. Apply an iodophor ointment and sterile dressing to the insertion site and tape it securely.

16. Return the patient to a flat position and remove the pillow or roll from the shoulders.

17. Perform chest x-ray examination to verify catheter position (if fluoroscopy was not used).

Subclavian vein. Cannulation of the subclavian vein for venous catheterization has grown in popularity since 1962, when Wilson et al. described their successful experience with subclavian insertion of central venous catheters. Percutaneous catheterization of the subclavian vein has become a common approach to insertion of central venous, PA, and pacing catheters. This approach has been very popular for long-term placement of catheters for parenteral nutrition because it is easier to secure the catheter and there is less interference with the patient's mobility. The subclavian vein is also the easiest vein to cannulate in patients with profound circulatory collapse.

ANATOMY. The subclavian vein begins at the lateral border of the first rib as the continuation of the axillary vein, and it ends at the medial border of the anterior scalene muscle. It joins the internal jugular vein behind the sternoclavicular joint to form the innominate vein (Fig. 4-5). The vein is separated from its artery by the anterior scalene muscle, which is approximately 10 to 15 mm thick. The vein crosses the first rib and lies anteroinferior to the artery (posterior to the middle third of the

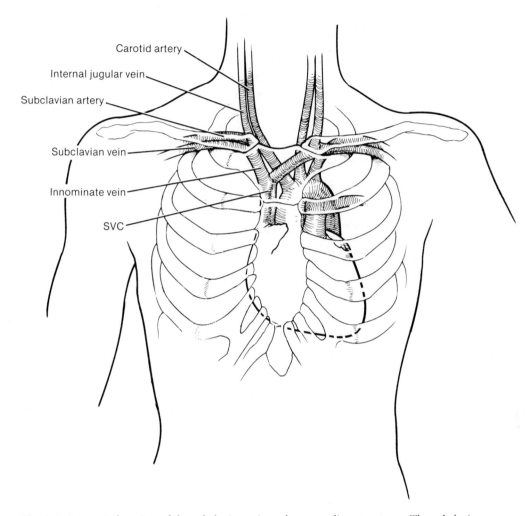

Carotid artery

Internal jugular vein

Subclavian artery

Subclavian vein

Innominate vein

SVC

Fig. 4-5. Anatomic location of the subclavian vein and surrounding structures. The subclavian vein joins the internal jugular vein to become the innominate vein at about the manubrioclavicular junction. The innominate vein becomes the superior vena cava (SVC) at about the level of the midmanubrium.

clavicle). The apical pleura lies approximately 5 mm posterior to the junction of the jugular and subclavian veins. The subclavian vein is a large vein with an inside diameter of 1.5 to 2.0 cm or more.

EQUIPMENT. The equipment required is the same as that for the internal jugular vein approach.

PATIENT PREPARATION. The patient first should be prepared as described on p. 53. Additional preparation consists of the following:
1. Place a rolled towel under the patient's back between the scapulae.
2. Turn the patient's head to the contralateral side.
3. Place the patient in a 15- to 25-degree Trendelenburg position.

PROCEDURE. The subclavian vein can be approached from either the superior or inferior direction. Overall success and complication rates of both methods are very similar. However, the supraclavicular approach offers several practical advantages:

there is a shorter distance between the vein and the skin (0.5 to 4 cm); it is a more direct path to the superior vena cava; it is more easily performed during CPR with minimal or no interruption of chest compression; and the rate of correct catheter tip location is greater than with the infraclavicular approach.

Practical advantages notwithstanding, the infraclavicular approach to percutaneous subclavian catheterization remains the most popular method, and discussion here is limited to this technique. Either the right or left subclavian vein may be cannulated, although the left subclavian vein may be preferred for catheter insertion because it gently curves into the innominate vein and no sharp bends of the catheter are required. However, the pleural dome is not as high on the right side as on the left side.

1. Identify the junction of the middle and medial thirds of the clavicle where the first rib proceeds beneath the clavicle. Needle insertion should be approximately 1 to 2 cm lateral and inferior to this location. A frequent error is use of a more lateral insertion site at the midclavicle area. Another means of identification is to palpate the inferior surface of the clavicle and locate a tubercle on the clavicle approximately one-third to one-half the length of the clavicle from the sternoclavicular joint. This tubercle marks the site of needle entry.

2. Make a small (3 mm) skin nick at the insertion site using a #11 blade, sharp side upward (or do this after guidewire insertion).

3. Depress the area 1 to 2 cm beneath the junction of the distal and middle thirds of the clavicle with the thumb of the nondominant hand and place the index finger of the same hand approximately 2 cm above the sternal notch.

4. Administer a local anesthetic and locate the vein via a small (21- or 25-gauge) needle directed toward the index finger above the notch and at a 20- to 30-degree angle with the thorax. (Direct the bevel of the needle inferiomedially to encourage guidewire passage into the innominate vein.)

5. Insert the needle under the clavicle at the point identified in step 1 (Fig. 4-6).

6. Advance the needle, "walking" it down until it slips beneath the clavicle while maintaining gentle negative pressure within the syringe.

7. When the vein is entered, remove the smaller needle and attach the 18-gauge needle to a syringe containing 5 to 10 ml of heparin or lidocaine and repeat steps 3 to 6 while maintaining negative pressure in the syringe.

8. When the vein is entered with the cannulating needle, ask the patient to hold his or her breath or hum while you quickly remove the syringe from the 18-gauge needle and immediately cap the needle hub with your thumb or index finger.

9. Insert the flexible tip of the guidewire 10 to 15 cm through the needle and remove the needle, maintaining gentle pressure on the puncture site. Instruct the patient to resume breathing.

10. With the sheath's side arm closed to the patient, advance the catheter introducer set (dilator and sheath) over the guidewire into the vein, using a slight twisting motion (the side arm is closed to the patient).

11. Remove the guidewire and dilator together from the sheath.

12. Aspirate and flush the side arm of the sheath and close its stopcock to the patient.

13. Insert the catheter of choice. Having the patient bring his or her ear to the shoulder on the side of the insertion site creates a sharp angle between the jugular

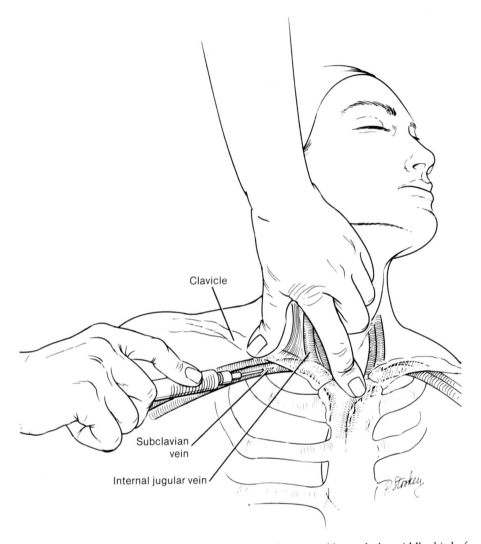

Clavicle

Subclavian
vein

Internal jugular vein

Fig. 4-6. Puncture of the subclavian vein with the needle inserted beneath the middle third of the clavicle at a 20- to 30-degree angle aiming medially.

and subclavian veins and helps prevent misdirection of the catheter into the internal jugular vein during advancement.

14. Advance and position the catheter in the heart.
15. Aspirate and flush the catheter and the side arm of the sheath and connect the side arm of the sheath and the hub of the catheter to a heparin IV infusion and pressure tubing.
16. Suture the sheath and catheter to the skin near the insertion site.
17. Apply an iodophor ointment and sterile dressing to the insertion site and tape it securely.
18. Return the patient to a flat position and remove the roll from his or her back.
19. Obtain a chest x-ray film to verify catheter position if fluoroscopy was not used.

Special precautions

PREVENTION OF GUIDEWIRE MISDIRECTION INTO THE JUGULAR VEIN. If guidewire passage is not entirely smooth, the wire may have entered the jugular vein. The patient may complain of an unpleasant sensation in the area of the ipsilateral ear. The guidewire location should be confirmed with fluoroscopy and the wire repositioned before the catheter is advanced over it. A caudal direction of the bevel of the needle and having the patient bring his or her ear down to the shoulder on the insertion side during guidewire passage are steps that may prevent guidewire misdirection into the jugular vein.

PASSAGE OF THE NEEDLE UNDER THE CLAVICLE. If it proves difficult to depress the needle sufficiently to pass under the clavicle into the vein, the needle may be bent smoothly over its entire length to form a gentle arc. The needle should then be inserted at a 45-degree angle under the clavicle, and following its 30-degree arc, it will usually enter the vein.

REDUCING THE RISK OF PNEUMOTHORAX. The operator can reduce the risk of pneumothorax by avoiding too lateral or too deep a needle insertion. Multiple attempts at cannulation should be avoided. Generally, if three attempts prove unsuccessful, another site should be chosen. Patients with chronic obstructive pulmonary disease with overinflated stiff lungs, especially patients receiving ventilatory support, are at a higher risk for pulmonary complications resulting from attempted subclavian cannulation. Thus subclavian vein cannulation is best avoided in these patients. If cannulation is attempted but unsuccessful, a chest radiograph should be obtained to rule out pneumothorax before contralateral insertion.

CORRECT AIM OF THE NEEDLE IN THE ELDERLY. In elderly patients the subclavian vein may be more inferior, requiring aiming of the needle toward the inferior margin of the sternal notch. These patients also may have a bony prominence beneath the medial portion of the clavicle, making cannulation difficult.

PREVENTION OF PUNCTURE OF THE SUBCLAVIAN ARTERY. The operator can avoid puncture of the subclavian artery by selecting a puncture site that is away from the most lateral course of the vein and by not angulating the needle too far posteriorly. If the subclavian artery is punctured, the needle should be removed and firm pressure applied over the puncture site for 10 minutes.

Venous or arterial vascular access can be achieved in less than optimal conditions with the use of the SmartNeedle™. This technology incorporates a Doppler flow probe within an 18- or 20-gauge needle to aid in identifying vessel location and in positioning the needle within the vessel.

1. Turn the SmartNeedle™ monitor on and note illumination of the indicator light.
2. Under sterile conditions flush the SmartNeedle™ with sterile saline or other IV solution to remove air from within the needle, which could interfere with the quality of the signal.
3. Following standard cannulation technique, insert the SmartNeedle™ subcutaneously at the estimated site of vessel entry.
4. Following subcutaneous entry, again flush the needle with approximately 0.5 ml sterile saline to remove any air bubbles from the tip of the needle, which would interfere with transmission of the Doppler signal.
5. Listen for the Doppler flow signal while advancing the catheter in the direction that

produces the strongest audible signal. (Arterial flow sound is sharper and higher-pitched than the lower-pitched venous flow sounds.)

6. Continue to advance the needle in the direction of the most intense signal until the needle punctures the vessel—as indicated by a distinct increase in the intensity and crispness of the signal.

7. Remove the Doppler flow probe from the needle and observe blood flow at the needle hub.

8. Follow standard guidewire and catheter insertion steps as outlined on p. 60.

This technology may be extremely useful for percutaneous cannulation of obese patients, patients with weak pulses, or patients with absent pulses secondary to occlusive disease. Under such conditions, the SmartNeedle™ may improve the speed and accuracy of vascular cannulation, as well as minimize complications.

Arm vein. Cannulation of a vein in the antecubital fossa used to be a popular technique for inserting central catheters with the lowest major complication rate. However, catheterization of the central veins has become more common since the advent of balloon flotation pulmonary artery (PA) catheters. When fluoroscopy is not used, improper positioning of central venous catheters from an arm vein occurs much more frequently than clinically suspected, with reported incidences of 36% to 52%. In addition, arm movement can cause catheter tip movement of several centimeters, increasing the risk of phlebitis and cardiac tamponade. With pacemakers, this movement may result in electrode dislodgment or right ventricle (RV) perforation.

A central venous line usually can be inserted through the median vein or the basilic vein distal to the antecubital fossa. The cephalic vein is an equally large vein, but its sharp angle at the shoulder makes it more difficult to navigate.

ANATOMY. Venous blood from the arm drains through two main intercommunicating veins—the basilic and the cephalic veins. The basilic vein is deeper and ascends along the ulnar surface of the forearm (Fig. 4-7). It is joined by the median cubital vein in front of the elbow and continues up along the medial side of the brachial artery to the lower border of the teres major, where it becomes the axillary vein. The cephalic vein ascends on the radial aspect of the forearm. It communicates with the basilic vein through the median cubital vein just in front of the elbow and ascends laterally until it curves sharply as it pierces the clavipectoral fascia, crosses the axillary artery, and passes beneath the clavicle to join the axillary vein, or occasionally the external jugular vein. Because of this anatomy, the cephalic vein is more difficult to catheterize, making the basilic vein preferable.

PATIENT PREPARATION. The patient is first prepared as described on p. 53. Additional specific preparation is conducted as follows:

1. Locate the vein. This may be easier if you temporarily apply a tourniquet above the antecubital fossa and the patient makes a fist to distend the veins.

2. Abduct the selected arm 30 to 45 degrees from the body and secure it on a flat, padded arm board.

3. For placement of a central venous catheter without fluoroscopy, estimate the length of catheter needed as described on p. 53.

PROCEDURE. This discussion will be limited to insertion of a PA catheter into an antecubital vein via the Seldinger technique.

1. Apply a venous tourniquet to the upper arm.

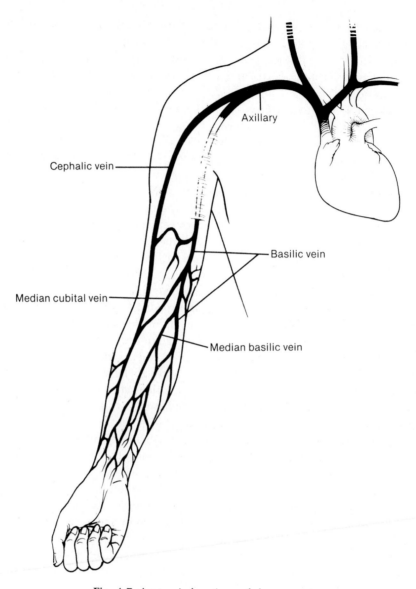

Fig. 4-7. Anatomic locations of the arm veins.

2. While retaining traction on the skin distal to the insertion with one hand, puncture the vein with the needle held bevel side upward at a 15- to 20-degree angle.
3. With the appearance of the backflow of blood into the needle, insert the guidewire into the vein approximately 2 to 4 cm beyond the tip of the needle.
4. Release the tourniquet and slowly continue to advance the guidewire several centimeters.
5. Withdraw the needle from the vein while firmly holding the guidewire in place in the vessel.
6. Wipe the guidewire with a sterile, moist gauze pad.

7. Insert the catheter of choice or a catheter introducer sheath over the guidewire into the vein.

8. Remove the guidewire. If a catheter introducer set is used, remove the inner dilator along with the guidewire, flush the sheath's side arm, and temporarily close the stopcock. Insert the catheter of choice into the sheath.

9. Aspirate and flush the catheter and connect both the catheter and side arm of the sheath to a heparinized flushing solution.

10. Position the catheter in the proper location.

11. Suture the catheter to the skin with 3-0 silk. (If a catheter sheath is used, suture the sheath and catheter separately to the skin.)

12. Apply an iodophor ointment and a sterile dressing to the insertion site and tape securely.

13. Immobilize the arm with an arm board.

14. Perform chest x-ray examination to verify the position of the catheter (if fluoroscopy was not used).

Special precautions

MEETING RESISTANCE. Do not force the catheter to advance. Withdraw the catheter 2 to 3 cm, rotate it slightly, and readvance it. Other maneuvers that may facilitate catheter passage include further abducting of the arm, having the patient move his or her shoulder anteriorly or posteriorly, having the patient inspire deeply, having the patient turn his or her head to the side of the venipuncture to prevent the catheter from entering the internal jugular vein, and partially inflating the balloon of the catheter, if available.

ENSURING VISIBILITY. Do not attempt placement of a central venous catheter into a vein that cannot be made visible or palpable by means of a tourniquet, warm compresses, or placement of the arm in a dependent position with opening and closing of the hand. Choose another site in such a case.

PA Catheter Insertion

The PA catheter should be connected to a fluid-filled transducer system before insertion to provide continuous pressure monitoring during advancement. When the catheter tip reaches the superior vena cava (SVC), the balloon of the catheter should be partially inflated to promote flotation into the RA (Fig. 4-8, *A* and *B*). When the tip of the catheter reaches the RA, as indicated by an RA waveform (Fig. 4-9) with marked respiratory variation, inflate the balloon with approximately 1 cc of air. The catheter then should float into the RV (Fig. 4-8, *C*), and an RV waveform will be displayed on the monitor (see Fig. 4-9). (Watch the ECG closely for signs of ventricular irritability when the catheter is in the RV.) Advance the catheter as quickly and smoothly as possible until the catheter resists advancement and a PA waveform is present on the monitor (see Fig. 4-9). Deflate the balloon, obtain a PA pressure recording, and slightly advance the catheter (Fig. 4-10). Slowly inflate the balloon until a pulmonary artery wedge (PAW) waveform appears on the screen (see Fig. 4-9). *Inflate only for a brief time and only enough to change the waveform from PA to PAW.* If there is a discrepancy between the PAW and PA diastolic pressures, repeat the measurements several times to verify. Ensure that the balloon is completely deflated after each inflation by removing the inflating syringe. Actively withdrawing the air back into the syringe is not recommended because it can damage the balloon.

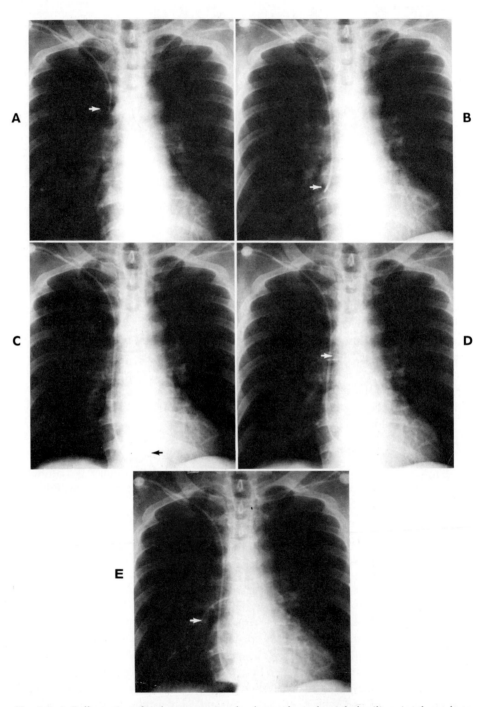

Fig. 4-8. A, Balloon-tipped catheter entering the thorax from the right basilic vein; the catheter tip is in the superior vena cava. **B,** Catheter tip is in the mid–right atrium. **C,** Catheter tip is in the right ventricle. **D,** Catheter tip is in the pulmonary artery. **E,** Catheter tip is advanced to a pulmonary artery wedge position.

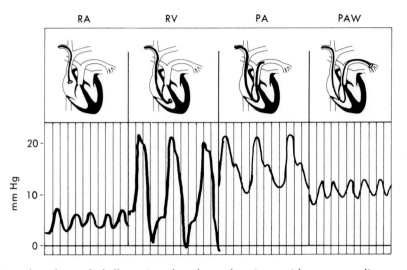

Fig. 4-9. Flow-directed, balloon-tipped catheter locations with corresponding pressure tracings.

From Schroeder JS, Daily EK: *Hemodynamic monitoring. Tampa Tracings slide series,* Tarpon Springs, Fla, 1976, Tampa Tracings.

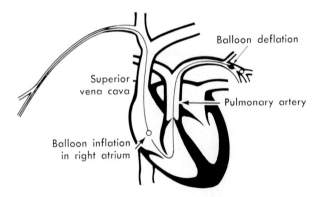

Fig. 4-10. Flow-directed, balloon-tipped catheter showing inflation of balloon in the right atrium and consequent "floating" of the catheter through the right ventricle and out to a distal pulmonary artery (PA) branch. The balloon is deflated, advanced slightly, and reinflated slightly to obtain a pulmonary artery wedge (PAW) pressure.

Complications

Complications common to all venous cannulation techniques include hematoma, thrombosis, phlebitis, sepsis, cellulitis, and air embolism. Other complications are specific to the site of insertion and are presented in Table 4-2, along with rates of successful insertion, central venous catheter malposition, and overall complications. Experience and meticulous attention to technique are the best safeguards against these complications. Even then, life-threatening complications may occur.

Venous air embolism. Venous air embolism is a rare but catastrophic complication of central venous catheter placement, with a mortality of approximately 50%. Lethal air embolism occurs with central injection of 200 to 300 cc of air at a rate of 70 to 150 cc per second, although as little as 20 cc of air may cause harm to a critically ill patient. The rate of air entry depends on both the inside diameter and the length of the tubing inserted. Air can enter a vein, particularly a large vein such as the internal jugular or subclavian, by one of three methods: (1) through a disconnection of or leak in the catheter, the infusion tubing, or any of the connecting sites; (2) through the needle or sheath at the time of insertion into the vein; or (3) along the formed track of a removed catheter that had been in place for a prolonged period, especially in a thin person with little subcutaneous tissue. This complication is more likely to occur

Table 4-2. Insertion success rate, central venous catheter malposition, overall complication rate, and specific complications associated with various venous insertion sites

Site	Insertion success rate (%)	Catheter malposition rate (%) (without fluoroscopy)	Overall complication rate (%)	Specific complications
Basilic	58-98	25-52	3-5	Thrombophlebitis Thrombosis Phlebitis/cellulitis
Internal jugular	80-94	0-6 (Right) 0-20 (Left)	< 1-13	Carotid artery puncture Myocardial perforation of pacing catheter Pneumothorax Hemothorax Air embolism Catheter embolism Nerve damage Thrombosis Horner's syndrome
Subclavian vein	85-98	20-33	< 1-17	Pneumothorax Subclavian artery puncture Sepsis Hemothorax Hydrothorax Air embolism Thrombophlebitis Thrombosis Catheter embolism Brachial plexus injury Phrenic nerve injury Sternoclavicular osteomyelitis
Femoral vein	89-95	—	4-20	Evidence of thrombus Infection Femoral artery puncture
External jugular vein	61-99	6	0-4	Hematoma Air embolism Thrombosis

---

Manifestations, prevention, and treatment of air embolism

MANIFESTATIONS

Acute respiratory distress, apnea, occasional wheezing
Sudden hypotension and syncope
Profound hypoxia, cyanosis
Audible machinery ("mill wheel") murmur
Elevated central venous pressure (CVP) or jugular venous pressure
Neurologic deficits (hemiplegia, aphasia) in presence of right-to-left shunt
Cardiac arrest with asystole or ventricular fibrillation

PREVENTION

Use meticulous insertion technique, occluding needle and catheter hub as necessary
Elevate venous pressure before insertion (Trendelenburg position; volume expansion,
   if venous pressure is low)
Use sheaths with pneumatic valve and check competency of valve before using
Use Luer-Lok connections
Securely tighten all central catheters and connections
Do not allow containers of IV solutions to completely empty
Secure vaseline gauze and occlusive dressing over insertion site after catheter removal

TREATMENT

Immediately place patient in left lateral Trendelenburg position
Have the patient perform the Valsalva maneuver, if possible
Administer 100% oxygen and ventilatory support
Aspirate air via CVP or pulmonary artery catheter
Administer hyperbaric oxygen treatment
Administer cardiopulmonary resuscitation if necessary

---

when the patient is in an upright position, takes a deep breath, or is in a state of hypovolemia with low central venous pressure.

Massive air embolism can cause obstruction of the right ventricular outflow tract and interfere with gas exchange, presenting with manifestations that are similar to those of pulmonary thromboembolism. The diagnosis of venous air embolism is primarily clinical; the condition should be suspected whenever sudden cardiovascular collapse occurs in patients with a central venous catheter in place or just recently removed. Two-dimensional echocardiography has been shown to be of value in the diagnosis of venous air embolism. High-resolution computed tomographic (CT) scanning and magnetic resonance imaging (MRI) are helpful in the diagnosis of arterial air emboli of the central nervous system. The clinical manifestations, as well as methods of prevention and treatment of venous air embolism, are listed in the box above.

ARTERIAL ACCESS

Catheterization of the arterial system is indicated for pressure measurements, angiography, cardiac output determination, and counterpulsation. In addition, continuous intraarterial pressure monitoring and multiple arterial blood sampling frequently are necessary in patients with unstable ischemic heart disease (with or without myocardial infarction), adult respiratory distress syndrome, severe arterial hypertension undergoing afterload-reducing therapy, hypotension or shock, and in patients who have undergone cardiac surgery.

Arterial Cannulation Sites

The arterial system can be cannulated either percutaneously or via a cutdown at several sites. If necessary, the arterial system also can be entered via cannulation of arterial grafts. To reduce complications and obtain the most accurate hemodynamic data, catheters preferably are placed in the large-diameter arteries. Listed in order of size, they are the femoral, axillary, brachial, and radial arteries. However, in clinical practice, cannulation of the axillary artery is used infrequently. Because of the poor collateral supply, cannulation of the brachial artery for long-term pressure monitoring is discouraged.

Table 4-3 lists some advantages and disadvantages of arterial insertion sites.

Percutaneous Cannulation

Percutaneous insertion of arterial catheters is the preferred method of cannulation because of its ease and speed of insertion, reduced infection rate, and fewer equipment requirements.

Patient preparation. Before cannulation of the radial artery, it is recommended to assess the adequacy of collateral blood flow to the hand. This can be done via a Doppler flow probe, a finger pulse monitor, or performance of the Allen test.

1. General patient preparation as described on p. 53.
2. Immobilize the patient's nondominant hand (if possible) palm side up on a padded arm board, providing approximately 60 degree extension of the wrist.
3. Secure a peripheral IV line or heparin lock.

Table 4-3. Advantages and disadvantages associated with percutaneous cannulation of radial and femoral artery sites

Site	Advantages	Disadvantages
Radial artery	Readily accessible Good collateral circulation Superficial location Collateral circulation can be assessed before the procedure (Allen test, Doppler flow test)	High risk of occlusion because of small size High rate of catheter malfunction In shock states with low blood pressure and peripheral vasoconstriction this site may not reflect central aortic pressure
Femoral artery	Large vessel easy to cannulate with decreased risk of occlusion Easier to cannulate in presence of vasoconstriction or hypotension Easy to compress after catheter removal	Reduced patient mobility Insertion site not as easily located in obese patients Risk of hematoma in very obese patients in whom direct compression may be difficult

Radial artery

Percutaneous cannulation of the radial artery traditionally is the most common means of arterial access in the critical care or emergency setting.

Anatomy. The radial artery is a small, superficially located terminal branch of the brachial artery (Fig. 4-11). It arises in the antecubital fossa and passes downward to the wrist along the radial side of the forearm. Its pulsations can be readily palpated at the wrist before the flexor carpi radialis tendon of the lateral anterior border of the radius.

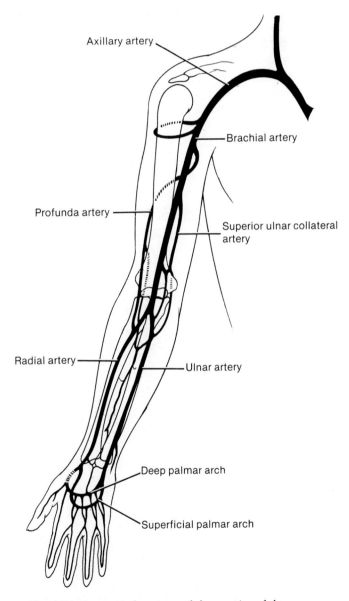

Fig. 4-11. Anatomic locations of the arteries of the arm.

The radial artery anastomoses with the ulnar artery in the hand, forming the deep palmar arch, the dorsal arch, and the superficial palmar arch.

Procedure

1. Palpate the radial artery to determine its exact location and direction.
2. Make a shallow 1- to 2-mm skin incision over the radial artery with a #11 scalpel.
3. Align a 20-gauge needle with stylet at a 20-degree angle over the radial artery approximately 3 to 4 cm proximal to the styloid process of the radius.
4. While palpating the pulse with one hand, insert the needle into and through the radial artery (Fig. 4-12).
5. Remove the inner stylet and slowly withdraw the needle until it is located in the artery; proper location is indicated by bright red blood pulsating from the needle hub.
6. Insert the soft flexible tip of an 0.018-inch (0.46-mm) guidewire 10 to 15 cm into the artery. While securely holding the wire in place, remove the needle. Wipe the guidewire with a moistened gauze pad. Insert a short (5-cm) 3-Fr catheter over the guidewire into the artery; remove the guidewire. Alternately, and more commonly, a catheter-over-needle is inserted into the radial artery for long-term monitoring. If a catheter-over-needle is used, remove the stylet and slowly withdraw the catheter and needle until bright red blood pulsates from the needle hub. Advance the Teflon catheter into the artery and simultaneously withdraw the needle.
7. Aspirate, discard the aspirate, and gently flush the catheter. Attach the heparinized IV solution and stopcock to the catheter.

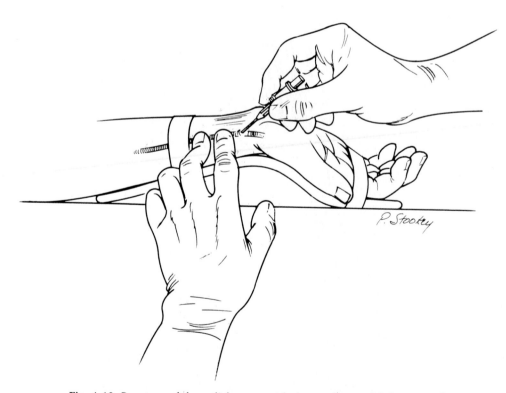

Fig. 4-12. Puncture of the radial artery with the needle at a 30-degree angle.

8. Suture the hub of the catheter to the skin with 3-0 silk.

9. Cleanse the area and apply an iodophor ointment and a sterile dressing secured with tape.

Special precautions

DIMINISHED RADIAL PULSE. Occasionally the radial artery pulse will diminish or disappear after infiltration with lidocaine. This usually is temporary. However, return of the pulse sometimes can be hastened by gentle massage of the surrounding tissues.

PULSATILE BLOOD CESSATION. If cessation of pulsatile blood occurs at any time during catheter advancement, slowly withdraw the catheter until blood flow resumes. Withdraw the catheter 1 to 2 mm more and then readvance the catheter. If no blood flow reappears during the second catheter withdrawal, remove the catheter entirely

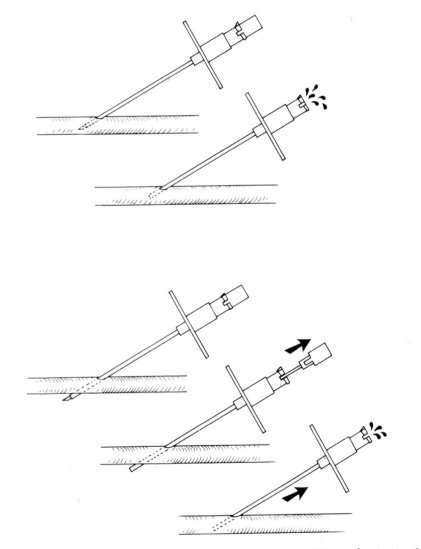

Fig. 4-13. Methods of arterial cannulation via **(A)** direct puncture or **(B)** transfixation in which both walls are punctured, after which the inner stylet is removed and the cannula is slowly withdrawn until blood flow appears at the hub.

and apply compression for 5 minutes before repuncturing the artery. If there never was evidence of blood flow, the artery probably was never punctured; in this case compression is not necessary before reattempting to puncture the artery.

METHODS OF CANNULATION (FIG. 4-13). Cannulation can be successfully performed by either direct threading or fixation, as described in step 5. Transfixation of the vessel by deliberate puncture of both the anterior and posterior wall of the artery is a commonly used method in the smaller arteries. Reports indicate no significant difference in the complication rates of these methods.

CIRCULATORY ASSESSMENT OF THE HAND. Circulation in the hand should be assessed every 4 hours and the catheter removed immediately upon any signs of circulatory compromise.

PREVENTION OF BLEEDING. Bleeding from the puncture site can be prevented by applying firm pressure for 5 to 10 minutes after catheter removal. The puncture site should then be observed for several minutes to assure the adequacy of hemostasis. This should be followed by application of a light pressure dressing and frequent evaluations of the radial pulse and blood flow to the hand.

A loose connection from the arterial line can quickly cause hemorrhage. For this reason, only Luer-Lok connections should be used. All connections should be secured tightly, and all connectors should be readily visible so that leaks can be detected immediately.

Complications

RADIAL ARTERY THROMBOSIS. The most significant determinants of radial artery thrombosis seem to be catheter size, shape, and composition and the length of time the catheter is left in the artery. For these reasons it is strongly recommended that the radial artery be cannulated with a nontapered Teflon catheter no larger than 20 gauge and that the catheter be removed as soon as clinically possible. Short-term cannulation

Table 4-4. Insertion success rate and specific complications associated with percutaneous cannulation of the radial and femoral arteries

Site	Insertion success rate (%)	Specific complications
Radial artery	85	Thrombosis
		Hematoma
		Emboli
		Infection
		Diminished pulse
		Distal ischemia
		Sepsis
		Bleeding
		Distal necrosis
		Pseudoaneurysm
Femoral artery	99	Hematoma
		Thrombosis
		Distal ischemia
		Emboli
		Sepsis

for less than 4 hours can be performed safely with little risk of thrombosis. The risk of arterial occlusion is also higher if the artery is punctured more than once during attempted cannulation. Despite the high rate of thrombotic complications with radial artery catheters, permanent damage occurs infrequently, with resolution of symptoms usually within 48 hours to 7 days of catheter removal. Therapeutic maneuvers that may improve distal blood flow include heparin infusion, administration of lidocaine, performance of a sympathetic nerve block, or thrombectomy via a Fogarty catheter. Careful attention to technique, use of a small, preferably nontapered Teflon catheter for short periods, and meticulous nursing care can markedly reduce the risk of serious complications. Other complications of arterial cannulation are listed in Table 4-4.

REFERENCES

Abrams HL: *Angiography,* Boston, 1983, Little, Brown.

Asimacopoulos PJ, Bagley FH, McDermott WF: A modified technique for subclavian puncture, *Surg Gynecol Obstet* 150:241, 1980.

Bedford RF, Wollman H: Complications of percutaneous radial artery cannulation in objective prospective study in man, *Anesthesiology* 38: 228-236, 1973.

Bernard RW, Stahl WM: Subclavian vein catheterizations: a prospective study. I. Non-infectious complications, *Ann Surg* 173:184, 1971.

Blitt CD et al: Central venous catheterization via the external jugular vein: a technique employing the J-wire, *JAMA* 229:817, 1974.

Brinkman AJ, Costley DO: Internal jugular venipuncture, *JAMA* 223:182, 1973.

Civetta JM, Gabel JC, Gemer M: Internal-jugular-vein puncture with a margin of safety, *Anesthesiology* 36:622, 1972.

Cooper MW: A simple method for insertion of multiple catheters through a single venipuncture site, *Cathet Cardiovasc Diagn* 8:305, 1982.

Daily PO, Griepp RB, Shumway NE: Percutaneous internal jugular vein cannulation, *Arch Surg* 101:534, 1970.

Davis FM: Methods of radial artery cannulation and subsequent arterial occlusion, *Anesthesiology* 56:331, 1982.

Dronen S et al: Subclavian vein catheterization during cardiopulmonary resuscitation: a prospective comparison of supraclavicular and infraclavicular percutaneous approaches, *JAMA* 247:3227, 1984.

Feliciano DV et al: Major complications of percutaneous subclavian vein catheters, *Am J Surg* 138:869, 1979.

Fergusson DJG, Kamada RO: Percutaneous entry of the brachial artery for left heart catheterization using a sheath, *Cathet Cardiovasc Diagn* 7:111-114, 1981.

Folland ED et al: Brachial artery catheterization employing a side arm sheath, *Cathet Cardiovasc Diagn* 10:55-61, 1984.

Goldfarb G, Lebrec D: Percutaneous cannulation of the internal jugular vein in patients with coagulopathies: an experience based on 1000 attempts, *Anesthesiology* 56:321, 1982.

Gottdiener JS et al: Detection of venous air embolism by 2D echocardiography: evidence for entry of air into intracardiac shunt, *Circulation* 72(suppl III):III-352, 1985.

Gurman GM, Krierman S: Cannulation of big arteries in critically ill patients, *Crit Care Med* 13:217-220, 1985.

Hales S: *Statistical essays: Hemostaticks,* vol 2, ed 3, London, 1738, W Innys & R Manby.

Huyghens L et al: Cardiothoracic complications of centrally inserted catheters, *Acute Care* 11:53-56, 1985.

Jacob AS, Schweiger MJ: A method for inserting two catheters, pulmonary arterial and temporary pacing, through a single puncture into a subclavian vein, *Cathet Cardiovasc Diagn* 9:611, 1983.

Johnston AOB, Clark RG: Malpositioning of central venous catheters, *Lancet* 2:1395, 1972.

Jones RM et al: The effect of the method of radial artery cannulation on post cannulation blood flow and thrombus formation, *Anesthesiology* 55:76-78, 1981.

Kaiser CW et al: Choice of route for central venous cannulation: subclavian or internal jugular vein: a prospective randomized study, *J Surg Oncol* 17:345, 1981.

Kashuk JL, Penn I: Air embolism after central venous catheterization, *Surg Gynecol Obstet* 159:249, 1984.

Kearns PJ, Haulk AA, McDonald TW: Homonymous hemaniopia due to cerebral air embolism from central venous catheters, *West J Med* 140:615, 1984.

Kelly J et al: Comparison of Allen test, Doppler and finger-pulse transducer to assess patency of ulnar artery, *Anesthesiology* 59(supp.):A178, 1983.

Legler D, Nugent M: Doppler locatization of the internal jugular vein facilitates its cannulation, *Anesthesiology* p. A179, 1983 (abstract).

Linos DA, Mucha P, Van Heerden JA: Subclavian vein, a golden route, *Mayo Clin Proc* 55:315, 1980.

O'Reilly MV: The technique of subclavian vein cannulation, *Can Med Assoc J* 108:63, 1973.

Pepine CJ, Von Gunten C, Hill JA: Percutaneous brachial catheterization using a modified sheath and new catheter system, *Cathet Cardiovasc Diagn* 10:637-642, 1984.

Rao TLK, Wong AY, Salem MR: A new approach to percutaneous catheterization of the internal jugular vein, *Anesthesiology* 46:362, 1977.

Rapoport S et al: Pseudoaneurysm: a complication of faulty technique in femoral arterial puncture, *Radiology* 154:529-530, 1985.

Russell JA et al: Prospective evaluation of radial and femoral artery catheterization sites in critically ill adults, *Crit Care Med* 11:936-939, 1983.

Schwartz AJ, Jobes DR, Gruchow E: Carotid artery puncture with internal jugular cannulation using the Seldinger technique: incidence, recognition, treatment, and prevention, *Anesthesiology* 51: S160, 1979.

Schwartz AJ, Jobes DR, Levy WJ: Intrathoracic vascular catheterization via the external jugular vein, *Anesthesiology* 56:400, 1982.

Seneff MG: Central venous catheterization: a comprehensive review (II). *J Intens Care Med* 2:218-232, 1987.

Simon RR, Brenner BE: Procedures and techniques in emergency medicine, Baltimore, 1984, Williams & Wilkins.

Skowronski GA, Pearson IY: A technique for insertion of two intravascular catheters via a single puncture, *Crit Care Med* 10:404, 1982.

Smith DC: Catheterization of prosthetic vascular grafts: acceptable technique, *AJR Am J Roentgenol* 143:1117-1118, 1984 (editorial).

Soderstrom CA et al: Superiority of the femoral artery for monitoring: a prospective study, *Am J Surg* 144:309-312, 1982.

Swanson RS et al: Emergency intravenous access through the femoral vein, *Emerg Med* 13:244, 1983.

Sznajder JI et al: Central vein catheterization: failure and complication rates by three percutaneous approaches, *Arch Intern Med* 146:259-261, 1986.

Thomas F et al: The risk of infection related to radial vs. femoral sites for arterial catheterization, *Crit Care Med* 11:807-81, 1983.

Valeix B et al: Selective coronary arteriography by percutaneous transaxillary approach, *Cathet Cardiovasc Diagn* 10:403-409, 1984.

Weinshelbaum A, Carson SN: Separation of angiographic catheter during arteriography through vascular graft, *AJR Am J Roentgenol* 134:583-584, 1980.

Weiss BM, Gattiker RI: Complications during and following radial artery cannulation: a prospective study, *Intens Care Med* 12:424-428, 1986.

Wilson JN, Grow JB, Demong C: Central venous pressure in optimal blood volume maintenance, *Arch Surg* 85: 563, 1962.

Yock PG et al: Use of the "SmartNeedle™" for internal jugular and subclavian vein cannulation, *JACC* 19:95A, 1992.

Zajko AB et al: Percutaneous puncture of venous bypass grafts for transluminal angioplasty, *AJR Am J Roentgenol* 137:799-801, 1981.

Chapter 5

Central Venous and Right Atrial Pressure Monitoring

Central venous catheters have been used widely in the coronary care unit for more than 20 years for administration of fluids, blood sampling for routine laboratory analysis, venous oxygen saturation determination, and central venous pressure (CVP) measurement. It was previously thought the CVP reflected changes in left ventricular (LV) function that would allow accurate assessment of the patient's hemodynamic status, response to therapy, or both. It has now been documented through further clinical experience that severe left-sided hemodynamic abnormalities may occur rapidly after myocardial infarction without significant changes in superior vena cava (SVC) pressures. However, CVP measurement does provide useful information about right ventricular (RV) function and cardiovascular status and frequently is used to monitor the volemic state and right heart function of patients who do not require pulmonary arterial (PA) pressure monitoring.

PHYSIOLOGIC REVIEW

The CVP is a reflection of the right atrial (RA) pressure and thus provides useful information about both the preload of the right side of the heart and the adequacy of venous return.

True preload of the right ventricle is really the end-diastolic myocardial fiber length produced by the end-diastolic volume. However, the clinical measurement of preload of the right side of the heart is the pressure during filling of the right ventricle (end-diastolic pressure). Except in tricuspid stenosis, the pressure in the RA *is* the preload or filling pressure of the RV. Thus right atrial pressure (RAP) or CVP is valuable clinically in assessing preload of the right side of the heart. Although the CVP eventually will reflect left-sided heart failure or other abnormalities, the timing and sequence of the pressure changes in the superior vena cava are less predictable.

Venous return, or the amount of blood returning to the heart, is determined by the difference between mean systemic pressure and the RA pressure. The greater the difference between the two pressures, the greater the volume of blood returning to the heart. Decreases in RAP or CVP at a constant mean arterial pressure (MAP) result in increased venous return until the CVP falls below zero, at which point the veins leading into the thorax tend to collapse. Likewise, increases in RAP or CVP above 7 mm Hg at a constant MAP result in reduced venous return and hence cardiac output.

CLINICAL APPLICATION

The CVP is most valuable in monitoring blood volume, adequacy of central venous return, and RV function. It is particularly helpful after surgery, during active bleeding, or in assessing dehydration, when it may be difficult to determine the true blood volume of the patient. The CVP actually reflects the pressure in the great veins as blood returns to the heart (Fig. 5-1). If blood return decreases, the pressure usually decreases. In general, a low pressure (less than 5 cm H_2O) indicates that additional fluid or blood can be given safely without overloading the intravascular space or the heart. This additional volume of blood or fluid causes increases in central venous return and the CVP. This increase in filling pressure contributes to an increase in cardiac output and systemic pressures, according to Starling's Law.

The CVP is useful also in differentiating right ventricular failure from left ventricular failure. With failure of the RV, usually following RV ischemia or infarction, the CVP is high because of decreased compliance of the RV, requiring higher filling pressures. The pulmonary artery wedge (PAW) pressure, however, is characteristically lower because of reduced volume filling the left side of the heart. The reverse hemodynamic picture frequently occurs with LV failure, in which the PAW pressure is elevated and the CVP may be normal or low.

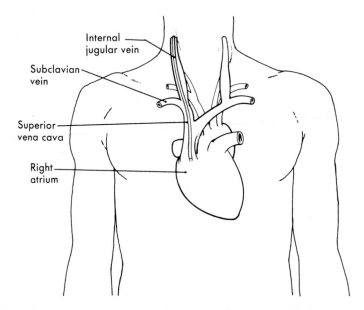

Internal jugular vein

Subclavian vein

Superior vena cava

Right atrium

Fig. 5-1. Central venous pressure (CVP) catheter properly positioned in the superior vena cava (SVC) just above the right atrial (RA) junction. The catheter has been inserted through the right internal jugular vein.

When PA pressure monitoring is not possible, the CVP may be used to monitor the patient with chronic right and left heart failure. In these patients the CVP *tends* to follow the PAW pressure, rising with increased LV failure and falling with certain treatments, such as diuresis.

Patient Example 1

A 54-year-old man was admitted to the coronary care unit with an anteroseptal myocardial infarction. On hospital day 2, he had recurrence of chest pain, suggesting an extension of the infarction. Shortly thereafter, he complained of increasing shortness of breath, but the CVP remained stable at 8 cm H_2O. A PA catheter was advanced to the pulmonary artery, showing a PA systolic pressure of 35, a PA diastolic pressure of 21, and a mean PAW pressure of 23 mm Hg.

In the absence of severe pulmonary emphysema, pulmonary vascular disease, or mitral valve disease, we can conclude that the patient was indeed in LV failure, with an elevated left ventricular end-diastolic pressure (LVEDP) leading to rises in the left atrial (LA), PAW, and PA pressures, as measured. The elevated PAW pressure caused additional fluid to shift into the patient's pulmonary alveolar space, accounting for his complaint of shortness of breath.

Patient Example 2

A 22-year-old man was brought to the emergency room with a pneumothorax and hemothorax after an automobile accident. Bleeding from the chest tube continued. After he had received 3 units of whole blood, his hematocrit reading was 38% despite a continuing decrease in arterial blood pressure and a decreasing urinary output. Was he developing hemorrhagic shock caused by blood volume depletion?

A CVP catheter was advanced to the superior vena cava through the right antecubital basilic vein. A fluid-filled manometer showed a pressure of 0 cm H_2O when the manometer zero level was held at midchest level. He was given 5 additional units of whole blood before the CVP showed a rise to 8 cm H_2O. Thus the additional fluid was given safely and resulted in a return of his cardiac output and systemic pressures to normal. Table 5-1 shows data charted on this patient.

Table 5-1. Patient data for Patient Example 2

	5 AM	6 AM	8 AM	Noon	6 PM
CVP (cm H_2O)	?	0	2	8	6
Blood pressure	90/60	85/60	100/65	115/75	112/83
Urine output (ml/hr)	30	22	54	125	115
Blood given (units)	3	—	2	3	—

NORMAL CVP WAVEFORM

Fig. 5-2 depicts a normal central venous waveform obtained using a pressure transducer. Its morphology is identical to an RA waveform. (See the following discussion of the components of the RA waveform.) The normal CVP ranges from 0

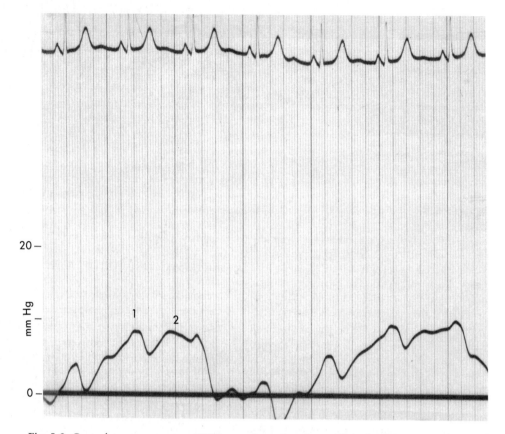

Fig. 5-2. Central venous pressure (CVP) waveform showing *a (1),* and *v (2)* waves and normal respiratory variation in a spontaneously breathing patient. The mean value of this pressure measured at end-expiration (just before the inspiratory drop) is approximately 7 mm Hg.

to 7 mm Hg (0 to 10 cm H_2O) with a normal average reported to be approximately 3 mm Hg (4 cm H_2O).

Pressure in the central veins is affected by changes in intrathoracic pressure. For this reason, the CVP falls during spontaneous inhalation and rises during spontaneous exhalation. To minimize the effects of these respiratory changes, the CVP should be measured at end-expiration whether the pressure is measured via a H_2O manometer or a transducer. This is also true whether the patient is breathing spontaneously or with mechanical ventilation.

NORMAL RA PRESSURE
Physiology and Morphology

The pressure changes produced by the right atrium are small and usually consist of two major and one minor positive waves—*a, c,* and *v*—followed by negative waves—*x, x^1, and y* descents (Fig. 5-3). The *a* wave is one of the two major waves and is produced by the action of atrial contraction. The decline in pressure that immediately follows the *a* wave is termed the *x descent* and reflects atrial relaxation (immediately following systole). The *c* wave is a minor wave that may appear as a distinct wave or as a notch on the *a* wave, or may be absent altogether. It reflects a

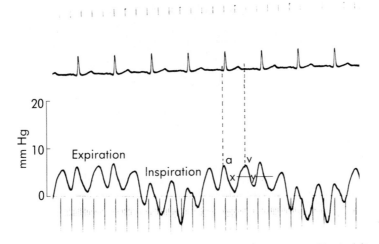

Fig. 5-3. Normal RA waveform in a spontaneously breathing patient. Vertical lines drawn show the *a* wave following the ECG P wave, and the *v* wave following the ECG T wave. Horizontal line indicates measurement of the mean right atrial (RA) pressure of approximately 4 mm Hg.

slight increase in pressure in the right atrium produced by closure of the tricuspid valve leaflets. The negative wave immediately following the *c* wave is termed the x^1 *descent*. It is produced by a downward pulling of the AV junction during ventricular systole. (If the *c* wave appears only as notch on the *a* wave, the single descent following the *ac* wave is termed the *x* descent.)

The *v* wave is an increase in atrial pressure produced by right atrial filling during concomitant right ventricular systole. The *y* descent immediately follows the *v* wave and is produced by the opening of the tricuspid valve and rapid emptying of the right atrium into the right ventricle.

Because the pressure rises produced during both atrial systole (*a* wave) and diastole (*v* wave) are nearly the same (usually within 3 to 4 mm Hg of each other), an average or a mean of both the pressure rises is obtained (Fig. 5-3). The normal resting mean right atrial pressure is 2 to 6 mm Hg. However, in instances in which either the *a* or *v* wave of the RA waveform is elevated more than 2 or 3 mm Hg above the other wave, it is necessary to determine the mean of only the RA *a* wave as a measurement of the right heart filling pressure (Fig. 5-4).

ECG Correlation

The RA *a* wave, which represents mechanical atrial systole, immediately succeeds electrical atrial depolarization, that is, after the P wave of the ECG. Because of the time required for the mechanical event to reach the sensing device (the transducer) and depending on the length of tubing used, the degree of delay varies between the recorded electrical event and the mechanical event. Nonetheless, the *a* wave of the RA pressure generally is seen 80 to 100 msec after the P wave or at some time within the PR interval of the ECG (see Fig. 5-3).

The *c* wave, reflecting closure of the tricuspid valve, corresponds to the RST junction of the ECG. Its timing following the *a* wave approximates the PR interval.

The *v* wave, occuring during ventricular systole, would naturally succeed electrical

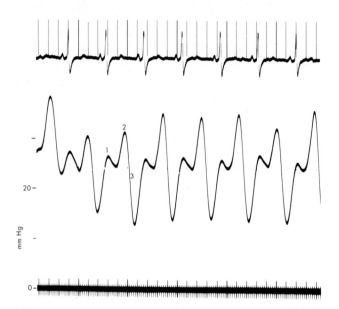

Fig. 5-4. Elevated right atrial (RA) pressure with exaggerated *v* wave *(2)* and rapid *y* descent *(3)* in a patient with tricuspid regurgitation as a result of acute right ventricular (RV) failure. The *a* wave *(1)* of approximately 26 mm Hg reflects an elevated right ventricular end-diastolic pressure (RVEDP) and RV failure.

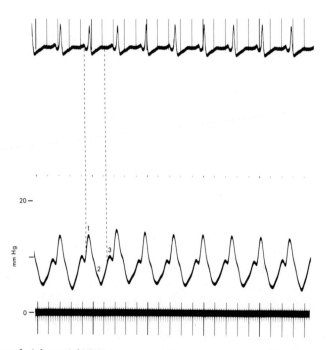

Fig. 5-5. Elevated right atrial (RA) pressure with exaggerated *a* wave *(1)* in a patient with right ventricular (RV) failure and increased resistance to ventricular filling. *(2, x* descent; *3, v* wave.)

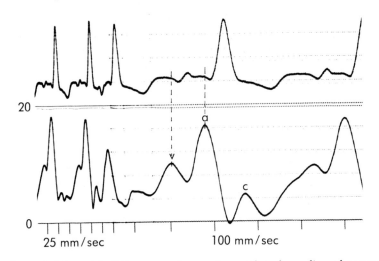

Fig. 5-6. Elevated right atrial (RA) pressure in a patient with tachycardia and premature beat making it difficult to discern actual components of the waveform. However, changing the paper speed to 100 mm/sec (right half of figure) clarifies identification of the *a* and *v* waves.

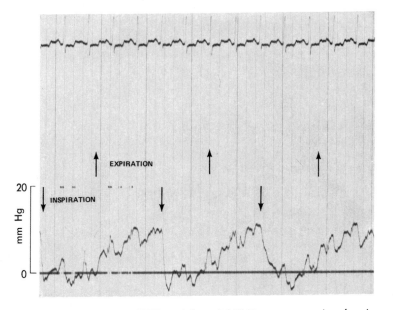

Fig. 5-7. Central venous pressure (CVP) or right atrial (RA) pressure tracing showing pressure variation during spontaneous respiration. At maximal inspiration there is actually a negative pressure in the thorax and right atrium in comparison with the rest of the body and atmospheric pressure. The pressure measured at end-expiration is approximately 8 mm Hg.

ventricular depolarization and can be observed near the end of the T wave or any time in the TP interval.

Proper measurement and identification of the RA waveform components require correlation with a simultaneously obtained ECG. Using a straight edge to draw lines from the electrical event down through the corresponding mechanical event is a useful way to identify the components and appropriately measure the pressure, particularly in conditions that alter the atrial waveform configuration (Fig. 5-5). However, even this technique may prove inadequate to determine waveform morphology when the heart rate is very rapid. In such circumstances, increasing the paper speed from 25 mm per second to 50 or even 100 mm/sec can be very helpful (Fig. 5-6).

Respiratory Correlation

With normal spontaneous inspiration, the height of the RA *a* and *v* waves declines and the *x* and *y* descents become more exaggerated, resulting in a lowered mean RA pressure. Pressures may even become negative during spontaneous inspiration in patients with low CVP or RA pressures (Fig. 5-7). To minimize the changing pleural pressure effects on the measured CVP or RA pressure, pressures should be measured consistently at end-expiration, when pleural pressure is at or near zero.

ALTERATIONS ASSOCIATED WITH DYSRHYTHMIAS
Atrial Fibrillation

Atrial fibrillation is characterized by the absence of uniform atrial depolarization and consequently results in absent P waves in the ECG and absent *a* waves in the CVP or right atrial pressure waveform (Fig. 5-8). For every QRS complex, there is one

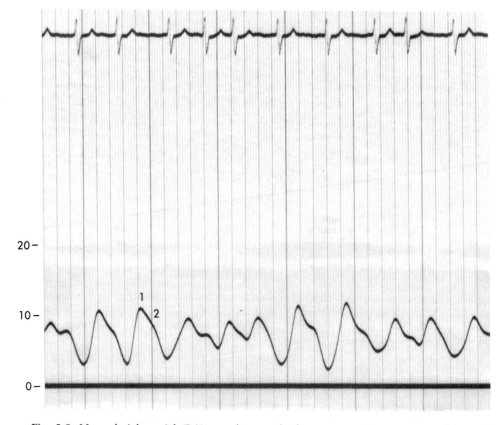

Fig. 5-8. Normal right atrial (RA) waveform with absent *a* waves in a patient with atrial fibrillation. (*1, v* wave; *2, v* descent.) Note the effect of varying RR intervals on the extent of the *y* descent reflecting changes in right ventricular (RV) filling (and RA emptying).

distinct pressure rise—the *v* wave. Frequently, however, it is possible to see small flutter or fibrillatory waves throughout the pressure tracing.

Measurement of the mean RA pressure in the absence of *a* waves, particularly if the *v* wave is dominant and elevated, is best done by simply measuring the corresponding pressure that occurs just following the QRS complex. This will provide the nearest approximation to end-diastolic pressure. This, of course, requires a two-channel paper recorder, which should be used for all pressure measurements.

Atrial Flutter

The RA waveform in *atrial flutter* typically demonstrates mechanical flutter waves that correspond to the rate of flutter activity. Often the RA waveform can be very useful in aiding the diagnosis of atrial dysrhythmias such as this.

Junctional Rhythm and AV Dissociation

In *junctional rhythm* or during certain beats of *AV dissociation* where the atria contract against a closed tricuspid valve, intermittent giant *a* or cannon *a* waves are seen in the right atrial pressure tracing (Fig. 5-9). Cannon *a* waves also can be seen following a premature ventricular contraction (PVC). Avoid measuring cannon *a* waves, if present, when determining the mean RA pressure, because they will artifactually elevate the pressure value. Rather, measure the mean pressure during a normally conducted beat.

Close scrutiny of the atrial waveform in conjunction with the ECG is also very helpful in determining the atrial activity associated with paroxysmal supraventricular tachycardia (PSVT) in which retrograde P waves may be disguised within the QRS complex. Reviewing the atrial waveform at a faster paper speed (50 mm/sec) facilitates correlation of the electrical and mechanical events of the heart.

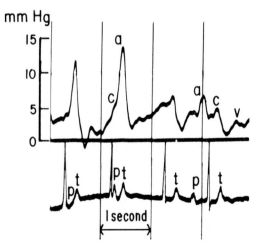

Fig. 5-9. Right atrial (RA) pressure waveform in a patient with AV dissociation showing the presence of cannon *a* waves as the atria contracts against a closed tricuspid valve. Note the change in the RA waveform with normal *a* and *v* waves when the patient converts to normal sinus rhythmn.

From Kory, RC, Tsagaris, TJ, Bustamente, RA: *A primer of cardiac catheterization*, Springfield, Ill, 1965, Charles C Thomas.

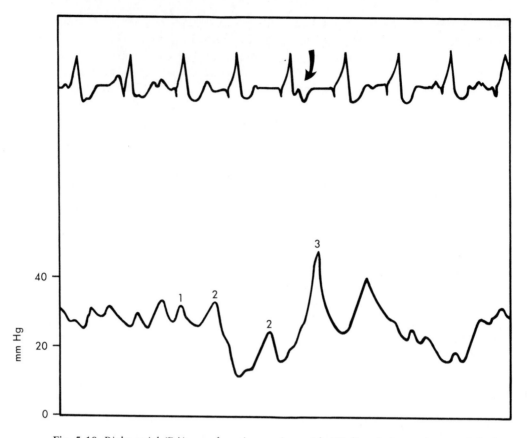

Fig. 5-10. Right atrial (RA) waveform in a patient with AV dissociation and a paced rhythm. *1, a* wave; *2, v* wave; *3,* cannon *a* wave following the retrograde P wave *(arrow)* as the atrium contracts against a closed tricuspid valve.

Pacemakers

Patients with a ventricular pacemaker may have absent *a* waves, occasional, random *a* waves, or even cannon *a* waves at times, depending on the underlying rhythm (Fig. 5-10). This is the result of absent or dissociated atrial activity that does not relate to the QRS.

Patients with an AV sequential pacemaker exhibit normal RA waveform morphology with an *a* wave following the paced atrial electrical activity and a *v* wave following the paced ventricular activity (Fig. 5-11).

ABNORMAL RA PRESSURES

Elevated RA pressures occur in the following conditions:
1. Right ventricular failure
2. Tricuspid stenosis and regurgitation
3. Cardiac tamponade
4. Constrictive pericarditis
5. Pulmonary hypertension (primary or secondary)

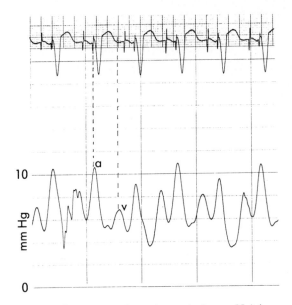

Fig. 5-11. Normal right atrial (RA) waveform (mean is 8 mm Hg) in a patient with an AV sequential pacemaker. The waveform is displayed at a low scale to illustrate the normal relationship of the electrical and mechanical events.

6. Chronic left ventricular failure
7. Volume overload

Elevated *a* Waves

The *a* wave of the RA pressure tracing is exaggerated and elevated in any condition that increases the resistance to right ventricular filling. These include tricuspid stenosis, RV failure, pulmonary hypertension, and pulmonic stenosis (see Fig. 5-5).

Elevated *v* Waves

The *v* wave of the RA pressure tracing is exaggerated and elevated in tricuspid regurgitation because of a reflux of blood into the right atrium through the insufficiently closed tricuspid valve during ventricular systole (see Fig. 5-4). Clinically, tricuspid regurgitation most commonly occurs secondary to acute RV failure and dilation. Flotation of the PA catheter into the RV and out to the PA often is very difficult in such situations.

Exaggerated and elevated *v* waves artifactually elevate the mean RA pressure if considered in the measurement process (as done by all monitor systems). Such a value does not reflect the actual filling pressure (preload) of the right heart. Therefore whenever the *v* wave is higher than the *a* wave (by more than a few millimeters of mercury, the mean value of just the *a* wave should be determined as a reflection of the diastolic filling pressure. This is done from a two-channel strip recording by (1) locating the *a* wave just following the ECG P wave and (2) calculating the average of its pressure from the peak of the *a* wave to the trough of the *x* descent. If a *c* wave is clearly evident on the *x* descent, this point may be used as a marker of the end-diastolic pressure.

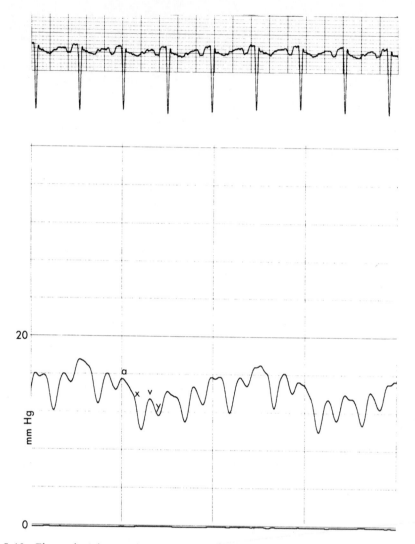
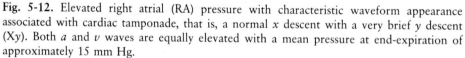

Fig. 5-12. Elevated right atrial (RA) pressure with characteristic waveform appearance associated with cardiac tamponade, that is, a normal x descent with a very brief y descent (Xy). Both a and v waves are equally elevated with a mean pressure at end-expiration of approximately 15 mm Hg.

Elevated a and v Waves

In cardiac tamponade both the a and v waves are equally elevated and reflect the elevated diastolic filling pressures in all chambers of the heart. The contour of the RA pressure tracing is distinct, however, showing a predominant x descent with a very short or absent y descent (Xy) (Fig. 5-12). The mean value of the RA pressure is elevated and approximates the PAW mean value, as well as the PA end-diastolic value (Fig. 5-13). Generally, the normal respiratory response is observed, with a decline in RA pressure during spontaneous inhalation and an elevation during exhalation.

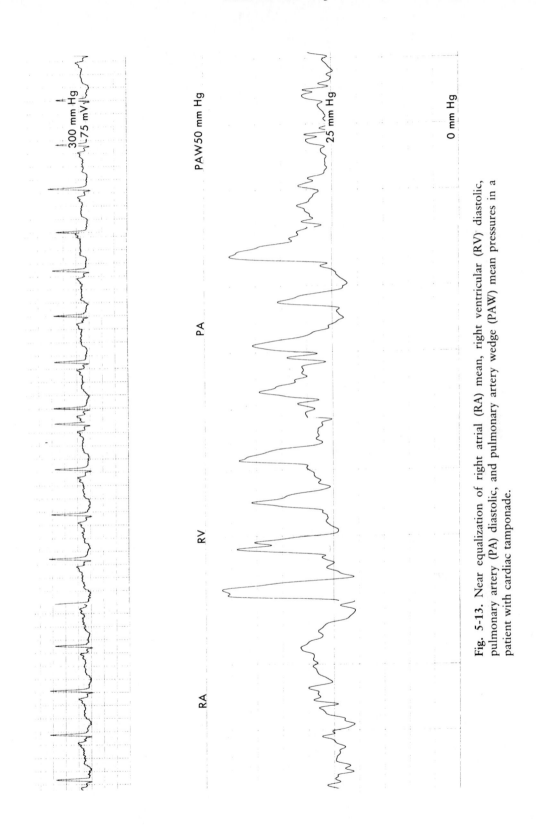

Fig. 5-13. Near equalization of right atrial (RA) mean, right ventricular (RV) diastolic, pulmonary artery (PA) diastolic, and pulmonary artery wedge (PAW) mean pressures in a patient with cardiac tamponade.

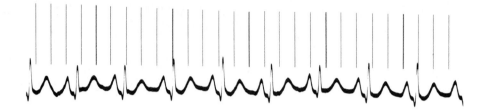

Fig. 5-14. Elevated right atrial (RA) pressure with characteristic waveform appearance associated with constrictive pericarditis, that is, a normal or brief *x* descent with an exaggerated *y* descent. The exaggerated *y* descent is a result of rapid ventricular filling (atrial emptying) during early diastole followed by an abrupt rise in pressure as the size of the heart is increased and compressed by the inelastic, constricted pericardium. The *a* and *v* waves are both equally elevated with a mean RA pressure of approximately 22 mm Hg. (*1, a* wave; *2, c* wave; *3, v* wave; *4, y* descent.)

In constrictive pericardial disease the *a* and *v* waves of the RA pressure tracing are also equally elevated, but the contour of the waveform differs from cardiac tamponade, showing either a predominant *y* descent or equally dominant *x* and *y* descents (Fig. 5-14). In addition, Kussmaul's sign (a *rise* rather than a fall in right atrial pressure during spontaneous inspiration) can be seen in constrictive disease but rarely, if ever, in cardiac tamponade. Kussmaul's sign and elevation of the RA waveform with an *xY* or *xy* pattern can be seen also in patients with acute right ventricular infarction in which an acutely dilated RV is restricted by the noncompliant pericardium. As in tamponade, the elevated RAP in patients with constrictive pericarditis or RV infarction usually equals the pulmonary artery end-diastolic pressure (PAEDP) and PAW pressure.

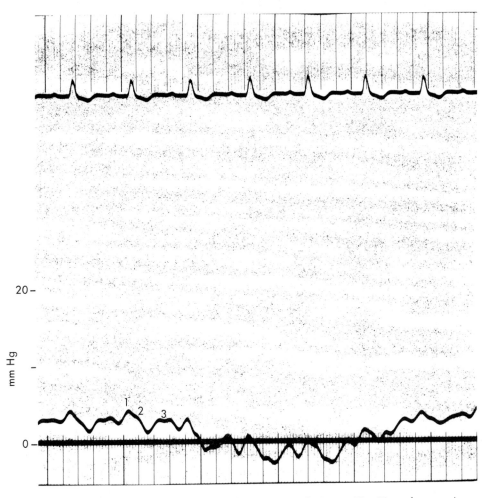

Fig. 5-15. A low right atrial (RA) pressure of approximately 3 mm Hg. Note the negative pressure during spontaneous inspiration. (*1, a* wave; *2, x* descent; *3, v* wave.)

Very low CVP or RA pressures occur with hypovolemia from any cause (Fig. 5-15).

METHODS OF MEASURING CVP OR RA PRESSURE

The CVP can be measured with a water manometer (the original technique) or with a transducer, as is more commonly used today. When the CVP is measured with a water manometer, its measurement is in centimeters of water (cm H_2O). When measured with the use of a pressure transducer, its measurement is in millimeters of mercury (mm Hg). These differences in units of measurement may cause some confusion, which can be avoided if the manometrically measured CVP is converted to mm Hg.

An easy way to make the conversion is to remember that mercury is 13.6 times heavier than water. Therefore 1 mm Hg equals 13.6 mm H_2O, which equals 1.36 cm H_2O. The saline manometer pressures are more commonly reported in centimeters of water. Centimeters of water can be converted to millimeters of mercury by dividing the centimeters of water by 1.36:

$$5 \text{ cm H}_2\text{O} = \frac{5 \text{ cm H}_2\text{O}}{1.36} = 3.7 \text{ mm Hg}$$

Perhaps an easier formula for conversion is 1 cm H_2O equals 0.74 mm Hg. Using this formula, centimeters of water are converted to millimeters of mercury by multiplying by 0.74:

$$5 \text{ cm H}_2\text{O} = 5 \text{ cm H}_2\text{O} \times 0.74 \text{ mm Hg} = 3.7 \text{ mm Hg}$$

Use of a Water Manometer

Use of a plastic disposable or glass manometer with a three-way stopcock is an easy method for measuring CVP and involves the following steps (Fig. 5-16):

1. Place the patient flat before setting the zero level of the manometer and for all subsequent CVP measurements. Place the zero level of the manometer at the

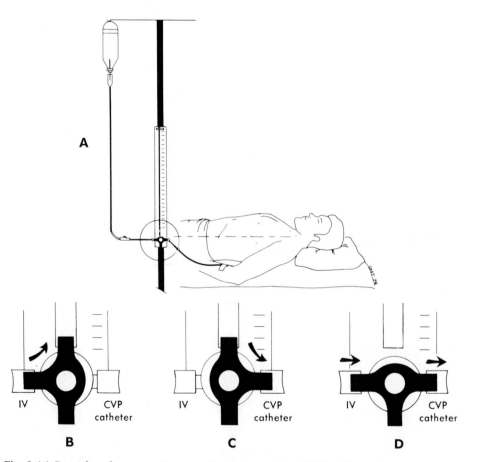

Fig. 5-16. Procedure for measuring central venous pressure (CVP) with water manometer. **A,** Manometer and IV tubing in place. **B,** Turn the stopcock so that the manometer fills with fluid above the level of the expected pressure. **C,** Turn the stopcock so that the intravenous (IV) flow is stopped and the manometer directs the flow to the patient. Obtain a reading after the fluid level stabilizes. **D,** Turn the stopcock to resume the IV flow to the patient.

patient's midchest level, which is the approximate level of the right atrium. The manometer may be secured to an IV pole. If the patient cannot tolerate lying flat, a mark can be made on the skin at midchest level; the zero level of the manometer is then always held at this mark for serial CVP measurements.

2. Connect the IV tubing to one side of the three-way stopcock; connect the manometer to the upper part; and connect the CVP catheter to the other side, using extension tubing if necessary. Different brands of stopcocks have varying methods of indicating the direction of flow. CVP measurement setups that are already properly connected are available commercially. See the package directions for specific instructions.

3. Check the catheter for patency by allowing the IV fluid to drip rapidly before taking the CVP measurement.

4. To obtain a CVP reading, turn the stopcock so that the manometer fills with fluid above the level of the expected pressure (see Fig. 5-16). Do *not* allow the manometer to overflow; overflowing may result in contamination.

5. Turn the stopcock so that the IV tubing is closed and the fluid in the manometer flows into the patient (see Fig. 5-16). The fluid column will then equalize to the hydrostatic pressure level at the tip of the catheter.

6. The fluid level in the manometer should fall rapidly and fluctuate with respiration. It will drop with inspiration as the intrathoracic pressure decreases and will rise with expiration. A reading may be taken when the fluid level stops falling and at end-expiration.

7. Turn the stopcock to resume the IV flow (see Fig. 5-16) after the measurement is obtained.

8. Record the pressure on the appropriate vital sign sheet.

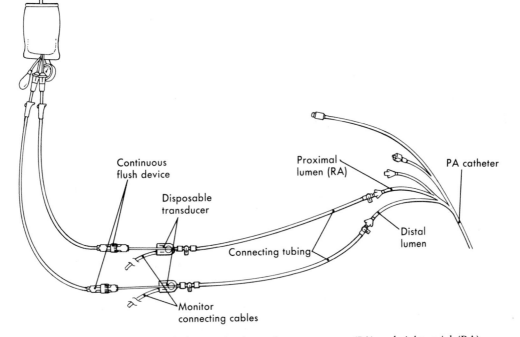

Fig. 5-17. An appropriate setup for monitoring pulmonary artery (PA) and right atrial (RA) pressures using disposable transducers and one IV solution bag.

Use of a Transducer

With the widespread use of hemodynamic monitoring via the PA catheter, use of a transducer to measure the CVP or RAP via the proximal port of the PA catheter has become the more common practice today. In addition to providing a more accurate measurement of the mean CVP or RAP, it permits observation and analysis of the actual waveform (see Fig. 5-2). Fluid-filled tubing and the transducer are attached to the proximal port of the PA catheter (Fig. 5-17) following the steps outlined on pp. 125-127. Transduced pressures also can be obtained from CVP catheters in the same manner.

As with all right heart pressure monitoring, the air-reference port of the transducer

Table 5-2. Problems encountered with CVP catheters

Problem	Cause	Prevention	Treatment
Pain and/or inflammation at insertion site	Mechanical irritation of catheter leading to sterile thrombophlebitis Bacterial infection ascending along catheter at insertion site	Prepare skin properly. Use sterile technique during insertion and dressing change. Insert catheter smoothly. Change dressing, stopcocks, and connecting tubing daily. Rotate insertion site every 48 to 72 hr.	Remove catheter. Apply warm compresses. Give pain medication as necessary.
Poor infusion of IV fluid	Partial clotting at catheter tip	Use continuous drip. Use 0.25 to 1 unit heparin/1 ml IV fluid. Occasionally hand flush or use fast flush. Flush with large volume after blood withdrawal.	Attach syringe to catheter and attempt to aspirate clot. Irrigate gently: *do not* forcibly flush catheter without consulting physician; remove catheter and reinsert at another site if it cannot be irrigated easily.
	Internal kinking of catheter	Coil and tape catheter carefully after insertion.	Remove dressing and check for possible kinking of catheter. Straighten catheter, retape, and apply new sterile dressing.
	Catheter tip against myocardium	Position catheter just above RA. Check chest x-ray film after catheter insertion.	Check for free backflow of blood from catheter. Reposition catheter.
Missing catheter tip when catheter is removed	Catheter cut or sheared	Never pull back catheter and readvance through needle. Use caution when using scissors near catheter.	Locate tip by palpation if in arm, or by chest x-ray film; may require venous cutdown if proximal end is in arm, or cardiac catheterization if proximal end is in thorax.

system should be positioned at approximately the RA level corresponding to the midchest position.

RISKS AND COMPLICATIONS

The risks and complications associated with CVP catheterization are basically those of PA catheterization (see the discussion on p. 127). A noteworthy difference, however, is the increased risk of cardiac perforation and tamponade with the use of CVP catheters. Most commonly, perforation by the catheter tip occurs in the RA, although perforations of the RV and SVC have been reported also. Perforation and tamponade may occur acutely after catheter insertion or from hours to days after insertion. When late tamponade occurs it is usually because of endocardial damage

Table 5-2. Problems encountered with CVP catheters—cont'd

Problem	Cause	Prevention	Treatment
Infection	Break in aseptic technique at insertion or system entry	Use aseptic technique during insertion or system entry. Apply sterile dead-ender caps each time system entered. Use single-lumen catheter.	Remove catheter (and obtain specimen for culture) or replace over guidewire. Begin antibiotic therapy.
	Colonization of catheter via skin/catheter interface or catheter hub	Prepare skin insertion site by clipping hair and scrubbing skin with antimicrobial agent(s). Do not use semipermeable transparent dressing. Apply iodophor ointment and sterile gauze dressing to site daily. Inspect site daily. Reassess need for catheter after 3 days.	
Venous air embolism	Air intake through *open* needle/catheter/sheath or skin tract when venous pressure < air pressure (deep inspiration, dyspnea, hypovolemia, upright position)	Occlude needle/catheter/sheath hub during insertion. Place patient in Trendelenburg position during insertion. Insert guidewire only during exhalation. Check all connecting sites frequently. Place patient in Trendelenburg during catheter removal. Apply vaseline and occlusive dressing to site after catheter removal.	Position patient on left side in Trendelenburg position. Perform closed-chest cardiac massage. Aspirate air from RV. Give 100% oxygen. Positive pressure ventilation. Hyperbaria.

and gradual erosion from catheter adherence. Such perforations are more likely to occur when CVP catheters are inserted through an arm vein, where subsequent movement of the extremity can cause the catheter to advance against the vessel or myocardial wall. The clinical signs of tamponade may occur slowly or dramatically and often can be misleading because of the similarity to other more common problems. However, because tamponade is associated with such high mortality, it is essential for the critical care nurse to be aware of its likelihood and diligently observe for any evidence of the development of tamponade. Cardiac tamponade should be suspected in any patient with a CVP catheter who develops unexplained hypotension. If the diagnosis of tamponade is confirmed, infusion through the CVP catheter should be discontinued immediately and aspiration of fluid attempted through the catheter to try to remove fluid from the pericardial sac. The CVP catheter should then be removed and pericardiocentesis performed.

Precautions to minimize cardiac perforation with CVP catheters include the following:

1. Position the CVP catheter tip just above (approximately 2 cm) the SVC/RA junction at the time of insertion (see Fig. 5-1).
2. Verify the position of the CVP catheter tip with a chest x-ray examination.
3. Suture the catheter securely to the skin.
4. Avoid CVP catheter insertion through the arm veins.
5. Use soft catheters without beveled edges.
6. Frequently (at least once per shift) check the ability to aspirate blood back from the catheter.

Table 5-2 identifies some other causes of problems encountered with CVP catheters, as well as appropriate preventions and interventions.

REFERENCES

Abbott N, Walrath JM, Scanlon-Trump E: Infection related to physiologic monitoring: venous and arterial catheters, *Heart Lung* 12:28-34, 1983.

Anderson PT, Herlevsen P, Schaumburg H: A comparative study of Op-Site and Nobecutan gauze dressings for central venous line care, *J Hosp Infect* 7:161-168, 1986.

Ansley DM et al: The relationship between central venous pressure and pulmonary capillary wedge pressure during aortic surgery, *Can J Anaesth* 34:594-600, 1987.

Chabanier A et al: Iatrogenic cardiac tamponade after central venous catheter, *Clin Cardiol* 11:91-99, 1988.

Cobb DK et al: A controlled trial of scheduled replacement of central venous and pulmonary-artery catheters, *N Engl J Med* 327:1062-1068, 1992.

Collier PE, Ryan JJ, Diamond DL: Cardiac tamponade from central venous catheters. Reports of a case and review of the English literature, *Angiology* 35:595-600, 1984.

Duntley P et al: Vascular erosion by central venous catheters: clinical features and outcome, *Chest* 101:1633-1638, 1992.

Edwards H, King TC: Cardiac tamponade from central venous catheters, *Arch Surg* 117:965-967, 1982.

Fitchie C: Central venous catheter–related infection and dressing type, *Intensive and Critical Care Nursing* 8:199-202, 1992.

Frog M et al: Pericardial tamponade caused by central venous catheters, *World J Surg* 6:138-143, 1982.

Hilton E et al: Central catheter infections: Single- versus triple-lumen catheters, *Am J Med* 84:667-672, 1988.

Hoffman KK et al: Transparent polyurethane film as an intravenous catheter dressing: a meta-analysis of the infection risks, *JAMA* 267:2072-2076, 1992.

Orebaugh SL: Venous air embolism: clinical and experimental considerations, *Crit Care Med* 20:1169-1177, 1992.

Recker D: Catheter-related sepsis: an analysis of the research, *Dim Crit Care Nursing* 11:249-265, 1992.

Thielen JB: Air emboli: a potentially lethal complication of central venous lines, *Focus Crit Care* 17:374-383, 1990.

Chapter 6

Pulmonary Artery and Pulmonary Artery Wedge Pressure Monitoring

T he flow-directed, balloon-tipped catheter presents the opportunity to indirectly acquire important diagnostic and therapeutic information about the function of the two pumps, the right ventricle (RV) and the left ventricle (LV). Although slightly different in structure, both pumps share equally in the responsibility of maintaining circulatory dynamics. Blood flow through the two pumps is equal and is determined by the heart rate, preload, afterload, and contractility. (See Chapter 1 for a complete discussion of these determinants.)

PHYSIOLOGIC REVIEW
Preload

Clinically the *preload* of the ventricles is assessed by *indirectly* measuring the filling pressure of each of the ventricles (Fig. 6-1). The right ventricular (RV) preload, or filling pressure, is the central venous pressure (CVP) or right atrial pressure (RAP) (except in patients with tricuspid stenosis). This pressure is measured by a CVP catheter or by the proximal lumen of the pulmonary artery (PA) catheter.

The indirect measurement of the preload, or filling pressure, of the LV is the left atrial (LA) pressure. This pressure, which sometimes is measured directly after cardiac surgery, is more commonly measured indirectly as the pulmonary artery wedge (PAW) pressure.

The PAW pressure is obtained by inflating the balloon of the catheter to occlude a branch of the pulmonary artery. This occlusion causes a cessation of forward blood flow in that branch of the pulmonary artery so that the catheter tip, which is beyond the inflated balloon, "sees" only the pressure ahead in the more distal pulmonary venous system. This pressure is a direct retrograde reflection of the LA pressure and

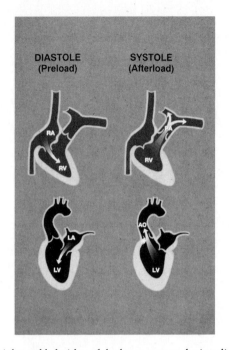

Fig. 6-1. Preload of the right and left sides of the heart occurs during diastolic filling as depicted on the left side of the figure. Clinically the direct or indirect right atrial (RA) pressure and the direct or indirect left atrial (LA) pressure are used to reflect right and left heart preload, respectively. Afterload occurs during systole (depicted on the right side of the figure). Clinically, pulmonary vascular resistance (PVR) and systemic vascular resistance (SVR) are used to reflect right and left heart afterload, respectively. (Right heart at top of figure; left heart at bottom.)

provides information about pressure events during LV diastole, that is, when the mitral valve is open (Figs. 6-2 and 6-3).

In the patient with normal pulmonary vascular resistance (PVR) and a normal mitral valve, the PA end-diastolic pressure also may be used to reflect the left ventricular end-diastolic pressure (LVEDP). At the end of diastole, just before the next systole, the mitral valve is still open and the left ventricle is filled with blood. At this point there is an equilibration of pressures between the left ventricle and the left atrium (in the absence of mitral valve disease). Because there are no valves in the pulmonary venous system, the pressure equilibrates between the pulmonary veins, pulmonary capillaries, and the pulmonary artery at end-diastole. Therefore, at this point, the PA end-diastolic pressure is equal to the LVEDP. Fig. 6-4 illustrates this correlation.

However, in situations that increase PVR, such as pulmonary embolism, hypoxia, or chronic lung disease, the PA pressure also increases, whereas the PAW pressure may remain normal. In these situations the PA pressure reflects the high PVR and not the LVEDP. For proper evaluation of the LVEDP in these instances, the PAW pressure must be monitored. Generally, however, the PA diastolic pressure is most suitable and it is safer to monitor.

Inasmuch as the PAW pressure is the pressure in the pulmonary capillary, it is also a critical determinant affecting the movement of fluid from the vascular bed to the

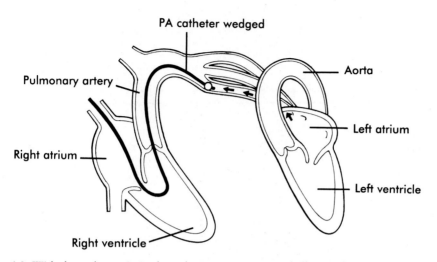

Fig. 6-2. With the catheter tip in the pulmonary artery (PA), balloon inflation causes forward flow to cease in that branch of the PA. The catheter tip beyond the balloon senses the pressure generated distally by the left atrium.

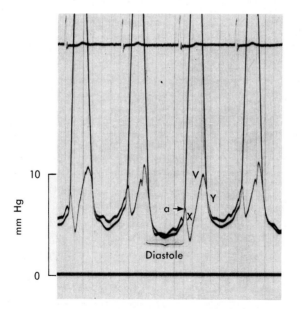

Fig. 6-3. Simultaneous recording of left ventricular (LV) and pulmonary artery wedge (PAW) pressures. Note the normal *a* and *v* waves with *x* and *y* descents. During diastole, the PAW pressure is barely 1 mm higher than the LV pressure when the mitral valve is open and blood is flowing from the left atrium to the left ventricle.

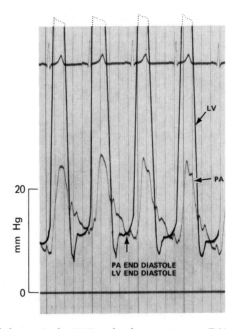

Fig. 6-4. Simultaneous left ventricular (LV) and pulmonary artery (PA) pressures. Note the close correlation between LV and PA at end-diastole. PA systolic pressure is 29 mm Hg; diastolic pressure is 12 mm Hg. LV systolic pressure is off scale; diastolic pressure is 12 mm Hg.

interstitial and alveolar spaces of the lung. Mild pulmonary congestion is usually evident when the PAW pressure is acutely elevated to 18 to 20 mm Hg. Acute pulmonary edema can occur with PAW pressure >30 mm Hg.

Afterload

Afterload, the resistance to flow from either ventricle during systole, is evaluated by the measurement of resistance (either systemic or pulmonary vascular resistance). On a broader scale, however, the systolic pressures generated by each ventricle reflect the afterload met by the ventricle. In the absence of aortic or pulmonic stenosis, the systolic systemic arterial pressure and the systolic PA pressure equal the LV and RV systolic pressures, respectively. Thus these pressures are used clinically to assess afterload, or the function of the ventricles in systole.

As illustrated in Fig. 6-1 and noted in Table 6-1, the PA catheter, along with the arterial catheter, permits on-line evaluation of both the diastolic and systolic function of both the right and left ventricles.

PA AND PAW HEART PRESSURES

The morphology and characteristics of the waveforms produced by the chambers and vessels of the right side of the heart are related to the underlying physiologic and electrophysiologic cardiac events. Pressure changes (increases as well as decreases) are reflections of physiologic changes in myocardial fiber tension (myocardial fibers are either contracting or relaxing) or changes in blood volume (blood is either entering

Table 6-1. Hemodynamic parameters used to assess ventricular preload and afterload

	Parameters	
Function	Right ventricle	Left ventricle
Preload (diastolic function)	RAm	LAm, PAWm, or PAEDP
Afterload (systolic function)	PA systolic pressure	Peripheral or central arterial systolic pressure

RAm, Right atrial mean; *LAm*, left atrial mean; *PAWm*, pulmonary artery wedge mean; *PAEDP*, pulmonary artery end-diastolic pressure; *PA*, pulmonary artery.

or exiting a chamber). Because cardiac electrical stimulation precedes mechanical activity, the ECG defines the timing of the corresponding mechanical response. A sound understanding of normal hemodynamic waveforms is essential in differentiation of abnormal waveforms from a variety of causes.

PA Pressure
Physiology and morphology

The pressure in the PA is similar to the systemic arterial waveform and is divided into two phases: systole and diastole. Systole begins with the opening of the pulmonic valve, resulting in rapid ejection of blood into the pulmonary artery. On the PA pressure waveform this is seen as a sharp rise in pressure, followed by a decline in pressure as the volume being ejected decreases (Fig. 6-5). When the RV pressure falls below the level of the PA pressure, the pulmonic valve snaps shut. This sudden closure of the valve leaflets produces a small notch on the downslope of the PA pressure and is termed the *dicrotic notch*. The systolic value referred to is the peak systolic pressure reached. Normal PA systolic pressure is 20 to 30 mm Hg (the same as the RV systolic pressure).

Diastole follows closure of the pulmonic valve. During this time, runoff to the pulmonary system occurs without any further blood flow from the right ventricle until the next systole. The PA diastolic value measured is the end-diastolic pressure just before the next systole. This value corresponds closely to the LV end-diastolic pressure (LVEDP) in the absence of pulmonary disease or mitral valve disease. Normal PA end-diastolic pressure is 8 to 12 mm Hg.

Respiratory correlation. Both the systolic and diastolic PA pressures decline during spontaneous inspiration. As with all hemodynamic pressures, PA readings should be obtained at end-expiration.

ECG correlation. The systolic phase of the PA pressure follows ventricular depolarization. However, catheter length and the amount of tubing used can delay this somewhat. Generally, PA systole occurs within the T wave of the ECG. The end-diastolic PA pressure, which immediately precedes the upstroke of the PA, corresponds with the QRS complex of the ECG.

Alterations associated with dysrhythmias

Atrial fibrillation. In atrial fibrillation the value of the PA pressure varies greatly (Fig. 6-6), depending on the RR intervals and length of time for ventricular filling. The

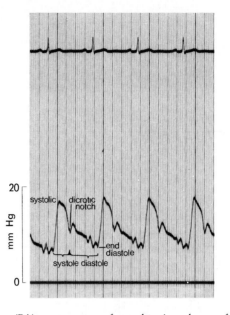

Fig. 6-5. Pulmonary artery (PA) pressure waveform showing phases of systole, dicrotic notch (pulmonic valve closure), and end-diastole. Normally, PA end-diastole closely represents left ventricular end-diastolic pressure (LVEDP).

shorter the RR interval, the shorter the ventricular filling time, the less stroke volume ejected, and the less the pressure in the subsequent PA waveform. The contour of the PA pressure tracing remains normal, however.

Ventricular ectopy. After a premature ventricular contraction (PVC), the PA pressure declines as a result of a decreased stroke volume. Pressure measurements should exclude these beats.

Abnormal PA pressures

Certain pathologic conditions alter the PA pressure. Elevation of PA systolic and diastolic pressures occurs in the following conditions:

1. Increased PVR, as in pulmonary diseases, pulmonary hypertension, or pulmonary embolus(i)
2. Increased pulmonary venous pressure, as in mitral stenosis and LV failure
3. Increased pulmonary blood flow, as in left-to-right shunt caused by an atrial or ventricular septal defect

Although these conditions alter the PA pressure values, the contour of the PA waveform remains unchanged.

Because of the increased risks associated with PAW pressure measurements, such as pulmonary infarction or even pulmonary rupture, monitoring the PA diastolic (PAd) pressure instead of the PAW is commonly used as a reflection of LVEDP. Normally, the PAd and PAW pressures are nearly the same (within 2 to 4 mm Hg) (Fig. 6-7). Situations in which this is not true, thus obviating the use of PAd pressure monitoring as a reflection of LVEDP, are listed in Table 6-2.

Elevations of the PVR, from whatever cause, elevate the PA pressure. However,

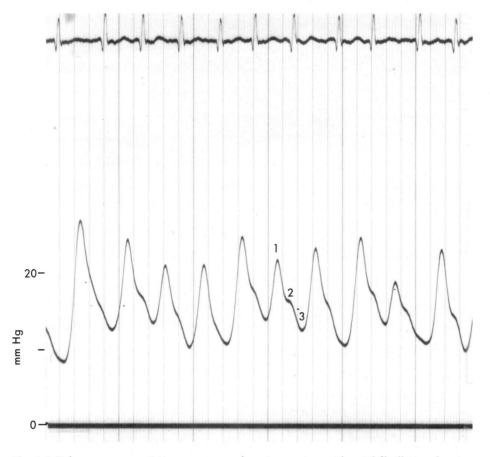

Fig. 6-6. Pulmonary artery (PA) pressure waveform in a patient with atrial fibrillation showing the varying systolic pressure values associated with varying RR intervals and length of time for diastolic filling. (*1,* PA systole; *2,* dicrotic notch; *3,* PA end-diastole.)

inflation of the balloon of the catheter stops the flow of blood in that branch of the PA. Thus the effects of increased resistance are no longer met, and the pressure obtained is a retrograde transmission of the pressure from the LA. For this reason, PAW pressure usually equals LA pressure, even in situations such as pulmonary disease and pulmonary embolus (Fig. 6-8).

Tachycardias (> 130 beats/min) abbreviate the duration of diastole and therefore falsely elevate the PAEDP and invalidate the usual relationship between the PAEDP and PAW or LVEDP (Fig. 6-9).

In addition to pathologic abnormalities, mechanical abnormalities frequently alter the PA pressure both in contour and value. "Fling" or "whip" in the PA pressure tracing (Fig. 6-10), consisting of exaggerated oscillations, can occur if excessive catheter coiling occurs in either the RA or the RV or if the catheter tip is located near the pulmonic valve, where blood flow is turbulent. These oscillations may become exaggerated if the monitoring system is suboptimally damped and the system's natural frequency is low (see discussion, p. 46). Patients with pulmonary hypertension and dilated pulmonary arteries frequently exhibit fling in the PA pressure tracing. In

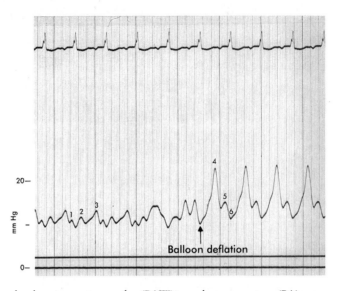

Fig. 6-7. Normal pulmonary artery wedge (PAW) to pulmonary artery (PA) pressure waveforms associated with deflation of the balloon of the PA catheter. Note the mean PAW pressure of approximately 11 mm Hg is closely related to the PA end-diastolic pressure of 12 mm Hg. Once this close correlation has been established, the pulmonary artery end-diastolic pressure (PAEDP) can be reliably used to monitor left heart filling pressures (LVEDP) and, thereby, avoid frequent balloon inflations. (*1,* PAW *a* wave; *2,* PAW *c* wave; *3,* PAW *v* wave; *4,* PA systolic, *5,* PA dicrotic notch; *6,* PA end-diastolic pressure.)

Table 6-2. Conditions in which the PAW pressure does not equal the PAEDP

↑ PVR	Pulmonary disease	↓ Diastole
Pulmonary embolus	COPD	↑ HR (>130 beats/min)
Hypoxia	ARDS	

PAW, Pulmonary artery wedge; *PAEDP,* pulmonary artery end-diastolic pressure; *PVR,* pulmonary vascular resistance; *COPD,* chronic obstructive pulmonary disease; *HR,* heart rate; *ARDS,* adult respiratory distress syndrome.

these situations accurate measurement of the PA pressure is difficult, and manipulation and repositioning of the catheter are necessary along with optimizing the system's dynamic response.

Damping of the PA pressure, resulting from a variety of causes, changes both the contour and the value of the PA waveform in a characteristic manner (Fig. 6-11). The entire waveform loses any sharp definition and becomes rather rounded out in appearance. Frequently the upstroke of the systolic pressure is slow and the dicrotic notch is absent or poorly defined. The value of the PA pressure is decreased considerably and as such is an inaccurate pressure. Most often fibrin at the tip of the catheter is the culprit when pressures become damped. Careful aspiration followed by gentle flushing usually corrects this problem, but occasionally catheter replacement is necessary. The tip of the catheter positioned against the wall of the vessel can also produce damped pressures and requires repositioning of the catheter. The presence of an air bubble (or bubbles) anywhere within the system also dampens the pressure

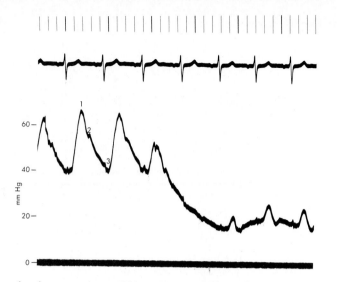

Fig. 6-8. Elevated pulmonary artery (PA) pressure (65/40) with a normal to mildly elevated pulmonary artery wedge (PAW) pressure (mean, 19 mm Hg). The wide disparity between the pulmonary artery end-diastolic pressure (PAEDP) and PAW mean pressures is due to chronic pulmonary disease and does not reflect the left heart filling pressures. Monitoring of left heart filling pressures in such situations requires measurement of the PAW pressure. (*1*, PA systole; *2*, dicrotic notch; *3*, PA end-diastole.)

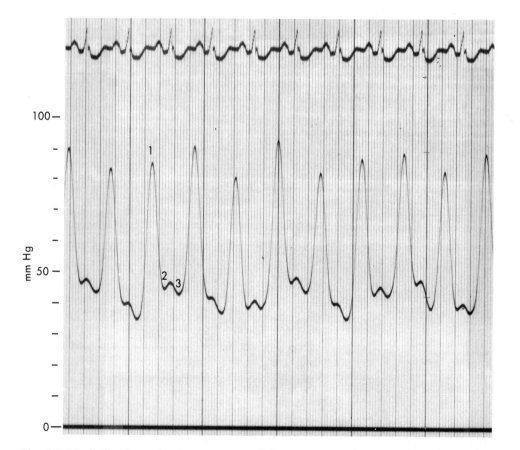

Fig. 6-9. Markedly elevated pulmonary artery (PA) pressure (90/42) in a patient with sinus tachycardia and pulmonary hypertension. Note the abbreviated diastolic period as a result of the rapid heart rate. (*1*, systole; *2*, dicrotic notch; *3*, end-diastole.)

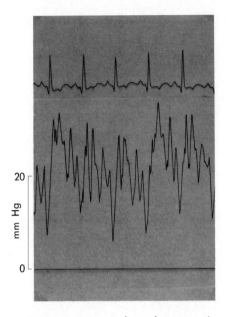

Fig. 6-10. Pulmonary artery (PA) pressure waveform demonstrating catheter fling caused by excessive catheter movement and/or inadequate damping of a system with a low natural frequency, making it impossible to accurately measure the pressure.

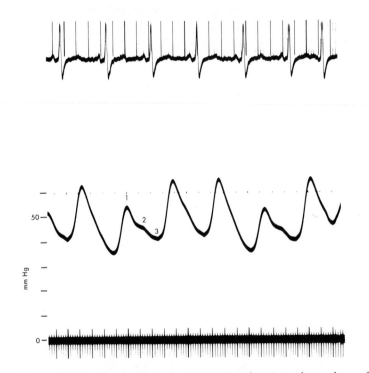

Fig. 6-11. Elevated pulmonary artery (PA) pressure (65/41) showing a damped waveform with poor definition and possible inaccurate measurement. (*1*, PA systole; *2*, dicrotic notch; *3*, PA end-diastole.)

waveform. Kinks in either the catheter itself or the extension tubing produce a dampened, lowered pressure waveform.

PAW Pressure

Physiology and morphology

When positioned in a small branch of the PA, with the balloon inflated, the catheter occludes flow in that segment of the pulmonary artery. The pressure obtained with balloon inflation is termed the *PAW*. This pressure is a backward reflection of the left atrial (LA) pressure and thus has similar contour and characteristics as the right atrial pressure (*a, c,* and *v* waves) inasmuch as the pressure is produced by the same physiologic events (Fig. 6-12). The *a* wave of the PAW pressure is produced by LA contraction and is followed by the *x* descent, reflecting LA relaxation following systole. The *c* wave that is produced by closure of the mitral valve frequently gets lost in retrograde transmission and often is not observed in the PAW pressure waveform although it sometimes can be seen. The *v* wave is produced by filling of the LA. The decline succeeding the *v* wave is the *y* descent, which represents opening of the mitral valve with a decrease in LA pressure and volume during passive emptying into the LV.

Although the contour of the PAW pressure is the same as the RA pressure, the value of the PAW pressure is normally higher. As with the RA pressure, the mean of the PAW pressure generally is recorded because the *a* and *v* waves are normally close to the same value. The normal resting PAW mean pressure is 4 to 12 mm Hg. If, however, either the *a* or the *v* wave is particularly dominant or elevated, it is not accurate to average the pressure rises. In those instances the mean value of the *a* wave should be measured as a reflection of the LV end-diastolic or filling pressure. However, the height of the *v* wave also should be noted.

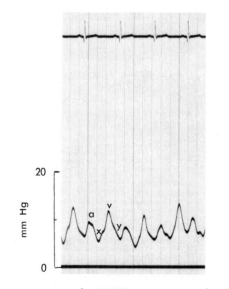

Fig. 6-12. Normal pulmonary artery wedge (PAW) pressure waveform showing *a* and *v* waves and *x* and *y* descents. The mean of this PAW pressure is about 8 mm Hg.

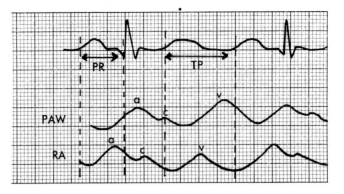

Fig. 6-13. The difference in timing of the right atrium (RA) and pulmonary artery wedge (PAW) waveform components relative to the ECG. Note the later appearance of the PAW *a* and *v* waves compared with the RA *a* and *v* waves.

ECG correlation. Timing of the electrical and mechanical events is the same as with the RA pressure; that is, the *a* wave follows the P wave of the ECG, and the *v* wave follows the T wave of the ECG. However, a greater time delay between electrical and mechanical events occurs with the PAW pressure inasmuch as it is a retrograde measurement of LA pressure. Thus the PAW *a* wave occurs later (approximately 200 to 240 msec) after the ECG P wave, whereas the *v* wave occurs well after the T wave, within the TP interval. Fig. 6-13 compares the timing of these events in both the RA and PAW waveforms.

Alterations associated with dysrhythmias

The effects of dysrhythmias on the PAW pressure are the same as those discussed with the RA pressure. In atrial fibrillation there are no *a* waves in the PAW pressure waveform, and only a *v* wave follows each QRS complex (Fig. 6-14). Junctional rhythm or AV dissociation can produce giant or cannon *a* waves.

Abnormal PAW pressures

Elevated PAW pressures occur in the following conditions:
1. LV failure
2. Mitral stenosis or regurgitation
3. Cardiac tamponade
4. Constrictive pericarditis
5. Volume overload

Elevated a waves. The *a* wave of the PAW pressure is exaggerated and elevated in any condition that increases the resistance to LV filling (Fig. 6-15). Elevation of the PAW *a* wave with LV failure reflects the increased filling pressure required with elevated LV diastolic pressures. In pure mitral stenosis the PAW *a* wave is dominant and elevated as a result of the resistance met at the narrowed mitral orifice. It represents the increased force of contraction required to eject blood through the stenotic valve. The *y* descent of the PAW pressure usually is prolonged in mitral stenosis, indicating increased resistance to passive filling of the LV. In the condition of mitral stenosis, the elevated PAW pressure does not reflect LVEDP.

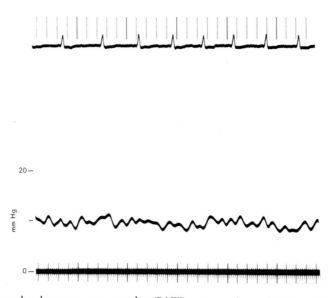

Fig. 6-14. Normal pulmonary artery wedge (PAW) pressure (mean is 10 mm Hg) in a patient with atrial fibrillation and absent *a* waves. Numerous small waves in this pressure tracing are likely a result of the fibrillatory activity of the atrium and make it difficult to identify the *v* wave.

Elevated v **waves.** The *v* wave of the PAW pressure is exaggerated and elevated with mitral insufficiency because of regurgitation of blood back into the LA during ventricular systole (Fig. 6-16). Mitral regurgitation can occur in varying degrees of severity and from a variety of causes. A mildly elevated and dominant *v* wave commonly is seen with LV failure and dilation. Rheumatic fever or bacterial endocarditis can cause destruction to the valve leaflets and thus produce chronic mitral regurgitation. Acute mitral regurgitation, with giant *v* waves, can occur with papillary muscle ischemia or rupture after myocardial infarction (Fig. 6-17).

In severe mitral regurgitation the appearance of the PAW becomes "ventricularized" and the *v* wave occurs sooner after the T wave than normal. When the PAW *v* wave is markedly higher than the *a* wave, the mean value, as measured by the monitoring system, will be artifactually elevated. To obtain a more accurate measurement of the LVEDP, the mean value of the *a* wave (or the *c* wave, if present) should be measured as the filling pressure (see Fig. 6-16). However, the *v* value also should be recorded to evaluate changes in the regurgitant volume that may occur after therapeutic interventions.

High *v* waves significantly elevate the pulmonary venous pressure, causing acute pulmonary edema. Often a giant *v* wave can be transmitted onto the PA waveform, producing a bifid appearance to the PA pressure wave (Fig. 6-18). Occasionally the *v* wave may even be higher than the PA systolic pressure, resulting in a PA waveform as seen in Fig. 6-19. Such an occurrence results in retrograde flow of blood and early closure of the pulmonic wave.

It is important to point out that not *all* elevations of the *v* wave of the PAW pressure result from mitral regurgitation. Increases in the *v* wave also can occur as a result of decreased compliance of the left atrium.

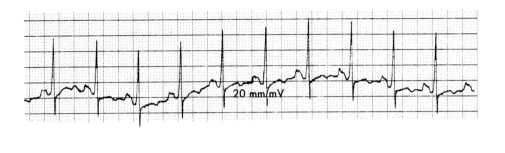

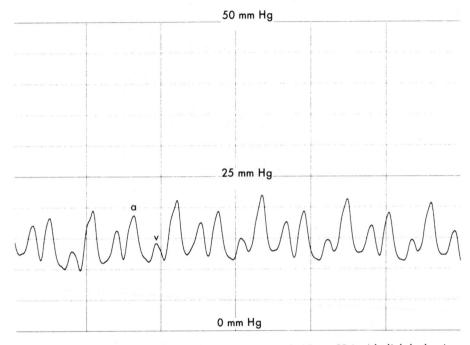

Fig. 6-15. Pulmonary artery wedge (PAW) pressure (mean is 15 mm Hg) with slightly dominant *a* wave as a result of left ventricle (LV) hypertrophy with decreased compliance during LV filling.

Abnormal elevations of the *v* wave of the PAW pressure may cause the PAW waveform to resemble a PA waveform (Figs. 6-17 and 6-20). This is particularly likely in patients with atrial fibrillation in whom the PAW waveforms consist solely of a large *v* wave. Such an error could result in permanent wedging of the PA catheter with the associated risks of pulmonary infarction or rupture. Close inspection of the timing of the PAW waveform in relation to the ECG (best done at fast paper speed) shows the *v* wave occurring after the T wave, whereas the upstroke of the PA systolic pressure usually occurs earlier and peaks with the T wave of the ECG.

If some doubt still exists as to whether the pressure is actually a PAW pressure or a damped PA pressure, obtaining a small blood sample while the balloon is inflated may confirm the location. If the catheter is indeed wedged, occluding forward blood flow, the blood sample obtained will be from the postcapillary vasculature and

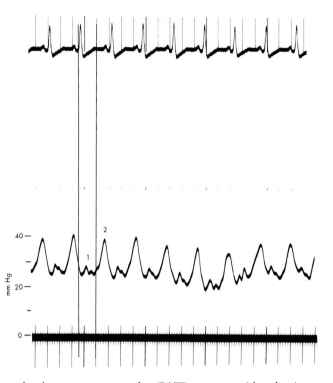

Fig. 6-16. Elevated pulmonary artery wedge (PAW) pressure with a dominant and elevated *v* wave (39 mm Hg) *(2)* as a result of mild mitral regurgitation. The *a* wave *(1)* also is elevated (25 mm Hg) indicating left ventricle (LV) failure. In this case the mitral regurgitation is likely functional second-degree LV failure and dilation. The first dark vertical line is drawn after the ECG P wave to identify the *a* wave. The second dark vertical line is drawn after the ECG T wave to identify the *v* wave.

therefore should be arterialized blood. If the catheter is not wedged, the blood sample obtained will be darker venous blood. These observations are generally made visually, although a small blood sample can be drawn and sent to the laboratory to determine oxygen saturation. After the blood sample is withdrawn from the PAW, it is essential to deflate the balloon before flushing the catheter to ensure that flushing is done in the PA and not in the PAW position.

Elevated a **and** *v* **waves.** In cardiac tamponade, constrictive pericardial disease, and hypervolemia the PAW *a* and *v* waves are both elevated. As with the RA waveform, in cardiac tamponade the *x* descent is prominent, whereas in constrictive pericarditis either the *y* descent is prominent or the *x* and *y* descents are equal, giving an M pattern to the PAW pressure waveform.

Low PAW pressure. Hypovolemia produces a low PAW pressure (Fig. 6-21). In the normal heart, PAW pressures less than 4 or 5 mm Hg indicate hypovolemia, whereas in the compromised heart, hypovolemia may be present despite higher PAW pressures.

Mechanical abnormalities

Mechanical abnormalities of the PAW pressure produce changes in both the value and the contour of the PAW pressure waveform. *Overwedging,* which is caused by

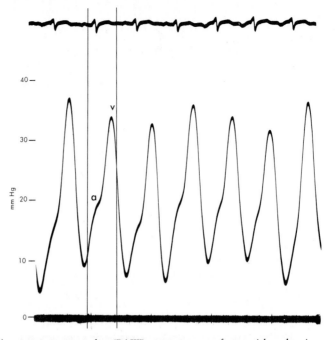

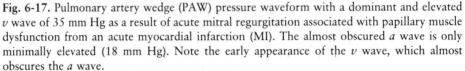

Fig. 6-17. Pulmonary artery wedge (PAW) pressure waveform with a dominant and elevated *v* wave of 35 mm Hg as a result of acute mitral regurgitation associated with papillary muscle dysfunction from an acute myocardial infarction (MI). The almost obscured *a* wave is only minimally elevated (18 mm Hg). Note the early appearance of the *v* wave, which almost obscures the *a* wave.

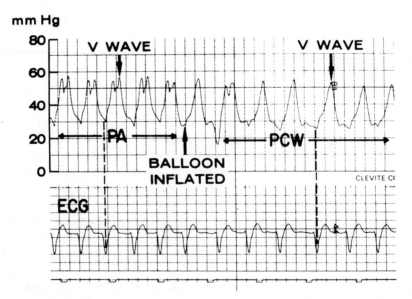

Fig. 6-18. Elevated pulmonary artery (PA) and pulmonary artery wedge (PAW) pressures showing a large *v* wave of the PAW that is reflected in the PA pressure, giving it a bifid (double-peaked) appearance. Careful examination of the mechanical events with the ECG reveals the PA systolic pressure occurring earlier in the cardiac cycle than the PAW *v* wave.

From Buchbinder N, Ganz W: *Anesthesiology* 45:146, 1976.

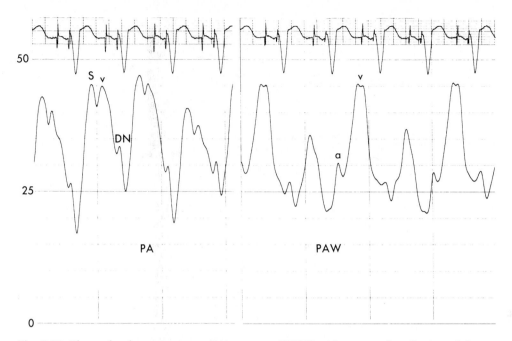

Fig. 6-19. Elevated pulmonary artery (PA) pressure (47/25) with retrograde reflection of the elevated v wave from the pulmonary artery wedge (PAW). In this case the v wave (46 mm Hg) is as high as the systolic *(S)* PA pressure. *(DN,* Dicrotic notch.) The PAW a wave averages approximately 27 mm Hg.

overinflation or eccentric inflation of the balloon of the catheter or an exceedingly distal location of the catheter tip, may produce an artifactually elevated, damped, and inaccurate PAW pressure (Fig. 6-22). In addition, there is usually a linear increase or decrease in the pressure waveform. (It resembles a line at an approximately 10- to 20-degree angle). Slow, careful, and accurate balloon inflation or, if the catheter is too distally positioned, withdrawal to a more proximal PA location may alleviate this problem.

Damping of the PAW pressure produces the same type of rounded-out appearance as with the PA pressure with lack of defined a and v waves (Fig. 6-23). The balloon should be deflated before the catheter is aspirated and then gently flushed. Never flush in the PAW position.

Occasionally a mixed PA/PAW pressure is obtained because of incomplete wedging of the catheter tip (Fig. 6-24). Sometimes the changes are directly related to respirations, with a PA pressure observed during expiration and a PAW pressure observed during inspiration. In this circumstance, slight advancement of the catheter is necessary to obtain an accurate PAW pressure.

The PAW mean pressure should be lower than the PA mean pressure, and a noticeable fall in pressure should occur as the balloon of the catheter is inflated (see Fig. 6-7). Similarly, there should be an abrupt rise in the systolic pressure as the balloon is deflated. The PAW pressure, like all hemodynamic pressures, should be measured at the end of expiration. Inasmuch as the digital display presents an average of the sweep, it is necessary to measure the pressure marking the end-expiratory phase of the respiratory cycle on a calibrated oscilloscope or graph paper.

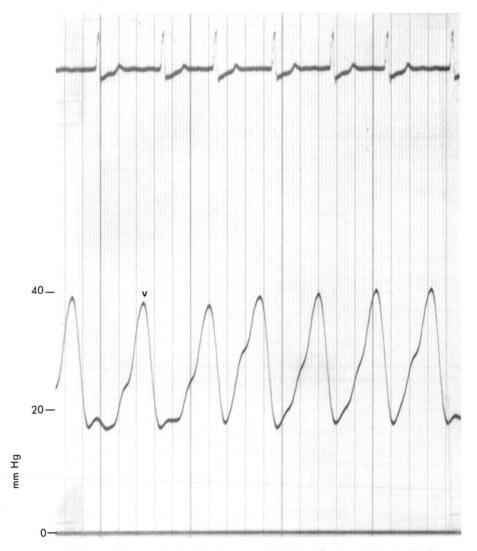

Fig. 6-20. Pulmonary artery wedge (PAW) pressure with elevated v wave (38 mm Hg) because of mitral regurgitation. Absent a waves in this waveform are a result of the underlying atrial fibrillation. The wide, triangular appearance of this PAW waveform could be mistaken for a pulmonary artery (PA) waveform. Differentiation can be achieved by obtaining a blood sample from the distal lumen of the catheter.

Left atrial pressure

Direct left atrial (LA) pressures sometimes are measured via a small catheter placed in the LA at the time of open heart surgery. Because the PAW pressure is an indirect measurement of LA pressure, both the contour and the value of the LA pressure are the same as the PAW pressure (Fig. 6-25). The LA a wave, produced by left atrial systole, is followed by the x descent, a decline in pressure as a result of reduced LA volume. The c wave is produced by closure of the mitral valve leaflets and may or may not be evident in the LA waveform. The v wave results from filling of the LA and bulging back of the mitral valve during ventricular systole. This is followed by

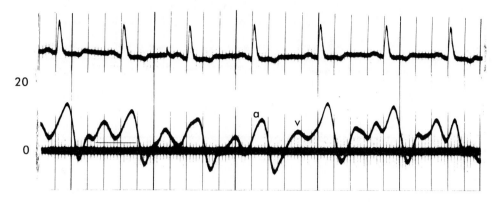

Fig. 6-21. Pulmonary artery wedge (PAW) waveform of normal contour but abnormally low value (mean is 4 mm Hg at end-expiration).

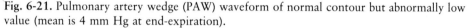

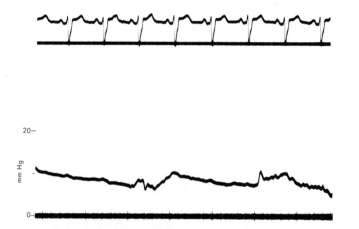

Fig. 6-22. Pulmonary artery wedge (PAW) pressure lacking the normal characteristics as a result of overwedging. Overwedging can occur when the balloon of the catheter is inflated with an excessive amount of air for the size of the vessel in which the catheter is positioned. Careful monitoring of the pressure waveform during balloon inflation, with immediate cessation of inflation when a PAW waveform is obtained, can prevent this problem.

the *y* descent, reflecting a decrease in LA volume during passive filling of the LV. The delay between electrical and mechanical events that one sees in the PAW pressure is less apparent with the direct LA pressure; for example, the LA *a* wave follows the P wave of the ECG more immediately than in the PAW.

Normal mean LA pressure is 4 to 12 mm Hg.

Limitations of PAW monitoring

PAW pressure unequal to LVEDP. Although the PAW pressure commonly is used as a reflection of the LVEDP, its limitations must be appreciated. Situations in which the PAW pressure *does not* equal or approximate the LVEDP include the following:
1. Mitral stenosis
2. Left atrial myxoma

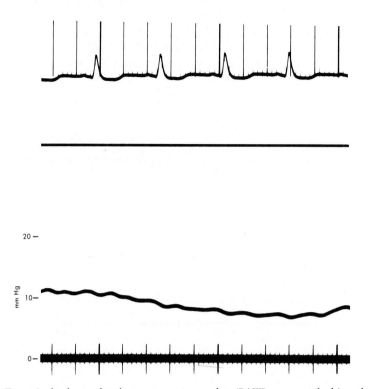

Fig. 6-23. Excessively damped pulmonary artery wedge (PAW) pressure lacking the normal characteristics and contour. After deflation to ensure the catheter is no longer wedged, the catheter should be aspirated and flushed.

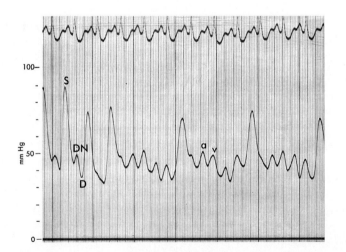

Fig. 6-24. Mixed pulmonary artery (PA) and pulmonary artery wedge (PAW) pressure waveforms as a result of spontaneous forward migration of the PA catheter tip. The change from PA to PAW appears to be cyclical and regular, indicating that the changes follow the respiratory pattern. Slight withdrawal of the catheter tip should eliminate this problem. (*S*, PA systolic; *DN*, dicrotic notch; *D*, PA diastolic; *a*, PAW *a* wave; *V*, PAW *v* wave.)

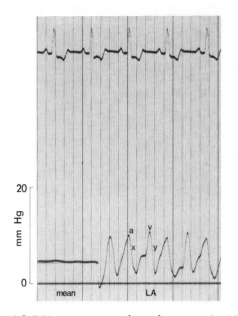

Fig. 6-25. Normal left atrial (LA) pressure waveform demonstrating similarity to pulmonary artery wedge (PAW) waveform.

3. Pulmonary venous obstruction
4. Increased pleural pressure
5. Placement of the catheter tip in a nondependent zone of the lung

The first three pathologic disorders cause an increase in the LA pressure and, therefore, the PAW pressure. However, the diastolic filling pressure of the left ventricle may be normal or even low as a result of reduced filling volume. Indirect assessment of LVEDP is not possible in these situations.

Increases in juxtacardiac and pleural pressures are transmitted to the cardiac chambers and vessels. PAW pressures obtained in patients with increased pleural pressure reflect the elevated juxtacardiac pressure rather than a high LVEDP. (See Chapter 15 for further discussion.)

When the tip of the PA catheter lies in nondependent lung zone I or II and the balloon of the catheter is inflated to measure the PAW pressure, the flow is interrupted and the vasculature beyond the catheter tip may partially or completely collapse. The recorded PAW pressure in such cases reflects the alveolar or airway pressure rather than the LVEDP. (This concept is discussed in greater detail in Chapter 15.)

PAW unequal to LVED volume. A major limitation of the ability to monitor the preload, or end-diastolic pressure of the LV, by monitoring the PAW pressure occurs in conditions that alter the diastolic pressure–volume relationship. The normal diastolic pressure–volume relationship of the LV can be altered by changes in ventricular compliance and geometry and by certain therapeutic interventions. Changes in ventricular compliance occur when the heart is prevented from expanding normally during ventricular filling. This can result from pericardial restriction or disease, positive end-expiratory pressure (PEEP), or myocardial disease, particularly myocardial ischemia.

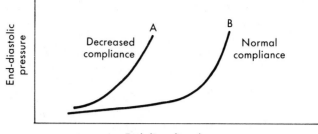

Fig. 6-26. Relationship between ventricular end-diastolic volume and end-diastolic pressure. With normal ventricular compliance, relatively large increases in end-diastolic volume are accompanied, up to a point, by relatively small increases in end-diastolic pressure *(curve B)*. In the noncompliant ventricle *(curve A)*, small increases in end-diastolic volume are associated with marked increases in end-diastolic pressure.

Fig. 6-26 illustrates the altered pressure-volume curve seen with decreased ventricular compliance. A higher filling pressure is required for the same amount of volume filling the ventricle. For this reason, a patient with a stiff, diseased left ventricle requires a higher filling pressure (in the range of 15 to 20 mm Hg) to maintain adequate stroke volume. In fact, in patients with decreased ventricular compliance from whatever cause, PAW pressures of normal value are likely to represent relative hypovolemia and to be accompanied by a low stroke volume. Administration of a fluid challenge may be necessary to increase the diastolic filling volume to improve stroke volume. The construction of individual ventricular function curves provides a helpful method to assess the patient's optimal PAW or filling pressure.

The possibility of such conditions affecting the PAW pressure measurement must be assessed before one clinically interprets an elevated PAW pressure. An elevated PAW pressure does not always mean the LVEDP or volume is elevated. It could be a result of increased surrounding pleural pressure, a noncompliant ventricle, or interruption of the fluid column between the catheter tip and the LA. Fig. 6-27 schematically illustrates the possible causes responsible for an elevation of the recorded PAW pressure.

Respiratory Effects on Hemodynamic Pressures

Because the heart lies between the lungs within the chest, an intimate relationship exists between the heart and the surrounding airway, esophageal, and pleural pressures. The cardiac as well as vascular structures within the thorax are constantly subjected to continually changing surrounding pressures of −2 to −7 mm Hg and even higher in certain disease states. Normally, however, the intrathoracic pressure changes are fairly small and constant from one respiratory cycle to another. For this reason it is common practice to reference intravascular pressures to atmospheric pressure rather than surrounding pleural pressure. However, this may not be appropriate when intrathoracic pressures are increased. In these situations, it is more accurate to measure the *transmural* intracardiac or intravascular pressures. Transmural pressures are determined by subtracting the intrapleural pressure from the measured hemodynamic pressure. Intrapleural pressure can be measured with

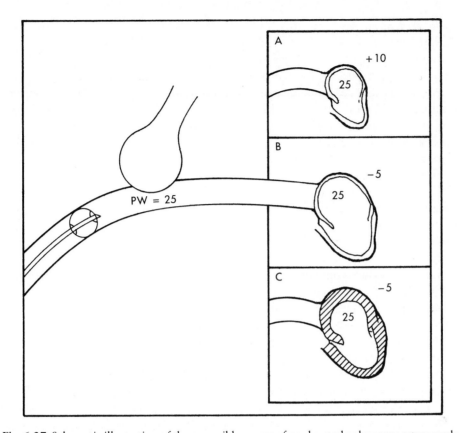

Fig. 6-27. Schematic illustration of three possible causes of an elevated pulmonary artery wedge (PAW) pressure: **A,** The PAW, left atrial (LA), and left ventricular end-diastolic (LVED) pressures are equally elevated as a result of increased pleural pressure (+10), although the end-diastolic ventricular volume (preload) is normal, or reduced. **B,** The left ventricular (LV), LA, and PAW pressures are all elevated as a result of increased LV preload and ventricular dilation, with normal compliance and normal pleural pressure. In this situation the PAW pressure accurately reflects the LVEDP and volume. **C,** Elevated LV, LA, and PAW pressures, with normal pleural pressure surrounding a noncompliant ventricle. In this case, the elevated PAW pressures, with normal pleural pressure surrounding a noncompliant ventricle, reflects the decrease in ventricular compliance and *not* the preload or end-diastolic volume of the ventricle, which is actually reduced. All three possible causes of elevated PAW pressures must be considered, when applicable, for accurate assessment of LV preload.

From Wiedemann HP, Matthay MA, Matthay RA: *Chest* 85:537-549, 1984.

esophageal catheters, although this method is difficult in the critically ill patient. More commonly, the intrapleural pressure is rather crudely estimated, as discussed in Chapter 15.

During spontaneous *inspiration,* lung volume increases and the pressure in the intrathoracic cavity becomes negative relative to atmospheric pressure. This decrease in intrathoracic pressure is transmitted to the structures in the thoracic cavity, causing a decrease in intravascular and intracardiac pressures during inspiration (see Fig. 5-7). Consequently, it is normal to observe falls in RA, PA, PAW, LA, and arterial pressures during normal, spontaneous inspiration. If, however, true transmural pressures were measured (i.e., the pressure within the heart chamber or vessel relative to the surrounding pleural pressure rather than the pressure in the atmosphere), the pressures would reflect the changes in volume that occur during the respiratory cycle. During inspiration, decreased intrapleural pressure causes venous return to increase, resulting in an increase in RA volume and, likewise, transmural RA pressure (relative to pleural pressure). Similarly, there is an increase in RV volume and end-diastolic pressure relative to pleural pressure. As a result of this increase in RV preload, pulmonary arterial outflow and therefore transmural PA pressure actually increase slightly during spontaneous inspiration.

The effects of inspiration on the left side of the heart are not as consistently explained as those of the right side of the heart. The inspiratory effect of increasing RV volume or preload causes an increase in RV size. Several studies have demonstrated that increasing RV size through the mechanism of ventricular interdependence may lead to decreased LV size, stiffening of the LV, and alterations in the LV pressure-volume curve. Decreases in LV filling pressures have been attributed to decreased pulmonary venous return as a result of pooling of blood in the lungs during inspiration. This distribution of blood in the pulmonary vasculature, which is thought to be caused by increased compliance of the pulmonary vasculature during inspiration, results in decreased LV filling. Evidence reveals increases in effective or transmural LV filling pressure during inspiration in some patients. This probably reflects the imposed alterations in the LV pressure-volume curve during inspiration as a result of decreased compliance of the LV.

The net result of these inspiratory effects on LV performance is a decrease in stroke volume. This decrease in stroke volume is caused not only by changes in LV preload but by increases in afterload that occur with decreased pleural pressure. Because stroke volume decreases during spontaneous inspiration, arterial pulse pressure falls.

During spontaneous expiration, intrathoracic pressure increases, resulting in increased pulmonary venous return to the LA, with increased filling of the LV and increased stroke volume. Therefore both intravascular and intracardiac pressures rise during spontaneous expiration.

Because the PA and PAW pressure can vary markedly as a result of intrathoracic pressure changes during respiration, all pressures should be measured at end-expiration, when intrathoracic pressure comes closest to atmospheric pressure.

PA and PAW Pressure Measurement

A pressure transducer, monitoring equipment, and an oscilloscope allow pressure monitoring during catheter insertion at the bedside. This technique permits location of the catheter tip position without fluoroscopy by means of the pressure measurement and the pressure waveform on the oscilloscope. The various types of transducers and monitoring equipment are described in Chapter 3.

Flotation PA catheters are now available to meet virtually every need in hemodynamic monitoring (Fig. 6-28 and Table 6-3). In addition to thermistors, which allow measurement of cardiac output and RV ejection fraction by the thermodilution technique, these catheters come equipped with fiberoptics for oxygen saturation measurement and pacing wires, as well as an additional RA port for the infusion of fluids or drugs.

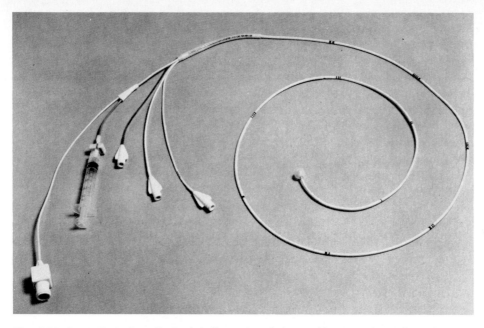

Fig. 6-28. Swan-Ganz flow-directed, balloon-tipped thermodilution catheter for pulmonary artery (PA) and right atrium (RA) pressure monitoring and cardiac output measurement. Syringe is used for inflating the balloon with air.

Courtesy American Edwards Laboratories, Santa Ana, Calif.

Table 6-3. Types of PA monitoring catheters

Type	Size (French)	Functions
Standard PA	5, 6, 7	PA and PAW monitoring
Standard thermodilution PA	5, 6, 7	RA, PA, PAW monitoring plus intermittent CO
Standard thermodilution PA with extra RA port	7.5	RA, PA, PAW, CO plus additional infusion port
Standard thermodilution PA with extra RA and RV ports	7.5, 8	RA, PA, PAW, CO plus two ports for infusions, temporary AV pacing, or intracardiac ECGs
Standard thermodilution PA with extra RV port	7.5	RA, PA, PAW, CO plus additional port for infusions, temporary ventricular pacing, or RV pressure monitoring
Standard thermodilution PA with atrial and ventricular electrodes	7	RA, PA, PAW, CO plus temporary pacing
Standard thermodilution PA with rapid response thermistor	7.5	RA, PA, PAW, CO plus RV volumes* and ejection fraction
Standard thermodilution PA with oximetric fiberoptics	7.5, 8	RA, PA, PAW, CO plus continuous Svo_2
Standard thermodilution PA with oximetric fiberoptics and rapid response thermistor	7.5	RA, PA, PAW, CO, continuous Svo_2 plus RV volumes* and ejection fraction
Standard thermodilution PA with oximetric fiberoptics and rapid response thermistor with extra RV port	8	RA, PA, PAW, CO continuous Svo_2 plus RV volumes* and ejection fraction, and temporary ventricular pacing
Standard thermodilution PA with extra RA port and thermal filaments	8	RA, PA, PAW, CO plus infusion port and continuous CO

PA, Pulmonary artery; *PAW*, pulmonary artery wedge; *RA*, right atrium; *CO*, cardiac output; *RV*, right ventricle; *AV*, atrioventricular; Svo_2, venous oxygen saturation.
*RV stroke volume, end-diastolic volume, and end-systolic volume.

The catheter is connected to the transducer by short stiff extension tubing and stopcocks (Fig. 6-29). The connecting tubing should be just long enough to connect the catheter to the transducer. Excessive tubing lengths cause distortion of the pressure waveforms. Ideally, the transducer should be connected directly to the catheter via a stopcock. The connector tubing must be flushed with IV fluid before it is connected to the catheter. To prevent a thrombus from forming at the catheter tip, 1 to 2 units heparin/1 ml IV fluid may be added and a continuous flush device is used.

Equipment

Hemodynamic monitoring of RA, PA, and PAW pressures requires the following equipment:
1. Catheter of choice
2. Catheter/sheath introducer
3. Sterile catheter sleeve
4. Pressure transducer
5. Electronic monitor and oscilloscope
6. Heparinized IV infusion fluid in a plastic bag
7. IV tubing with pediatric drip chamber
8. Pressure tubing
9. Three-way stopcocks
10. Continuous flush device

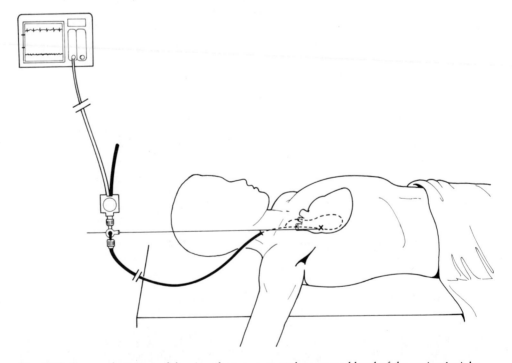

Fig. 6-29. Proper placement of the air-reference port at the assumed level of the patient's right atrium, which corresponds closely to the patient's midchest.

11. Pressurized IV cuff or pump
12. Fluoroscope (optional)
13. Paper recorder
14. Cardiopulmonary resuscitation equipment

Setting up equipment

1. Plug transducer cable into the monitor.
2. Select appropriate scale on the monitor.
3. Activate monitor power switch to "on."
4. Add heparin to IV solution in a collapsible bag and label solution bag (if not prepackaged and labeled).
5. Remove all air from the IV bag via a 22-gauge needle inserted into the medication port.
6. Remove protective cap from the drip chamber and insert into outlet port of IV bag. If desired, a second drip chamber can be inserted into the medication port of the IV bag, thus using only one IV bag for two monitoring lines. A single drip chamber distally divided into three monitoring lines is also available, allowing the use of one IV bag for three monitoring lines.
7. Open the IV roller clamp and lightly squeeze the drip chamber. Do not fill the drip chamber more than 0.5 cm, because the fluid level increases when pressure is applied to the bag.

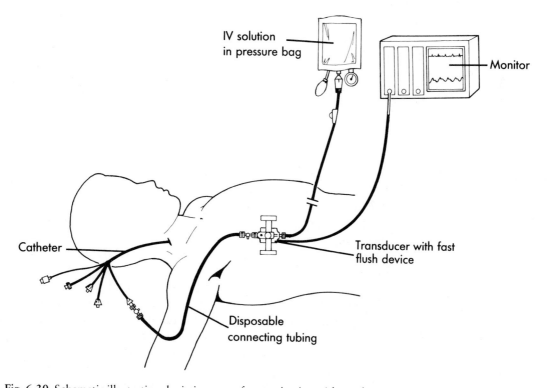

Fig. 6-30. Schematic illustration depicting setup for monitoring with a pulmonary artery (PA) catheter inserted in the internal jugular vein. Note placement of the transducer and air-reference port directly onto the patient's chest at the midchest position.

8. Close the IV roller clamp, insert the IV bag into a pressure administration cuff, and hang the pressure cuff.
9. Replace all vented caps with dead-ender caps on the sideports of all stopcocks.
10. Attach the IV set to the designated female end of the continuous flush device.
11. Attach a venting stopcock to one port of the transducer dome (if not preassembled).
12. Attach a Luer-Lok stopcock to the remaining port of the transducer dome.
13. Attach the female end of the continuous flush device to the Luer-Lok stopcock on the transducer dome.
14. Open the transducer venting stopcock to air.
15. Open the IV roller clamp, pull the fast flush device, and allow the IV solution to completely fill the tubing, the stopcocks, the flushing device, and the transducer dome. (It may be necessary to rotate the dome while fast-flushing to purge all air bubbles from the dome.)
16. Close the transducer venting stopcock.
17. Remove dead-ender cap at patient end of the connecting tubing; attach a Luer-Lok stopcock (if not preassembled) and close off its sideport.
18. Pull fast flush device and slowly flush entire monitoring line (using gravity pressure only), taking special care to ensure that no air is trapped in any stopcocks.
19. Pressurize cuff to 300 mm Hg. (Make sure the drip chamber does not completely fill.)
20. Hold the catheter hub end in a downward position below the heart level, and allow blood to completely fill the hub.
21. While pulling the fast-flush device, attach the IV line to the hub of the catheter, securing tightly.
22. Check drip rate to ensure flow of 1 to 5 ml/hr.
23. Check all connecting sites.
24. Place transducer air-reference stopcock at patient's midchest level and secure in this position (either directly on patient's arm or chest or on IV pole holder) (Fig. 6-30).
25. Open the air-reference stopcock to air.
26. Turn zero control knob on monitor to obtain a zero reading.
27. Push calibration knob and recheck monitor calibration; adjust if necessary.
28. Close the transducer venting stopcock to air.

Before any hemodynamic pressure measurements are obtained, the air-reference port of the transducer must be set level to the patient's phlebostatic axis or midchest height, which approximates the level of the RA (Fig. 6-31). With the reference stopcock open to room air, the zero dial on the monitor is set and the electrical calibration is checked. Although maintaining the same positional relationship between the patient's midchest and the air-reference port of the transducer is mandatory for consistency and accuracy of measurement, the patient's position may be changed, as necessary. It is not necessary to place the patient in a flat supine position to measure hemodynamic pressures. In fact, patients may be kept in backrest elevations up to 60 degrees, or in lateral recumbent positions, without compromising accuracy of pressure measurements, *as long as the air-reference port is leveled to the patient's midchest level* (which should be marked on the patient's chest). To ensure this practice, some clinicians tape the air-reference port onto

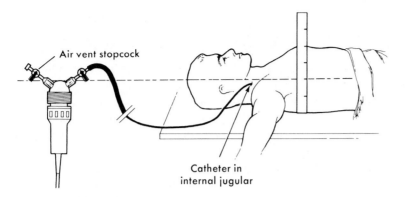

Fig. 6-31. The patient's midchest position is measured, marked, and used as an external anatomic reference point for placement of the air-reference port.

the patient's chest wall, at the marked midchest level, or phlebostatic axis. Before all hemodynamic pressure measurements are obtained, the system should be properly rezeroed to ensure that no hydrostatic pressure differences affect the hemodynamic measurement.

PROBLEMS AND COMPLICATIONS ENCOUNTERED WITH BALLOON-TIPPED CATHETERS

Although the relative ease of catheter insertion and the information obtained make PA pressure monitoring a valuable diagnostic tool, it is not without hazard. Reported overall complications rates for PA catheters are as high as 75%. This high rate, however, relates to the frequent occurrence of transient and clinically benign dysrhythmias. Most complications that occur with PA catheterization are minor, although fatalities may be associated with major complications. Potentially life-threatening complications have been reported to occur in approximately 4% of patients who have undergone PA catheterizations.

Cardiac Dysrhythmias

Either atrial or ventricular dysrhythmias frequently occur during right heart catheter insertion and usually are transient and benign, subsiding with completion of catheter passage out to the PA. Transient PVCs and nonsustained ventricular tachycardia are the most common dysrhythmias, but occasionally sustained ventricular tachycardia develops, requiring drug therapy or prompt cardioversion, or both. Rarely, ventricular fibrillation may occur and is treated by immediate defibrillation. The occurrence of ventricular dysrhythmias is highly correlated with the presence of shock, acute myocardial ischemia or infarction, hypokalemia, hypocalcemia, hypoxemia, acidosis, and prolonged catheter insertion times.

The sudden appearance of ventricular ectopy after the catheter is in place mandates an immediate evaluation of the pressure from the distal lumen of the catheter. If the pressure waveform is that of an RV (Fig. 6-32), or mixed RV and PA (Figs. 6-33 and 6-34), the ectopy is the result of mechanical irritation of the RV by the catheter tip. Immediate inflation of the balloon provides two benefits: (1) it

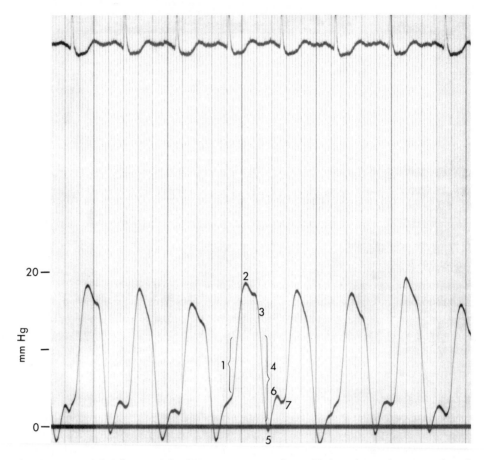

Fig. 6-32. Normal right ventricle (RV) pressure waveform. (*1*, isovolumetric contraction; *2*, rapid ejection; *3*, reduced ejection; *4*, isovolumetric relaxation; *5*, early diastole; *6*, atrial systole; *7*, end-diastole.) Note rapid upstroke and return to below-zero baseline pressure.

cushions the catheter tip and prevents it from irritating the ventricular wall and (2) it propels the catheter tip out to the PA. This maneuver usually successfully terminates the ventricular ectopy.

Right bundle branch block may occur during manipulation of the catheter in the right ventricle. This generally is not a problem unless the patient has preexisting left bundle branch block (LBBB), resulting in complete AV block. In patients with preexisting LBBB, it may be prudent to insert a PA catheter with pacing electrodes to prevent ventricular asystole. If a pacing catheter is not inserted, transvenous or transcutaneous pacing equipment should be readily available.

The best prevention of the development of any cardiac dysrhythmia or conduction abnormality is rapid placement of the catheter tip in the PA with minimal manipulation in the right ventricle or right atrium. In addition, the balloon should be fully inflated before entering the right ventricle to prevent catheter tip–induced dysrhythmias.

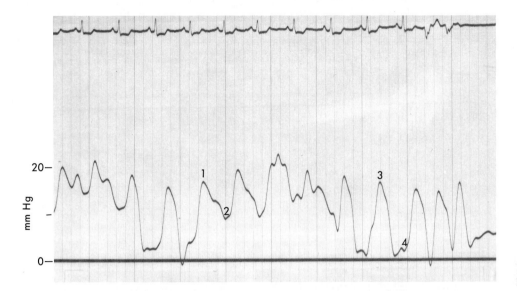

Fig. 6-33. Pressure tracing obtained from the distal lumen of the pulmonary artery (PA) catheter, with the catheter tip moving back and forth across the pulmonic valve producing intermittent PA and right ventricle (RV) pressure waveforms. It is not in a safe location for monitoring purposes (note the occurrence of premature ventricular contractions [PVCs]). It also would be impossible to obtain a pulmonary artery wedge (PAW) pressure with the catheter tip in this location. Frequently, inflation of the balloon will float the catheter tip distally to the PA, although it may not float distally enough to obtain a PAW pressure. (*1*, PA systole; *2*, PA end-diastole; *3*, RV systole; *4*, RV end-diastole.)

Thrombus Formation

Although thrombus formation may occur with any intravascular catheter, the polyvinylchloride material of the PA catheter has been shown to be highly thrombogenic, with formation of a fibrin sleeve around the catheter within 60 to 130 minutes after catheter insertion. Lange and colleagues found small thrombi with erosion of the endothelium of the vein, endocardium, or valves along the course of the catheter on autopsy. This same study reported a significant increase of blood vessel thrombosis (from 41% to 79%) after 2 days of catheterization despite anticoagulation.

Thrombus also can develop at the insertion site. In venographic autopsy examination, Chastre et al. found thrombosis of the internal jugular veins (the catheter insertion site) in 66% of patients despite lack of clinical evidence of thrombosis. The presence of a PA catheter has been shown to correlate with a continuing reduction in platelet count, likely caused by increased platelet consumption associated with aggregation along the catheter. The platelet count usually returns to normal within 2 to 4 days after catheter removal.

The incidence of thrombus formation is increased in patients with low cardiac output, disseminated intravascular coagulation, or congestive heart failure.

Reduction of the risk of thrombosis may occur with a continuous flush of heparinized saline or use of a catheter bonded with heparin. Use of a Teflon sheath

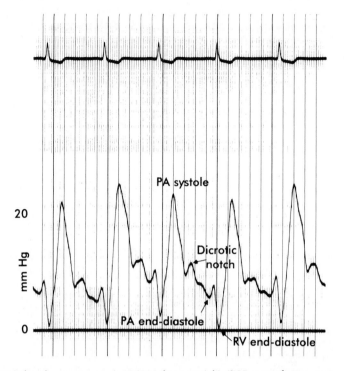

Fig. 6-34. Mixed pulmonary artery (PA)/right ventricle (RV) waveforms as a result of the catheter tip moving back and forth across the pulmonic valve. Note the decline in diastolic pressure to near zero level as the catheter tip falls into the RV during diastole. Inflation of the balloon of the catheter should allow the catheter to float out to the PA and avoid the inducement of ventricular dysrhythmias.

From Daily EK, Schroeder JS: *Hemodynamic waveforms: exercises in identification and analysis,* ed 2, St Louis, 1990, Mosby–Year Book.

with a side arm for continuous infusion also may reduce thrombus formation. Manual flushing of either the PA or arterial catheter should always be preceded by aspiration to remove any clots, if present. Flushing should then be performed gently with a small volume of fluid.

Pulmonary Infarction

Pulmonary infarction may occur as a result of embolization of thrombus from the catheter or as a result of catheter migration and prolonged wedging. Forward migration of the catheter occurs primarily during the first 24 hours as the catheter loop tightens with repeated RV contractions.

Prevention of this complication includes a review of a chest radiograph in the first 12 hours, continuous display of the pressure from the distal lumen of the catheter, wedging of the catheter only for a very brief time, monitoring of the PAEDP rather than PAW pressure (if a close correlation is established), and, perhaps, use of heparin-bonded catheters to reduce thrombolic occlusions. Chest radiographs should be repeated if catheter migration is suspected.

Infection

Infection secondary to the use of a PA catheter can range from contamination to colonization to sepsis. Contamination, with a positive culture of the catheter tip, or colonization, with growth of the same organisms from both the catheter tip and another site (for example, sputum, urine), has been reported to occur in 5% to 22% of cases. Most catheter-related infections involve the catheter introducer.

Colonization with bacteria (most commonly coagulase-negative staphylococci) has been associated more frequently with polyvinylchloride PA catheters than with Teflon intravascular CVP catheters. Sepsis, in which the same pathogen is grown from the blood and the catheter tip, has been reported to occur in 1% to 8% of PA catheter placements. Septic endocarditis involving the right side of the heart is a rare complication of prolonged PA catheterization.

Prevention of infection includes meticulous skin preparation and aseptic technique during catheter insertion, daily care of the insertion site (including cleansing with a bactericidal agent and application of iodophor ointment and a new sterile gauze dressing), and a short duration of catheter placement. Catheters left in place longer than 3 days are associated with a higher incidence of infection. Thus reassessment of the need for PA/PAW monitoring should be made after 3 days. To reduce the incidence of infection the Centers for Disease Control (CDC) recommends changing the IV solution, tubing, stopcocks, and transducer dome every 48 hours, using nonglucose IV solutions, and removing and replacing the catheter, if necessary, after 4 days. A bacteriologic evaluation of disposable pressure transducers showed no increase in contamination rates of disposable transducers changed every 4 days or every 2 days. Advancement of PA catheters after initial placement should be done only if the proximal portion of the catheter has been maintained sterile inside a sleeve. In one study, short-term sterility was provided by catheter sleeves for only 1 to 2 days if inserted under meticulous aseptic technique. All intravascular catheters should be removed immediately if colonization or sepsis develops, and appropriate antibiotic therapy instituted.

Pulmonary Artery Rupture

Rupture of the PA is a dramatic and usually fatal complication that occurs infrequently with the use of PA catheters. Because this complication often is associated with pulmonary hypertension, advanced age (>60 years), anticoagulation, and cardiopulmonary bypass surgery, PAWP measurements should be performed with caution in these subgroups of patients. During balloon inflation in all patients, PAWP should be measured with continuous waveform visualization. Inflation should be discontinued immediately on visualization of a PAW waveform. Should the PAW waveform become nonphasic, the balloon should be deflated immediately because this may represent overinflation or eccentric inflation, with the balloon extending around the catheter tip.

Although pulmonary hypertension, per se, may not render the arteries more fragile, the higher PA pressure tends to drive the catheter distally into smaller vessels, thereby increasing the risk of perforation. Changes in the vessel wall that occur in patients older than 60 years of age also result in lower rupturing pressures. The use of hypothermia, which stiffens the catheter, and manipulation of the heart during cardiac surgery also increase the risk of PA rupture. Four mechanical causes of PA rupture include distal migration of the catheter tip, overinflation of the balloon, eccentric inflation of the balloon, and manual flushing of a wedged catheter.

To prevent this frequently fatal complication, the following procedures should be performed:

1. Monitor the distal lumen pressure continuously.
2. Radiographically confirm catheter tip location in the central PA.
3. Inflate the balloon slowly, using only that amount of air necessary to achieve a PAW waveform, while constantly monitoring the pressure. Although the recommended balloon capacity of the 7-Fr catheter is 1.5 cc of air, an inflation volume of 0.8 to 1.0 cc of air is often sufficient.
4. Perform infrequent balloon inflations (monitor PAEDP, if in close agreement with PAW).
5. Always fully deflate the balloon before performing a manual flush. If necessary, withdraw the tip of the catheter slightly to prevent forceful flushing in the wedge position.
6. Never inflate the balloon with an excessive volume of air (greater than the recommended volume of air). If a PAW waveform is obtained with less than the usual volume of air, check the catheter position for distal migration.
7. Never inflate the balloon with fluid. Carefully identify infusion ports before injections to avoid injecting fluid into the balloon lumen.

Fig. 6-35 illustrates the radiographic findings associated with the rupture of a branch of the PA caused by excessive balloon inflation. Although only 1.5 cc of air was injected, the distal location of the catheter tip in a small vessel caused pulmonary artery rupture during balloon inflation.

If PA rupture is small, as indicated by a small amount of hemoptysis, the patient should be placed in a lateral recumbent position with the affected side down and closely monitored and observed. Anticoagulation should be stopped and reversed. Hemoptysis of 15 to 30 ml should prompt consideration of a "wedge" angiographic study to determine the amount and location of extravasation of dye. Massive hemoptysis can be controlled with insertion of a double-lumen endotracheal tube to prevent bleeding into the unaffected lung and aid ventilation. Prompt surgical repair may be necessary, along with pneumonectomy or lobectomy.

Cardiac Tamponade

Cardiac perforation resulting in cardiac tamponade can occur during manipulation of any catheter placed in the heart. This rare complication is associated with central venous (RA) catheters more commonly than PA catheters and may occur anywhere from minutes to days after catheterization. Clinical manifestations of cardiac tamponade in conjunction with low cardiac output and elevated RA and CVP pressures in patients with a right heart catheter should prompt suspicion of this complication.

Catheter Coiling or Knotting

Coiling or knotting of the PA catheter during catheter insertion often is associated with prolonged insertion time. This occurrence is considered a complication because it prevents correct catheter tip positioning and it can cause dysrhythmias or

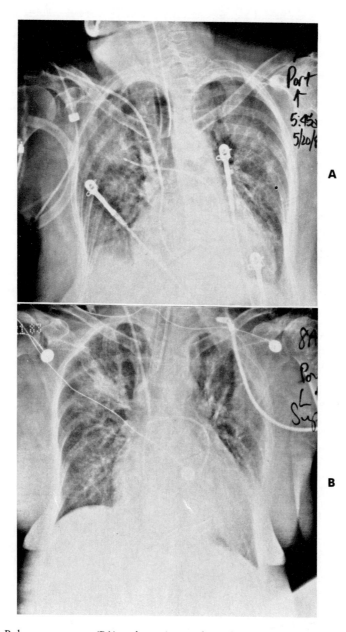

Fig. 6-35. A, Pulmonary artery (PA) catheter inserted via the right internal jugular vein in a patient with congestive heart failure and pulmonary edema. Note that the catheter tip has migrated distally into the upper lobe branch of the right PA with the beginning appearance of a wedge-shaped pulmonary infarction. **B,** Evolving right upper lobe pulmonary infarction is apparent in this same patient despite withdrawal of the catheter tip into the right PA.

Table 6-4. Problems encountered with PA catheters

Problem	Cause	Prevention	Treatment
Phlebitis or local infection at insertion site	Mechanical irritation or contamination	Prepare skin properly before insertion. Use sterile technique during insertion and dressing change. Insert smoothly and rapidly. Use Teflon-coated introducer. Attach silver-impregnated cuff to introducer. Change dressings, stopcocks, and connecting tubing every 24 to 48 hr. Remove catheter or change insertion site every 4 days.	Remove catheter. Apply warm compresses. Give pain medication as necessary.
Ventricular irritability	Looping of excess catheter in right ventricle	Suture catheter at insertion site; check chest film.	Reposition catheter; remove loop.
	Migration of catheter from PA to RV	Position catheter tip in main right or left PA.	Inflate balloon to encourage catheter flotation out to PA.
	Irritation of the endocardium during catheter passage	Keep balloon inflated during advancement; advance gently.	Advance rapidly out to PA.
Apparent wedging of catheter with balloon *deflated*	Forward migration of catheter tip caused by blood flow, excessive loop in RV, or inadequate suturing of catheter at insertion site	Check catheter tip by fluoroscopy; position in main right or left PA. Check catheter position on x-ray film if fluoroscopy is not used. Suture catheter in place at insertion site.	Aspirate blood from catheter; if catheter is wedged, sample will be arterialized and obtained with difficulty. If wedged, slowly pull back catheter until PA waveform appears. If not wedged, gently aspirate and flush catheter with saline; catheter tip can partially clot, causing damping that resembles damped PAW waveform.

PA, Pulmonary artery; *RV*, Right ventricle; *PAW*, pulmonary artery wedge; *ET*, endotracheal tube; *PAd*, pulmonary artery diastolic; *LVEDP*, left ventricular end-diastolic pressure.

Table 6-4. Problems encountered with PA catheters—cont'd

Problem	Cause	Prevention	Treatment
Pulmonary hemorrhage or infarction, or both	Distal migration of catheter tip Continuous or prolonged wedging of catheter Overinflation of balloon while catheter is wedged Failure of balloon to deflate	Check chest film immediately after insertion and 12-24 hr later; remove any catheter loop in RA or RV. Leave balloon deflated. Suture catheter at skin to prevent inadvertent advancement. Position catheter in main right or left PA. Pull catheter back to pulmonary artery if it spontaneously wedges. Do not flush catheter when in wedge position. Inflate balloon slowly with only enough air to obtain a PAW waveform. Do not inflate 7-Fr catheter with more than 1-1.5cc air. Do not inflate if resistance is met.	Deflate balloon. Place patient on side (catheter tip down). Stop anticoagulation. Consider "wedge" angiogram. Intubate with double-lumen ET. Surgery, if severe hemorrhage.
"Overwedging" or damped PAW	Overinflation of balloon Eccentric inflation of balloon	Watch waveform during inflation; inject only enough air to obtain PAW pressure. Do not inflate 7-Fr catheter with more than 1-1.5 cc air. Check inflated balloon shape before insertion.	Deflate balloon; reinflate slowly with only enough air to obtain PAW pressure. Deflate balloon; reposition and slowly reinflate.
PA balloon rupture	Overinflation of balloon Frequent inflations of balloon Syringe deflation damaging wall of balloon	Inflate slowly with only enough air to obtain a PAW pressure. Monitor PAd pressure as reflection of PAW and LVEDP. Allow passive deflation of balloon. Remove syringe after inflation.	Remove syringe to prevent further air injection. Monitor PAd pressure.
Infection	Nonsterile insertion techniques Contamination via skin	Use sterile techniques. Use sterile catheter sleeve. Prepare skin with effective antiseptic (chlorhexidine). Apply iodophor ointment and sterile gauze dressing daily. Do not use clear semipermeable dressing. Inspect site daily. Reassess need for catheter after 3 days. Avoid internal jugular approach.	Remove catheter. Use antibiotics.

Continued.

Table 6-4. Problems encountered with PA catheters — cont'd

Problem	Cause	Prevention	Treatment
Infection (cont'd)	Contamination through stopcock ports or catheter hub	Use sterile dead-ender caps on all stopcock ports. Change IV solution, stopcock, and tubing every 24-48 hr. Do not use IV solution that contains glucose.	
	Fluid contamination from transducer through cracked membrane of disposable dome	Check transducer domes for cracks. Change transducers every 48 hr. Change disposable dome after countershock. Do not use IV solution that contains glucose.	
	Prolonged catheter placement	Change catheter insertion site every 4 days.	
Heart block during insertion of catheter	Mechanical irritation of His bundle in patients with pre-existing left bundle branch block	Insert catheter expeditiously with balloon inflated. Insert transvenous pacing catheter before PA catheter insertion.	Use temporary pacemaker or flotation catheter with pacing wire.

endocardial trauma. Coiling can occur in either an enlarged RA or in the RV. If advancement of 15 cm of catheter does not result in a pressure change either from RA to RV or from RV to PA, the catheter should be slowly withdrawn and then readvanced to prevent knotting. Stiffening of the catheter by immersing it in or flushing it with iced saline or inserting a 0.025-inch (0.64 mm) guidewire may decrease the tendency for catheter coiling and enhance forward passage.

Knotting of the catheter can be handled in a variety of ways. Surgical removal may at times be necessary if intracardiac structures are involved in the knot.

Balloon Rupture

Balloon rupture after catheter insertion is usually a minor and infrequent complication that occurs as a result of improper technique. This may include overinflation of the balloon (more than 1.5 cc air for a 7 Fr catheter), inflation of the balloon with fluid instead of air, and frequent active rather than passive deflation of the balloon. The balloon should be passively deflated by removing the syringe and allowing the balloon to deflate. If the balloon air is actively withdrawn into the syringe, the latex of the balloon may be pulled into the side holes of the catheter, thus damaging the balloon.

Rupture of the balloon is indicated by a lack of any feeling of resistance during inflation, failure of the bevel of the inflation syringe to spring back during passive inflation, and the inability to obtain a PAW waveform after inflation. The appearance of blood in the balloon lumen also indicates balloon rupture. Should this occur, the stopcock of the air lumen should be turned off, tape placed over the stopcock, and

Table 6-5. Inaccurate pressure measurements

Problem	Cause	Prevention	Treatment
Damped waveforms and inaccurate pressures	Partial clotting at catheter tip	Use continuous drip with 1 unit heparin/1 ml IV fluid. Hand flush occasionally. Flush with large volume after blood sampling. Use heparin-coated catheters.	Aspirate, then flush catheter with heparinized fluid (*not* in PAW position).
	Tip moving against wall	Obtain more stable catheter position.	Reposition catheter.
	Kinking of catheter	Restrict catheter movement at insertion site.	Reposition to straighten catheter. Replace catheter.
Abnormally low or negative pressures	Incorrect air-reference level (above midchest level)	Maintain transducer air-reference port at midchest level; re-zero after patient position changes.	Remeasure level of transducer air-reference and reposition at midchest level; re-zero.
	Incorrect zeroing and calibration of monitor	Zero and calibrate monitor properly.	Recheck zero and calibration of monitor.
	Loose connection	Use Luer-Lok stopcocks.	Check all connections.
Abnormally high pressure reading	Pressure trapped by improper sequence of stopcock operation	Turn stopcocks in proper sequence when two pressures are measured on one transducer.	Thoroughly flush transducers with IV solution; re-zero and turn stopcocks in proper sequence.
	Incorrect air-reference level (below midchest level)	Maintain transducer air-reference port at midchest level; recheck and re-zero after patient position changes	Check air-reference level; reset at midchest and re-zero.
Inappropriate pressure waveform	Migration of catheter tip (e.g., in RV or PAW instead of in PA)	Establish optimal position carefully when introducing catheter initially. Suture catheter at insertion site and tape catheter to patient's skin.	Review waveform; if RV, inflate balloon; if PAW, deflate balloon and withdraw catheter slightly. Check position under fluoroscope and/or x-ray after reposition.
No pressure available	Transducer not open to catheter Amplifiers still on *cal, zero,* or *off*	Follow routine, systematic steps for pressure measurement.	Check system, stopcocks.
Noise or fling in pressure waveform	Excessive catheter movement, particularly in PA	Avoid excessive catheter length in ventricle.	Try different catheter tip position.
	Excessive tubing length	Use shortest tubing possible (<3 to 4 feet).	Eliminate excess tubing.
	Excessive stopcocks	Minimize number of stopcocks.	Eliminate excess stopcocks.

PAW, Pulmonary artery wedge; *RV*, right ventricle; *PA*, pulmonary artery.

the message "do not inflate" inscribed on the tape. Table 6-4 summarizes the complications of PA monitoring, along with causes, preventive measures, and appropriate interventions.

Inaccurate Hemodynamic Pressures

Multiple technical considerations affect the accuracy of hemodynamic pressure measurements. The onus of responsibility for obtaining the *most* accurate measurements in a standard, consistent manner rests with the nurse caring for the patient. Following strict guidelines for setup and troubleshooting can enhance the benefits and reduce the risks of hemodynamic monitoring. Table 6-5 lists several potential causes of inaccurate hemodynamic pressure measurements, as well as ways that possibly may prevent and/or manage the problem.

NURSING DIAGNOSES

Nursing diagnoses, as well as expected outcomes and interventions for patients undergoing invasive hemodynamic monitoring, are located in Appendix D.

REFERENCES

Ahrens TS, Taylor LA: *Hemodynamic waveform analysis,* Boston, 1992, WB Saunders Co.

Alderman E, Glantz S: Diastolic pressure-volume curves in man, *Circulation* 54:665-670, 1976.

Alpert JS: Hemodynamic monitoring: the basics, *Primary Cardiol* pp. 113-126, May 1981.

Baciewicz BJ, Gallucci A: Pulmonary artery catheter induced pulmonary artery rupture in patients undergoing cardiac surgery, *Can Anaesth Soc J* 32:258-264, 1985.

Baele P et al: Clinical use and bacteriologic studies of catheter contamination sleeves, *Intens Care Med* 10:297-300, 1984.

Baigrie RS, Morgan CD: Hemodynamic monitoring: catheter insertion techniques, complications and trouble-shooting, *Can Med Assoc J* 121: 885-892, 1979.

Band JD, Maki DG: Safety of changing intravenous delivery systems at longer than 24-hour intervals, *Ann Intern Med* 91:173-178, 1979.

Barash PG et al: Catheter-induced pulmonary artery perforation: mechanisms, management and modifications, *J Thorac Cardiovasc Surg* 82:5-12, 1981.

Berryhill RE, Benumof JL, Rauscher LA: Pulmonary vascular pressure reading at the end of exhalation, *Anesthesiology* 49:365-368, 1978.

Bodai BI, Holcroft JW: Use of the pulmonary arterial catheter in the critically ill patient, *Heart Lung* 11:406-416, 1982.

Bolton E: Procedural guidelines for the use of balloon-tipped, flow-directed catheters, *Crit Care Nurse* 1:33-40, 1981.

Boyd KD et al: A prospective study of complications of pulmonary artery catheterization in 500 consecutive patients, *Chest* 84:245-249, 1983.

Brandstetter RD, Gitter B: Thoughts on the Swan-Ganz catheter, *Chest* 89:5-6, 1986.

Buchbinder N, Ganz W: Hemodynamic monitoring: invasive techniques, *Anesthesiology* 45:146-155, 1976.

Calvin MP et al: Pulmonary damage from a Swan-Ganz catheter, *Br J Anaesth* 47:1107-1109, 1975.

Campbell ML, Greenberg CA: Reading pulmonary artery wedge pressure at end-expiration, *Focus Crit Care* 15:60-63, 1988.

Cason CL, Lambert CW: Position and reference level for measuring right atrial pressure, *Crit Care Nurse Q* 2:77-86, 1990.

Cengiz M, Crapo RO, Gardner R: The effect of ventilation on the accuracy of pulmonary artery and wedge pressure measurements, *Crit Care Med* 11:502-507, 1983.

Centers for Disease Control: Guidelines for prevention of infections related to intra-vascular pressure-monitoring systems, *Infect Control* 3:68, 1982.

Chastre J et al: Thrombosis as a complication of pulmonary artery catheterization via the internal jugular vein, *N Engl J Med* 306: 278-281, 1980.

Chulay M, Miller T: The effect of backrest elevation on pulmonary artery and pulmonary capillary wedge pressures in patients after cardiac surgery, *Heart Lung* 13:138-140, 1984.

Ciaccio JM: Measurements of hemodynamics in side-lying positions: a review of the literature, *Focus Crit Care* 17:250-254, 1990.

Cobb DK et al: A controlled trial of scheduled replacement of central venous and pulmonary artery catheters, *N Engl J Med* 327:1062-1068, 1992.

Conahan TJ et al: Valve competence in pulmonary artery catheter introducers, *Anesthesiology* 58:189-191, 1983.

Connors AF Jr et al: Evaluation of right-heart catheterization in the critically ill patient without acute myocardial infarction, *N Engl J Med* 308:262-267, 1983.

Connors AF Jr et al: Complications of right heart catheterization, *Chest* 88:567-572, 1985.

Damen J: Ventricular arrhythmias during insertion and removal of pulmonary artery catheters, *Chest* 88:190, 1985.

Disposable pressure transducers, *Health Devices* 13:268-289, 1984.

Dobbin K et al: Pulmonary artery pressure measurement in patients with elevated pressures: effect of backrest elevation and method of measurement, *Am J Crit Care* 1:61-69, 1992.

Drobac M et al: Giant left atrial v-waves in post-myocardial infarction ventricular septal defect, *Ann Thorac Surg* 27:347-349, 1979.

Duncan JW, Powner DJ: Complications associated with the use of pulmonary artery catheters, *Ariz Med* 39:433-435, 1982.

Eaton RJ, Taxman RM, Avioli LV: Cardiovascular evaluation of patients treated with PEEP, *Arch Intern Med* 143:1958-1961, 1983.

Elliott CG et al: Complications of pulmonary artery catheterization in the care of the critically ill patients, *Chest* 76:647-652, 1979.

Engel PT, Wayne D: Spontaneous cyclic severe mitral regurgitation, *Cathet Cardiovasc Diagn* 18:102-107, 1989.

Farber DL et al: Hemoptysis and pneumothorax after removal of persistently wedged pulmonary artery catheter, *Crit Care Med* 9:494-495, 1981.

Fisher ML et al: Assessing left ventricular filling pressure with flow-directed (Swan-Ganz) catheters, *Chest* 68:542-547, 1975.

Flores ED, Lange RA, Hillis LD: Relation of mean pulmonary arterial wedge pressure and left ventricular end-diastolic pressure, *Am J Cardiol* 66:1532-1533, 1990.

Foote GA et al: Pulmonary complications of the flow-directed balloon-tipped catheter, *N Engl J Med* 290:927-931, 1974.

Forrester JS et al: Filling pressures in the right and left sides of the heart in acute myocardial infarction, *N Engl J Med* 285:190-193, 1971.

Fromm RE et al: The craft of cardiopulmonary profile analysis. In Snyder JV, Pinsky MR: *Oxygen transport in the critically ill,* Chicago, 1987, Mosby–Year Book.

Geer RT: Interpretation of pulmonary-artery wedge pressure when PEEP is used, *Anesthesiology* 46:383-384, 1977.

Goldberg RJ: Risks and benefits of pulmonary artery catheterization, *J Intensive Care Med* 3:69-70, 1988.

Gomez-Arnau J et al: Retrograde dissection and rupture of pulmonary artery after catheter use in pulmonary hypertension, *Crit Care Med* 10:694-695, 1982.

Groom L, Frisch SR, Elliot M: Reproducibility and accuracy of pulmonary pressure measurement in supine and lateral positions, *Heart Lung* 19:147-151, 1990.

Hannan AT, Brown M, Bigman O: Pulmonary artery catheter-induced hemorrhage, *Chest* 85:128-131, 1985.

Hardy JF , Taillefer J: Inflating characteristics of Swan-Ganz catheter balloons: clinical considerations, *Anesthesiology* 62:363-364, 1983.

Hardy JF et al: The pathophysiology of pulmonary artery ruptures by pulmonary artery balloon tipped catheters, *Anesthesiology* 59:A127, 1983.

Hardy JF et al: Pathophysiology of rupture of the pulmonary artery by pulmonary artery balloon-tipped catheters, *Anesth Analg* 62:925-930, 1985.

Heard SO et al: Influence of sterile protective sleeves on the sterility of pulmonary artery catheters, *Crit Care Med* 15:499-502, 1987.

Hoar PF et al: Heparin bonding reduces thrombogenicity of pulmonary artery catheters, *N Engl J Med* 305:993-995, 1981.

Horst HM et al: The risks of pulmonary arterial catheterization, *Surg Gynecol Obstet* 159:229-232, 1984.

Iberti TJ et al: Ventricular arrhythmias during pulmonary artery catheterization in the intensive care unit, *Am J Med* 78:451-454, 1985.

Ishizawa Y, Dohi S: Alteration of pulmonary oxygenation by pulmonary artery occluded pressure measurements in intensive care patients, *Anesthesiology* 73:A250, 1990.

Jesudian MCS, Fabian JA, Chen J: An unusual complication of a pulmonary artery catheter, *J Cardiovasc Surg* 28:345-346, 1987.

Johnston WE et al: Short-term sterility of the pulmonary artery catheter inserted through an external plastic shield, *Anesthesiology* 61:461-464, 1984.

Johnston WE et al: Influence of balloon inflation and deflation on pulmonary catheter tip location, *Anesthesiology* 65:A23, 1986.

Katz JD et al: Pulmonary artery flow-guided catheters in the perioperative period, *JAMA* 237:2832-2834, 1977.

Kaye W: Catheter- and infusion-related sepsis: the nature of the problem and its prevention, *Heart Lung* 11:221-228, 1982.

Keating D et al: Effects of sidelying positions on pulmonary artery pressures, *Heart Lung* 15:605-610, 1986.

Kern MJ: Interpretation of cardiac pathophysiology from pressure waveform analysis: the left-sided *v* wave, *Cathet Cardiovasc Diagn* 23:211-218, 1991.

King EG: Influence of mechanical ventilation and pulmonary disease on pulmonary artery pressure monitoring, *Can Med Assoc J* 121:901-904, 1979.

Komadina KH et al: Interobserver variability in the interpretation of pulmonary artery catheter pressure tracings, *Chest* 100:1647-1654, 1991.

Kronberg GM et al: Anatomic locations of the tips of pulmonary artery catheters in supine patients, *Anesthesiology* 51:467-469, 1979.

Lalli SM: The complete Swan-Ganz, *RN* 41:65-77, 1978.

Lange HW, Galliani CA, Edwards JE: Local complications associated with indwelling Swan-Ganz catheters: autopsy study of 30 cases, *Am J Cardiol* 52:1108, 1983.

Lantiegne KC, Civetta JM: A system for maintaining invasive pressure monitoring, *Heart Lung* 7:610-621, 1978.

Levine SC: A review of the use of computerized digital instrumentation to determine pulmonary artery pressure measurements in critically ill patients, *Heart Lung* 14:473-477, 1985.

Maki DG, Band JD: A comparative study of polyantibiotic and iodophor ointments in prevention of vascular catheter-related infection, *Am J Med* 70:739-744, 1981.

Marini JJ et al: Estimation of transmural cardiac pressures during ventilation with PEEP, *J Appl Physiol* 53:384-391, 1982.

Marini JJ: Pulmonary artery occlusion pressure: clinical physiology, measurement and interpretation, *Am Rev Respir Dis* 128:319-326, 1983.

McDonald DH, Zaidan JR: Pressure-volume relationships of the pulmonary artery catheter balloon, *Anesthesiology* 59:240-243, 1983.

Meister SG et al: Potential artifact in measurement of left ventricular filling pressure with flow-directed catheters, *Cathet Cardiovasc Diagn* 2:175-179, 1976.

Mermel LA et al: The pathogenesis and epidemiology of catheter-related infection with pulmonary artery Swan-Ganz catheters: a prospective study utilizing molecular subtyping, *Am J Med* 91(suppl 3B):197S-202S, 1991.

Michel L, March HM, McMichan JC: Infection of pulmonary artery catheters in critically ill patients, *JAMA* 245:1032-1036, 1981.

Mitchell MM et al: Accurate, automated, continuously displayed pulmonary artery pressure measurement, *Anesthesiology* 67:294-300, 1987.

Muller BJ, Gallucci A: Pulmonary artery catheter induced pulmonary artery rupture in patients undergoing cardiac surgery, *Can Anaesth Soc J* 32:258-264, 1985.

Myers ML, Austin TW, Sibbald WJ: Pulmonary artery catheter infections: a prospective study, *Ann Surg* 201:237-241, 1985.

Nemens EJ, Woods SL: Normal fluctuations in pulmonary artery and pulmonary capillary wedge pressures in acutely ill patients, *Heart Lung* 11:393-405, 1982.

Nikolajski PY: Implementing pulmonary artery pressure monitoring, *Crit Care Choices* 92:46-51, 1992.

Noone J: Troubleshooting thermodilution pulmonary artery catheters, *Crit Care Nurse* 8:68-76, 1988.

Pace NL: A critique of flow-directed pulmonary arterial catheterization, *Anesthesiology* 47:455-465, 1977.

Paulson DM et al: Pulmonary hemorrhage associated with balloon flotation catheters, *J Thorac Cardiovasc Surg* 80:453-458, 1980.

Pichard AD et al: Large *v* waves in the pulmonary capillary wedge pressure tracing without mitral regurgitation: the influence of the pressure/volume relationship on the *v* wave size, *Clin Cardiol* 6:534-541, 1983.

Pinilla JC et al: Study of the incidence of intravascular catheter infection and associated septicemia in critically ill patients, *Crit Care Med* 11:21-25, 1983.

Raper R, Sibbald SJ: Misled by the wedge? The Swan-Ganz catheter and left ventricular preload, *Chest* 89:427-434, 1986.

Reeves JG: Cardiac physiology and monitoring, *Can Anaesth Soc J* 32:S1-S11, 1985.

Robotham JL et al: Effects of respiration on cardiac performance, *J Appl Physiol* 44:703-709, 1978.

Rosenblum WE et al: Pulmonary artery dissection induced by a Swan-Ganz catheter, *Cleve Clin J Med Q* 51:671-675, 1984.

Rowley KM et al: Right-sided infective endocarditis as a consequence of flow-directed pulmonary artery catheterization: clinopathologic study of 55 autopsied patients, *N Engl J Med* 311:1152-1156, 1984.

Salmenpera M, Peltola K, Rosenberg P: Does prophylactic lidocaine control cardiac arrhythmias associated with pulmonary artery catheterization? *Anesthesiology* 56:210-212, 1982.

Scharf SM: Mechanical effects of respiratory system on cardiocirculatory function, *Isr J Med Sci* 17:715-720, 1981.

Schermer L: Physiologic and technical variables affecting hemodynamic measurements, *Crit Care Nurse* 8:33-41, 1988.

Shah KB et al: A review of pulmonary artery catheterization in 6,245 patients, *Anesthesiology* 61:271-275, 1984.

Sharkey SW: Beyond the wedge: clinical physiology and the Swan-Ganz catheter, *Amer J of Med* 83:111-120, 1987.

Shasby MD et al: Swan-Ganz catheter location and left atrial pressure determine the accuracy of the wedge pressure when positive end-expiratory pressure is used, *Chest* 80:666-670, 1981.

Sheth NK et al: Colonization of bacteria on polyvinylchloride and Teflon intravascular catheters in hospitalized patients, *J Clin Microbiol* 18:1061-1063, 1983.

Shin B et al: Pitfalls of Swan-Ganz catheterization, *Crit Care Med* 5:125-127, 1977.

Shinn JA et al: Effect of intermittent positive pressure ventilation upon pulmonary artery and pulmonary capillary wedge pressures in acutely ill patients, *Heart Lung* 8:322-327, 1979.

Sise MJ, Hollingsworth P, Brimm JE: Complications of the flow-directed pulmonary artery catheter: a prospective analysis in 219 patients, *Crit Care Med* 9:315-317, 1981.

Skarvan K, Hasse J, Wolff G: Myocardial transmural pressure in ventilated patients, *Intensive Care Med* 7:277-283, 1981.

Smith P et al: Cardiovascular effects of ventilation with positive airway pressure, *Ann Surg* 195:121-130, 1982.

Sommers MS, Baas LS, Beiting AM: Nosocomial infections related to four methods of hemodynamic monitoring, *Heart Lung* 16:13-19, 1987.

Sprung CK et al: Prophylactic use of lidocaine to prevent advanced ventricular arrhythmias during pulmonary artery catheterization, *Am J Med* 75:906-910, 1983.

Stone JG, Khambatta HJ, McDaniel DD: Catheter induced pulmonary artery trauma: can it always be averted? *J Thorac Cardiovasc Surg* 86:146-155, 1983.

Swan HJC: Guidelines for use of balloon-tipped catheter, *Am J Cardiol* 34:119-120, 1974.

Swan HJC: Balloon flotation catheters: their use in hemodynamic monitoring in clinical practice, *JAMA* 233:865-867, 1975.

Swan HJC, Shah PK: The rationale for bedside hemodynamic monitoring, *J Crit Illness* 1:24-28, 1986.

Takkunen OS, Kalso EA: Catheter-induced pulmonary artery perforation associated with an unusual wedge pressure tracing, *Can J Anaesth* 34:168-171, 1987.

Thomson IR et al: Right bundle-branch block and complete heart block caused by the Swan-Ganz catheter, *Anesthesiology* 51:359-362, 1979.

Tooker J, Huseby J, Butler J: The effects of Swan-Ganz catheter height on the wedge pressure–left atrial pressure relationship in edema during positive-pressure ventilation, *Am Rev Respir Dis* 117:721-726, 1978.

Tuchschmidt J, Sharma OP: Impact of hemodynamic monitoring in a medical intensive care unit, *Crit Care Med* 15:840-843, 1987.

Tuchschmidt J et al: Elevated pulmonary capillary wedge pressure in a patient with hypovolemia, *J Clin Mtrg* 3:67-69, 1988.

Vender JS: Invasive cardiac monitoring, *Crit Care Clin* 4:455-477, 1988.

Weed HG: Pulmonary "capillary" wedge pressure not the pressure in the pulmonary capillaries, *Chest* 100:1138-1140, 1991.

West JB, Dollery CT, Naimark A: Distribution of blood flow in isolated lung: relation to vascular and alveolar pressures, *J Appl Physiol* 19:713-724, 1964.

Whalley DG: Hemodynamic monitoring: pulmonary artery catheterization, *Can Anesth Soc J* 32:299-305, 1985.

Wiedmann HP, Matthay MA, Matthay RA: Cardiovascular-pulmonary monitoring in the intensive care units, *Chest* 85:537-549 and 656-668, 1984.

Williams WH et al: Use of blood gas values to estimate the source of blood withdrawn from a wedged flow-directed catheter in critically ill patients, *Crit Care Med* 10:636-640, 1982.

Woods S, Grose L, Laurent-Bop D: Effect of backrest on pulmonary artery pressures in critically ill patients, *Cardiovasc Nurs* 18:19-24, 1982.

Yang SS et al: *From cardiac catheterization data to hemodynamic parameters*, Philadelphia, 1972, FA Davis Co.

Chapter 7

Arterial Pressure Monitoring

In 1733 the Reverend Stephen Hales cannulated the femoral artery of a horse and recorded the first direct intraarterial pressure measurement. With the use of a short piece of goose windpipe attached to a 12-foot brass pipe, he measured the height to which the blood rose (8 feet 3 inches, which is equivalent to 190 mm Hg). This manometrically measured pressure represented the mean femoral arterial pressure. Although numerous other techniques for measurement of arterial blood pressure were developed after that time, they all measured only the mean arterial pressure. It was not until the beginning of the twentieth century that Otto Frank, a German scientist, developed an optical-recording system that was able to measure the high-fidelity components of the pulsatile arterial pressure (systole, diastole, dicrotic notch). Today, intraarterial measurement of blood pressure has become a cornerstone in the care and management of critically ill patients. Directly measured arterial pressure is not only more accurate, but the ability to visually assess the arterial pulse waveform often can provide important diagnostic information. In addition, quick access to arterial blood significantly facilitates assessment of blood gases.

PHYSIOLOGIC REVIEW

The arterial blood pressure is generated by the ejection of blood into the arterial vasculature from the left ventricle (LV). The amount of pressure generated is determined by the volume of blood ejected as well as the resistance to ejection within the systemic vascular network. This is best expressed as:

$$\text{Pressure} = \text{Flow} \times \text{Resistance}$$

As blood is ejected into the proximal portion of the aorta, the vessel wall stretches and distends to accommodate the increase in volume. This stretching of an aortic segment is transmitted peripherally along adjacent segments of the aorta, producing a pulse wave that is transmitted through the arterial circulation and felt peripherally as a pulse. The rate at which the pulse wave travels down the aorta is determined by the compliance or distensibility of the arterial system. Decreases in compliance (as seen in elderly patients with arteriosclerosis) result in a rapid transmission of pulse wave. (In a completely rigid tube, the velocity or speed of pulse wave transmission would be extremely fast—approximately the speed of sound in blood!)

As the pulse wave travels peripherally from the central aorta, it changes in shape as well as value. This occurs as a result of reflected waves that summate on the primary systolic wave. (This is somewhat analogous to the phenomenon of dropping a stone in a shallow pond and producing ripples or waves that travel peripherally to the shore. Waves that have already reached the shore are reflected backward and on encountering a forward wave, summate it, resulting in a somewhat amplified wave.) Consequently, arterial pressures measured in the femoral or radial artery are higher than pressures measured in the brachial artery or the aorta. This difference is *amplified* in patients with increased vascular distensibility or compliance (as occurs in vasodilation) and *reduced* in patients with decreased compliance (as occurs in elderly patients and patients with hypertension or vasoconstriction). Such differences, particularly in the systolic component of the pressure wave, account for some of the disparities between the pressure measured by use of a sphygmamonometer cuff at the brachial artery and the pressure measured directly by means of a catheter in the radial artery. (See p. 170 for a discussion of other factors that affect these disparities.)

An important exception to the normal central/peripheral artery pressure relationship exists immediately after cardiopulmonary bypass. In this instance the radial artery pressure is *lower* than the aortic pressure to a variable extent. Possible causes of this change include increased sympathetic tone, resulting in reduction in the size of large conduit arteries, or in decreased regional blood flow to the hands. This condition reverts to the normal pattern of peripheral arterial pressure amplification approximately 15 to 45 minutes after bypass. Awareness of this phenomenon is clinically important and use of the peripheral measurement as the basis for administering pharmacologic agents to increase blood pressure should be avoided. Such action could result in aortic hypertension, a highly undesirable occurrence in this setting.

ARTERIAL PULSE WAVEFORM

The arterial pressure waveform resembles the pulmonary artery (PA) pressure waveform in contour inasmuch as the same basic physiologic events produce it. However, the PA and systemic artery waveform are not exactly alike because of corresponding ventricular characteristics and arterial impedance. In addition, the value of the arterial pressure is about six times greater on the left side of the heart. The arterial pressure wave is divided into two phases that correspond with the cardiac cycle: systole and diastole (Fig. 7-1). Arterial systole begins with the opening of the aortic valve and rapid ejection of blood into the aorta. This is followed by run-off of blood from the proximal aorta to the peripheral arteries. On the arterial pressure waveform this is seen as a sharp rise in pressure followed by a decline in pressure. As the pressure falls, the aortic valve snaps shut, causing a small change in arterial pressure that appears as a dip on the downslope and is termed the *incisura* in central aortic pressures and the *dicrotic notch* in peripheral artery pressures. This marks the end of the ejection period. The *peak systolic pressure* (which reflects LV systolic pressure) is normally 100 to 140 mm Hg. Children 10 years old and younger have lower systolic blood pressures of less than 100 mm Hg.

Diastole follows closure of the aortic valve and continues until the next systole.

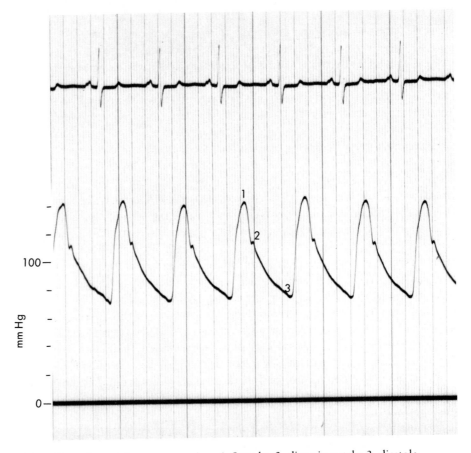

Fig. 7-1. Normal arterial pressure tracing. *1,* Systole; *2,* dicrotic notch; *3,* diastole.

From Daily EK, Schroeder JS: *Hemodynamic waveforms: exercises in identification and analysis,* ed 2, St Louis, 1990, Mosby–Year Book.

During this time, run-off to the peripheral arteries occurs without further flow from the LV. On the peripheral arterial pressure waveform this is seen as a gradual decrease in pressure. The lowest point of diastole (actually, end-diastole) is referred to as the *arterial diastolic pressure* and is normally 60 to 80 mm Hg.

Secondary Waves

Secondary waves, or reflected waves, occur on the arterial waveform as a result of the wave transmission process. Because of differences in wave transmission between the upper and lower portions of the body, these secondary waves differ according to the site of measurement. In the radial artery a secondary, or reflected, wave may appear in late systole, resulting in a second, separate systolic peak that is lower than the first peak (Fig. 7-2). In addition, another reflected wave that follows the dicrotic notch may appear in diastole (Fig. 7-3). In contrast, the femoral artery pressure wave exhibits one single, smooth systolic wave, with usually only one secondary wave in diastole.

The mean arterial pressure represents the average arterial pressure during systole

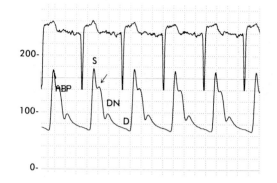

Fig. 7-2. Radial artery waveform with secondary systolic wave *(arrow)*. *(S,* Systole [170 mm Hg]; *DN,* dicrotic notch; *D,* diastole [70 mm Hg]; *ABP,* arterial blood pressure.)

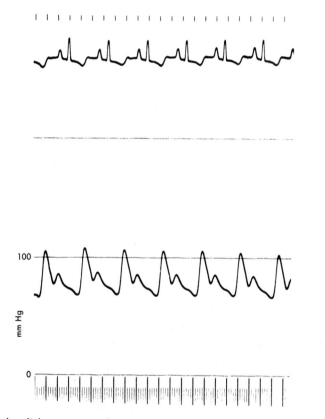

Fig. 7-3. Normal radial artery waveform with reflected diastolic waves appearing after the dicrotic notch.

and diastole. Normal mean arterial pressure (MAP) is 70 to 90 mm Hg. MAP depends on two factors: (1) the blood flow through the vessel (cardiac output) and (2) the elasticity or resistance of the vessels (systemic vascular resistance). This interrelation can be expressed as follows:

MAP = Cardiac output (CO) × Systemic vascular resistance (SVR)

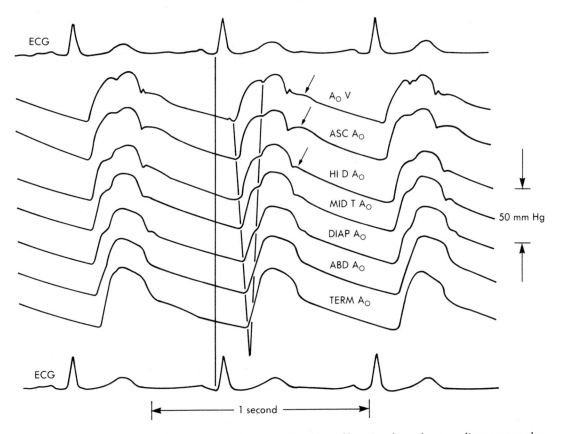

Fig. 7-4. Arterial pressure waveforms as a function of location from the ascending aorta to the iliac bifurcation in one patient. Figure constructed from single or pairs of pulses selected from cardiac cycles with equal RR intervals and from similar phases of respiration. *AoV,* Sensor just above aortic valve; *Asc Ao,* ascending aorta; *HI D Ao,* high descending aorta; *Mid T Ao,* midthoracic aorta; *Term Ao,* terminal abdominal aorta just before iliac bifurcation.

From Murgo JP et al: *Circulation* 62:105-116, 1980.

The pulse pressure is the difference between the systolic and diastolic pressures and is largely reflective of the stroke volume and arterial compliance. Wide pulse pressures are associated with large stroke volumes, whereas a narrow pulse pressure is seen in patients with low stroke volume.

    The arterial pressure differs in both contour and value in various arterial locations (Fig. 7-4). As mentioned previously, the systolic pressure is higher in the femoral artery than in the radial or brachial artery, by as much as 25 to 50 mm Hg. Generally, the diastolic and mean values remain nearly the same. In addition, the more distal the location of the arterial catheter, the sharper and later the upstroke and the less defined the dicrotic notch (Fig. 7-5).

Changes in the Arterial Pulse of Elderly Persons

    Figs. 7-6 and 7-7 depict changes in the arterial waveform associated with aging. In addition to an increase in the pulse pressure (higher systolic pressure and lower diastolic pressure), the arterial pulse wave of the older person typically reveals a late

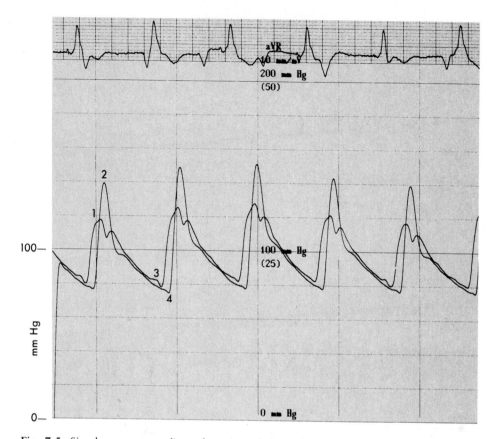

Fig. 7-5. Simultaneous recording of aortic and femoral artery pressure, showing normal discrepancy between amplitude and waveform configuration. (*1,* Aortic systolic pressure [118 mm Hg]; *2,* femoral artery systolic pressure [140 mm Hg]; *3,* aortic diastolic pressure [80 mm Hg]; *4,* femoral artery diastolic pressure [75 mm Hg]).

From Daily EK, Schroeder JS: *Hemodynamic waveforms: exercises in identification and analysis,* ed 2, St Louis, 1990, Mosby–Year Book.

systolic peak and a smooth diastolic pressure drop without secondary diastolic waves. These normal changes are attributed to arterial stiffening with increased pulse wave velocity.

ECG Correlation

The arterial pressure rise occurs immediately after ventricular depolarization, that is, after the QRS complex on the ECG. As the initiation of the upstroke occurs slightly later at more peripheral sites (see Fig. 7-4), it is difficult to define end-diastole in terms of exact timing. In addition, there may be some delay, depending on the catheter location and length of tubing used. Generally, end-diastole is measured just before the upstroke, shortly after the QRS complex. The dicrotic notch occurs after the T wave of the ECG.

In bracycardia, in which systolic ejection is prolonged, the arterial pressure wave may exhibit a secondary prominent wave, or shoulder, in late systole, that is followed by a smooth pressure decline during diastole (Fig. 7-8). Usually the timing associated

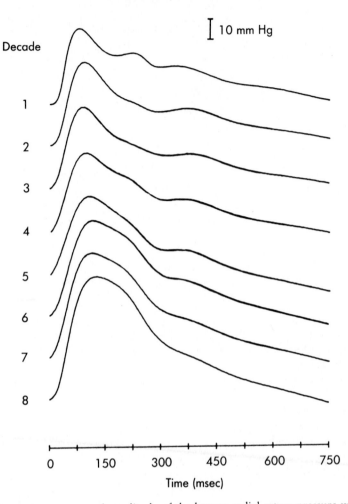

Fig. 7-6. Change in contour and amplitude of the human radial artery pressure with age.
From Kelly RP et al: *Circulation* 80:1652-1659, 1989.

with normal heart rates places this reflected wave in the diastolic period, after the dicrotic notch.

Abnormal Findings

Monitoring of the arterial pressure pulse provides valuable information, not only in terms of its pressure value but also in terms of shape and contour. In addition to undergoing changes as it travels distally, or in association with certain dysrhythmias, the arterial pulse wave can exhibit changes that are related to specific underlying pathologic conditions.

Aortic insufficiency

The arterial pressure waveform with aortic insufficiency classically reveals a rapid upstroke and decline with a wide pulse pressure, an elevated systolic pressure,

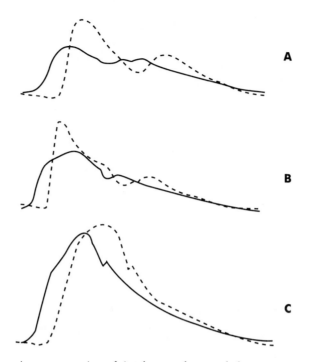

Fig. 7-7. Diagrammatic representation of simultaneously recorded pressure waves in the aorta *(solid line)* and radial artery *(dashed line)* of a young adult **(A)**, a middle-aged adult **(B)**, and an elderly person **(C).**

Redrawn from O'Rourke MF, Kelly RP, Avolio AP: *The arterial pulse,* Philadelphia, 1992, Lea & Febiger.

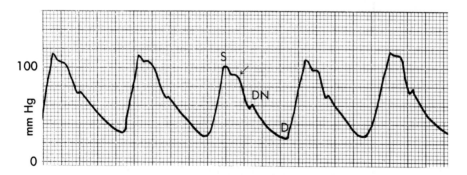

Fig. 7-8. Arterial pressure waveform in a patient with bradycardia. Arrow indicates prominent late systolic shoulder from forward reflection of the pulse wave from the lower body. With faster heart rates this reflection occurs during diastole. (*S,* Systole; *DN,* dicrotic notch; *D,* diastole.)

and a lowered diastolic pressure (Fig. 7-9). This is a result of rapid ejection of a large stroke volume (the normal stroke volume plus the regurgitant volume), with regurgitation of blood across the incompetent aortic valve during diastole. Also, the dicrotic notch on the downslope of the arterial pressure is usually absent.

Aortic stenosis

In aortic stenosis a pressure gradient develops between the left ventricle and aorta during ejection (Fig. 7-10). Both the contour and the value of the arterial pressure pulse are altered with aortic stenosis. Because of the increased resistance to ejection of blood through the narrowed aortic valve orifice, the upstroke of the arterial pressure

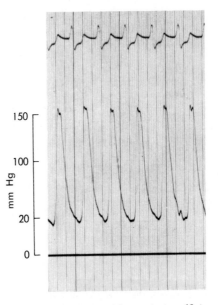

Fig. 7-9. Arterial pressure tracing in patient with aortic insufficiency. Note the wide pulse pressure with high systolic pressure of 150 mm Hg and low diastolic pressure of 20 mm Hg.

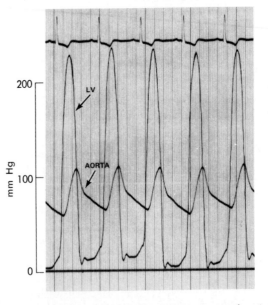

Fig. 7-10. Simultaneous left ventricular (LV) and aortic pressures showing marked pressure difference during systole because of severe aortic stenosis. Note the slow upstroke of the aortic pressure tracing.

Arterial Pressure Monitoring

waveform is slow and appears to rise at an angle rather than straight up (Fig. 7-11). This pulse is frequently referred to as *anacrotic* in reference to a notch observed on the upstroke of the pulse wave. Often the dicrotic notch is not well defined and may appear only as a "bend" on the downslope of the arterial pressure waveform. This is caused by the stiff closing movement of diseased aortic valve leaflets, which fail to produce a rise in pressure. The value of the arterial pressure is low with a narrow pulse pressure, indicating a low stroke volume. The contour of a damped arterial waveform closely resembles the arterial waveform of aortic stenosis (see Fig. 7-11).

Shock

In cardiogenic as well as hypovolemic shock, the arterial pressure is low, with a small pulse pressure as a result of low stroke volume. The arterial waveform typically exhibits a dicrotic, or even tricrotic, contour (Fig. 7-12). The exaggerated secondary diastolic waves may obscure the dicrotic notch, which may cause difficulty in correctly timing aortic counterpulsation. The high peripheral resistance that accompanies cardiogenic and hypovolemic shock causes greater than normal amplification of the peripheral arterial pressure, belying the true central aortic pressure. In general, in patients in cardiogenic or hypovolemic shock, one should assume that the central aortic pressure is always substantially lower than the pressure measured in the radial or brachial artery. Thus, even marginally low radial or brachial arterial pressures should prompt a "red flag" regarding central hypotension.

In septic shock the arterial pressure is, likewise, low; however, in this condition it is due to vasodilation rather than low stroke volume. As a result of the vasodilation there is less amplification of the peripheral arterial pressure and less wave reflection. Consequently the peripheral artery waveform in septic shock often appears damped. In contrast to cardiogenic or hypovolemic shock, however, its value more closely approximates the central aortic pressure.

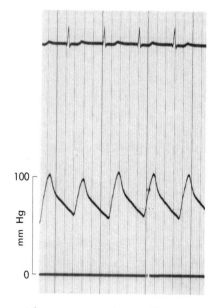

Fig. 7-11. Overdamped arterial pressure waveform with poor upstroke and loss of dicrotic notch. Note similarity to pressure waveform of aortic stenosis.

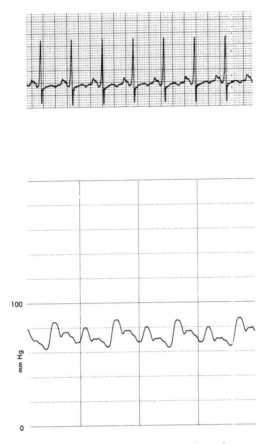

Fig. 7-12. Arterial pressure waveform demonstrating pulsus alternans, pulsus parvus, and diastolic waves in a patient in shock following an acute myocardial infarction (MI).

Dysrhythmias

Alterations in the cardiac rhythm can affect both the value and the contour of the arterial pressure wave. *Tachydysrhythmias* usually produce a low arterial pressure as a result of shortened ejection period and filling period. The waveform may exhibit a damped appearance. The value and appearance of the arterial pressure wave can be helpful in discerning the origin of the dysrhythmia (Fig. 7-13).

The separation of electrical and mechanical cardiac activity, *electromechanical dissociation* (EMD), is readily apparent on inspection of the simultaneously recorded ECG and arterial pressure waveform, which reveals an electrical impulse without an associated arterial pressure wave (Fig. 7-14). EMD may occur with pericardial tamponade, tension pneumothorax, ventricular rupture, severe acidosis, hypoxia, and hypovolemia.

In *atrial fibrillation* the arterial pressure value varies considerably (Fig. 7-15), depending on the RR intervals and length of time for ventricular filling. However, the normal characteristics of the waveform are still present.

When a *premature ventricular contraction* (PVC) occurs, ventricular systole is initiated early, before the LV has had time to fill with blood. This results in a

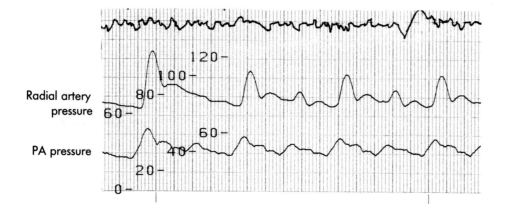

Fig. 7-13. The alarming ECG pattern in this patient clearly is the result of artifact (and not ventricular fibrillation), since arterial pressure waves continue. (Note also the presence of pulsus alternans in both the radial and pulmonary artery waveforms in this patient with severe biventricular failure.)

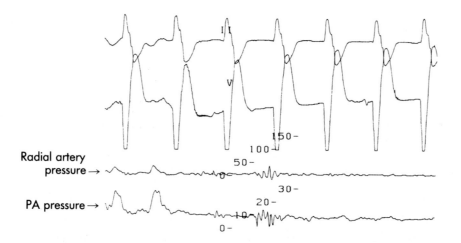

Fig. 7-14. Radial artery and pulmonary artery (PA) pressures in a patient with pulseless electrical activity (also known as electromechanical dissociation) illustrating the diminution followed by the absence of pulse waves.

diminished stroke volume and lowered arterial pulse pressure generated by the extrasystolic beat (Fig. 7-16). Isolated PVCs are usually well compensated for by a pause and an increase in stroke volume and arterial pressure with the succeeding contraction. Runs of PVCs, however, can be devastating, because there is virtually no opportunity for LV filling and therefore stroke volume and arterial pressure fall precipitously (Fig. 7-17).

Pulsus bisferiens

The term *pulsus bisferiens* is derived from the Latin "bisferiere" or "twice beating" and describes an arterial pulse with two distinct systolic peaks (Figs. 7-18 and 7-19). Either the first or second peak may be highest, or the peaks may be of equal

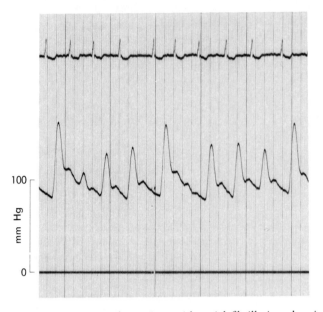

Fig. 7-15. Arterial pressure tracing of a patient with atrial fibrillation showing the marked beat-to-beat variation in peak systolic pressure, dependent on the length of the previous RR interval.

height. This characteristic feature occurs in patients with mixed aortic regurgitation and aortic stenosis or, more commonly, hypertrophic cardiomyopathy. The first peak is produced by rapid, forceful ejection of blood into the aorta in early systole. The pressure then declines slightly and is followed by a second pressure rise produced by forward flow in late systole.

Pulsus alternans

Pulsus alternans refers to a regular, alternating pattern of changes in pressure pulse amplitude, with every other pulse being slightly greater than the previous one (Figs. 7-12 and 7-20). Typically, the systolic pressure alternates by ≥ 20 mm Hg. Generally it is a result of alternating ventricular contractility and subsequent stroke volume, and it commonly accompanies severe LV failure. Pulsus alternans also can occur transiently after dysrhythmic episodes and rapid atrial pacing, as well as myocardial ischemia (Fig. 7-12). The regular electrical rhythm of pulsus alternans differentiates it from pulsus bigeminus, in which the rhythm is bigeminal.

Pulsus paradoxus

Pulsus paradoxus was first described by Kussmaul as a paradoxic disappearance of peripheral arterial pulsations during inspiration despite continued regular heartbeats. It represents an exaggeration of the normal fall in systolic blood pressure that occurs during spontaneous inspiration. When the systolic arterial pressure declines more than 10 mm Hg during normal spontaneous inspiration, pulsus paradoxus is said to exist (Fig. 7-21). (This phenomenon is observed most easily from the displayed intraarterial pressure; however, it also can be obtained, although less easily, from the

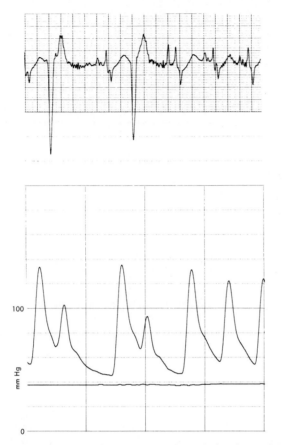

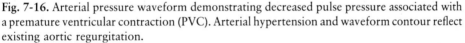

Fig. 7-16. Arterial pressure waveform demonstrating decreased pulse pressure associated with a premature ventricular contraction (PVC). Arterial hypertension and waveform contour reflect existing aortic regurgitation.

noninvasive indirect blood pressure measurement.) Pulsus paradoxus is classically seen in cases of cardiac tamponade (about 70% to 80%) but also can occur in patients with obstructed airway disease and, less commonly, in hypovolemic shock and pulmonary embolism.

Reversed pulsus paradoxus

Reversed or positive pulsus paradoxus is a phenomenon characterized by an exaggerated *rise* in systolic arterial pressure (>10 mm Hg) during inspiration in patients receiving positive pressure ventilation (Fig. 7-22). This variation in systolic pressure is thought to be a sensitive reflection of hypovolemia in patients receiving positive pressure ventilation and usually disappears with appropriate volume therapy.

Effects of Drugs

Certain drugs alter the arterial pressure wave in both value (amplitude) and contour through their action on cardiac output or vascular resistance, or both. Pharmacologic agents that produce *vasoconstriction* generally exaggerate the peak

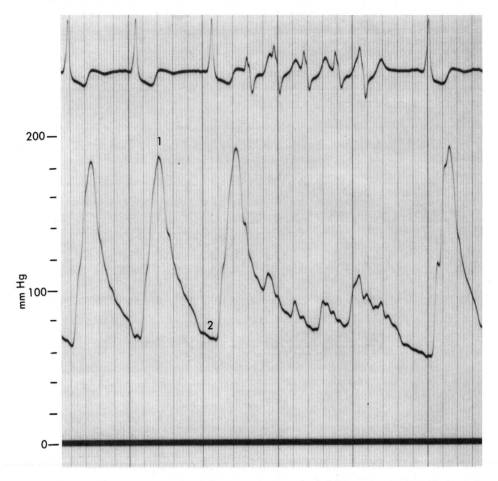

Fig. 7-17. Arterial pressure waveform demonstrating marked reduction in stroke volume and pulse pressure associated with a run of ventricular ectopy. (*1,* Systole; *2,* end-diastole.)

systolic pressure, although the mean arterial pressure may change only a little. Vasoconstrictors also increase the pulse wave velocity, producing a more rapid upstroke of the arterial wave.

Pharmacologic *vasodilation* of the vascular bed reduces wave reflection at the aorta and results in a decrease in peak aortic pressure with less diastolic fluctuation in the arterial waveform. This, along with reduced pulse wave velocity, contributes to the overall damped appearance of the arterial waveform in patients receiving vasodilator therapy. As mentioned earlier, however, the *peripheral* arterial pressure may not reflect the degree of these changes and therefore inadequately reflects the actual reduction in ventricular afterload, as well as the possible existence of aortic hypotension. This phenomenon, which is particularly common with the use of the nitrate preparations, also may be observed with the use of angiotensin converting enzyme (ACE) inhibitors, beta-adrenergic blockers, and calcium channel blockers (see O'Rourke, Kelly, Avolio reference). However, the reduction of aortic systolic pressure can be inferred if the late systolic shoulder on the peripheral artery waveform declines or completely disappears after initiation of vasodilator therapy (Fig. 7-23).

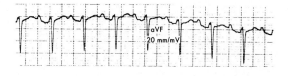

aVF
20 mm/mV

200 mm Hg

100 mm Hg

0 mm Hg

Fig. 7-18. Arterial pressure waveform demonstrating bisferiens or "double-peaked" systolic waveform in a patient with hypertrophic cardiomyopathy.

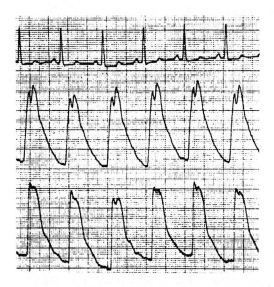

Fig. 7-19. Bisferiens pulse in a 51-year-old man with combined aortic stenosis and incompetence. The biphasic systolic peak is more readily apparent in the carotid pulse *(above)* than in the radial pulse *(below)*. Arterial pressure is 185/45 mm Hg. Heart rate is 70/min.

From O'Rourke MF, Kelly RP, Avolio AP: *The arterial pulse,* Philadelphia, 1992, Lea & Febiger.

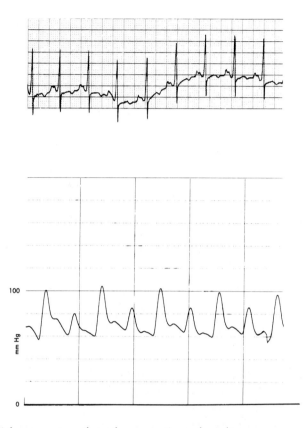

Fig. 7-20. Arterial pressure waveform demonstrating pulsus alternans as a result of alternating stroke volume in a patient with severe left ventricular failure.

Mechanical Effects

Abnormalities of the arterial pressure waveform may result from mechanical causes of damping, fling, or whip or inaccurate zeroing or calibrating. Damping produces an arterial pressure waveform similar to that of aortic stenosis, that is, a slow upstroke, rounded appearance, poorly defined dicrotic notch, and narrow pulse pressure (see Fig. 7-11). A clot at the tip of the catheter or lodging of the catheter tip against the vessel wall is usually the cause, and gentle flushing with a small volume or repositioning the catheter tip eliminates this problem. Fling or whip in the arterial pressure waveform may be a result of excessive movement of the catheter tip or an underdamped monitoring system.

Because of the high-frequency components within the arterial pulse wave, distortion caused by inadequate dynamic response characteristics of the monitoring system is the *major* reason for inaccuracies in direct arterial pressure monitoring. This becomes emphasized in the presence of tachycardia, which further increases the frequency response requirements of the monitoring system. Because the resonant or natural frequency and the damping coefficient of the monitoring system can be assessed in such a practical and simple way at the bedside (see the discussion in

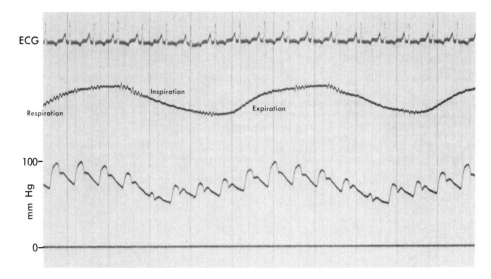

Fig. 7-21. Brachial artery pressure tracing of a patient with constrictive pericarditis during normal respiration. Systolic pressure falls from 100 mm Hg during expiration to 70 mm Hg during inspiration. This exaggerated fall in pressure is termed *pulsus paradoxus.*

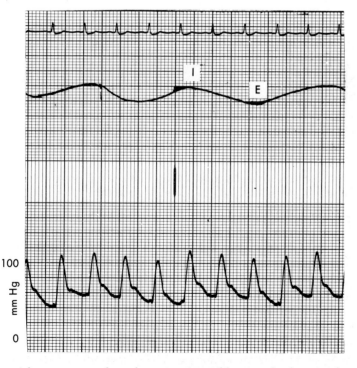

Fig. 7-22. Arterial pressure waveform demonstrating mild reversed pulsus paradoxus with an increase of approximately 14 mm Hg during *mechanical inhalation.* (Note pneumotachograph on upper portion of tracing indicating inhalation *[I]* and exhalation *[E].*)

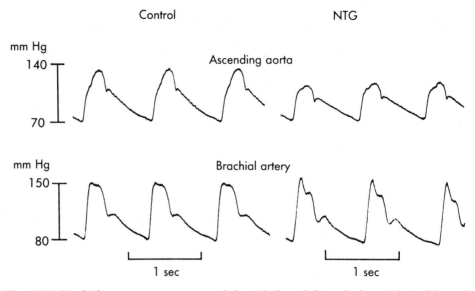

Fig. 7-23. Brachial artery pressure waves (below) before (left) and after (right) sublingual nitroglycerin together with ascending aortic pressure waves (above).

From O'Rourke MF et al: *The arterial pulse*, Philadelphia, 1992, Lea & Febiger.

Chapter 3), it is highly recommended that frequent checks of the system be performed.

Fling occurs in the pressure waveform when there is excessive catheter movement in the artery or, more commonly, when the catheter tip faces "upstream" into the flow. It also can occur when excess tubing is used, when the heart rate is very rapid, or when the rate of pressure rise (dP/dT) is rapid. Fling is characterized by rapid, sharp negative or positive waves, particularly during systole. Fling usually can be reduced or eliminated by moving the catheter tip, reducing the tubing length, or using a damping device.

Table 7-1 describes some causes of inaccurate arterial pressure measurement.

CLINICAL APPLICATIONS

Data obtained from direct arterial pressure provide important information regarding cardiac performance as well as vascular conditions.

Systolic Pressure

In the absence of aortic stenosis, the peak systolic arterial pressure reflects the maximum pressure generated by the LV (Fig. 7-24). In addition, *systolic pressure* frequently is used to monitor ventricular *afterload*. Afterload is defined as LV wall tension during systole. The two principal determinants are systolic pressure and the radius of the left ventricle. During hemodynamic monitoring, the radius, or size of the left ventricle (related to LV volume) is assumed to remain relatively constant, and therefore the systolic arterial pressure is the parameter used to clinically monitor afterload.

Table 7-1. Inaccurate arterial pressure measurements

Problem	Cause	Prevention	Treatment
Damped pressure tracing	Catheter tip against vessel wall	Usually cannot be avoided.	Pull back, rotate, or reposition catheter while observing pressure waveform.
	Partial occlusion of catheter tip by clot	Use continuous drip under pressure. Briefly "fast flush" after blood withdrawal (<2-4 ml) Add 1 unit heparin/1 ml IV fluid.	Aspirate clot with syringe and flush with heparinized saline (<2-4 ml).
	Clot in stopcock or transducer	Carefully flush catheter after blood withdrawal and reestablish IV drip. Use continuous flush device.	Flush stopcock and transducer; if no improvement, change stopcock and transducer.
	Air bubbles in transducer or connector tubing	Carefully flush transducer and tubing when setting up system and attaching to catheter.	Check system; flush rapidly; disconnect transducer and flush out air bubbles.
	Compliant tubing	Use stiff, short tubing.	Shorten tubing or replace softer tubing with stiffer tubing.
Abnormally high or low readings	Change in transducer air-reference level	Maintain air-reference port of transducer at midchest and/or catheter tip level for serial pressure measurements.	Recheck patient and transducer positions.
No pressure available	Transducer not open to catheter Settings on monitor amplifiers incorrect—still on *zero, cal,* or *off*	Follow routine, systematic steps for setting up system and turning stopcocks.	Check system—stopcocks, monitor, and amplifier setup.
	Incorrect scale selection	Select scale appropriate to expected range of physiologic signal.	Select appropriate scale.

Diastolic Pressure

The *diastolic arterial pressure* reflects both the velocity of run-off and the elasticity of the arterial system. The elastic properties of the vessels affect the arterial system's ability to change luminal dimensions as the blood volume changes. Heart rate also affects the diastolic pressure because it determines the duration of diastole in the cardiac cycle. The longer the period of diastole (bradycardia), the further the diastolic pressure declines. Conversely, the shorter the diastolic period (with tachycardia), the higher the diastolic pressure.

The diastolic arterial pressure is also important in determining coronary artery perfusion, particularly to the left ventricle, where most flow occurs during diastole. Coronary artery perfusion pressure (CPP) of the left ventricle is calculated as follows:

$$CPP = \text{Arterial diastolic pressure} - \text{LVEDP (or PAW pressure)}$$

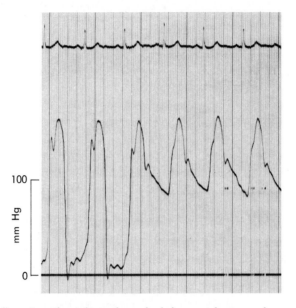

Fig. 7-24. Pullback tracing of a catheter from the left ventricle across the aortic valve into the aorta. Note that the systolic pressures are the same and that there is no left ventricle (LV)–aortic pressure gradient.

Normal coronary artery perfusion pressure is 60 to 80 mm Hg. Perfusion pressures below 50 mm Hg threaten myocardial perfusion. Efforts to maintain adequate CPP include increasing the arterial diastolic pressure or decreasing the PAW pressure, or both. In most institutions the CPP is not a commonly monitored hemodynamic parameter. This is likely due to the assumption that the mean arterial pressure (MAP) is a sufficient reflection of perfusion pressure. However, as can be reasoned from the aforementioned CPP formula, elevations of the PAW pressure (reflecting LVEDP) could result in a fall in CPP that would not be apparent in the MAP. For example, if a patient's arterial pressure was 114/70, the MAP would be approximately 85 mm Hg and would likely be assumed to be adequate. If, however, the patient's mean PAW pressure was 30 mm Hg, the perfusing pressure to the left ventricle would only be 40 mm Hg (70 mm Hg − 30 mm Hg)! This is an inadequate pressure to maintain coronary perfusion, particularly in a patient with coronary artery stenosis. If invasive hemodynamic monitoring is performed, all the available data should be derived from the monitoring tool to optimize its benefit to the patient. This means that in patients with elevated PAW pressure, the CPP should be a parameter that is calculated and carefully monitored.

Mean Pressure

The *mean arterial pressure* represents the average pressure within the arterial system. Because diastole typically lasts approximately two thirds of the entire cardiac cycle, the mean pressure value is closer to the diastolic value than the systolic value. Although the arterial pressure pulse is amplified as it travels away from the heart, the MAP remains relatively unchanged, highlighting its value as a general reflection of overall perfusion. Monitoring systems automatically compute the MAP. If necessary, however, the MAP can be mathematically estimated by means of the following equation:

$$MAP = \frac{\text{Systolic pressure} + (\text{Diastolic pressure} \times 2)}{3}$$

Mean arterial pressure is determined by flow and resistance in the following way:

$$MAP = \text{Cardiac output (CO)} \times \text{Systemic vascular resistance (SVR)}$$

On the basis of this formula, it is clear that a change in flow or CO without a change in SVR will cause a corresponding change in mean arterial pressure. This is true whether the increase in CO is accomplished by an increase in stroke volume or an increase in heart rate, or both.

Systemic Vascular Resistance

According to Poiseuille's law, resistance is determined by length, viscosity, and the reciprocal of the radius raised to the fourth power (R^4) as follows:

$$SVR = \frac{8 \text{ length} \times \text{Viscosity}}{\pi R^4}$$

Inasmuch as length does not alter after completion of growth and—except in hemorrhage, polycythemia, or marked temperature changes—viscosity remains relatively constant, the radius of the arterial vessels remains the primary determinant of changes in vascular resistance. The formula for mean arterial pressure can, therefore, be rewritten as follows:

$$MAP = CO \times \text{Viscosity} \times (L/R^4)$$

Even very small changes in the diameter of the major resistance vessels (the arterioles) result in large changes in pressure. For example, doubling the radius of the arterial vessels (with an arterial vasodilator) would decrease the mean arterial pressure by a factor of 16 if the CO remained constant.

Direct measurement of the SVR is not possible but can be simply calculated using the previous formula rewritten as follows:

$$SVR = \frac{MAP}{CO} \times 80$$

Rapid adjustment of the SVR in response to changes in position, activity, and stress normally maintains a narrow range of blood pressure. However, in the patient with cardiac disease, as the left ventricle fails and cardiac output falls, stimulation of the baroreceptors causes vasoconstriction and the SVR rises in an attempt to maintain adequate blood pressure. This increase in afterload or impedance to LV ejection can aggravate the failing heart and further decrease the stroke volume. With pharmacologic afterload reduction, a decrease in resistance may allow an increase in stroke volume without a significant fall in blood pressure, as shown in the following example:

EXAMPLE: If the patient's CO is 5 L/min and MAP is 100 mm Hg, the SVR is 1600 dynes/sec/cm^{-5}.

$$SVR = MAP \text{ (mm Hg)} \div CO \text{ (L/min)} \times 80$$
$$1600 = (100 \text{ mm Hg} \div 5 \text{ L/min}) \times 80$$

with afterload reduction therapy, SVR decreased to 1200 dynes/sec/cm^{-5} and increased CO to 7 L/min, resulting in a MAP of 105 mm Hg, essentially unchanged from the original MAP of 100 mm Hg.

$$105 \text{ mm Hg} = 7 \text{ L/min} \times (1200 \div 80)$$

A more accurate calculation of SVR is obtained when the pressure difference between the proximal and distal ends of the cardiovascular system (arterial and venous) is divided by the CO. The formula is as follows:

$$SVR = \frac{MAP - RAm}{CO} \times 80$$

Because the right atrial (RA) pressure is generally quite low, the venous pressure is usually not included in calculating SVR. If, however, the RA pressure is significantly elevated, it should be subtracted from the MAP to obtain a true driving pressure.

NORMAL VALUES FOR SVR: **900 to 1400 dynes/sec/cm^{-5}**

The systemic arterial pressure determines the perfusion of the body tissues, including not only muscle, skin, and extremities but more critical organs such as the brain, heart, and kidneys. By varying the degree of vasoconstriction or vasodilation, some organs can partially regulate the amount of blood flow through them. More than 70% of the coronary blood flow occurs during diastole. Because of this and because the heart tissues have a very high extraction ratio of oxygen from hemoglobin, the heart is quite sensitive to hypotension. There are no clinically applicable bedside techniques presently available for monitoring the amount or sufficiency of coronary blood flow. Renal blood flow and perfusion may be partially monitored by urinary flow, but renal autoregulation of this flow does not allow a direct correlation between the two. Thus the health of the body tissues depends on an adequately functioning heart and vascular system to supply an appropriate flow *and* perfusion pressures that are sufficient to deliver blood throughout the body.

INTRAARTERIAL PRESSURE MEASUREMENT

Direct measurement of arterial pressure can be obtained via a transducer connected to a small Teflon catheter inserted into a peripheral artery. Transduced pressures provide systolic, diastolic, and mean values as well as a displayed arterial waveform. As described previously, much valuable information can be obtained from observation of the contour of the arterial pressure wave.

Equipment preparation and setup for intraarterial pressure monitoring is the same as for PA monitoring (see p. 125). Ideally, the transducer should be placed as close to the catheter as is practically possible, limiting the length and complexity of the fluid-filled monitoring lines. Special attention also should be paid to carefully remove even the smallest of air bubbles from the system. This not only prevents the inadvertent injection of air into the arterial system but also improves the dynamic response of the monitoring system. Even a very tiny air bubble can reduce the resonant

Table 7-2. Problems encountered with arterial catheters

Problem	Cause	Prevention	Treatment
Hematoma after withdrawal of needle	Bleeding or oozing at puncture site	Maintain firm pressure on site during withdrawal of catheter and for 5-15 min (as necessary) after withdrawal. Apply elastic tape (Elastoplast) firmly over puncture site. For femoral arterial puncture sites, leave a sandbag on site for 1-2 hr to prevent oozing. If patient is receiving heparin, discontinue 2 hr before catheter removal.	Continue to hold pressure to puncture site until oozing stops. Apply sandbag to femoral puncture site for 1-2 hr after removal of catheter.
Decreased or absent pulse distal to puncture site	Spasm of artery	Introduce arterial needle cleanly, nontraumatically.	Inject lidocaine locally at insertion site and 10 mg into arterial catheter.
	Thrombosis of artery	Use 1 unit heparin/1 ml IV fluid	Arteriotomy and Fogarty catheterization both distally and proximally from the puncture site result in return of pulse in more than 90% of cases if brachial or femoral artery is used.
Bleedback into tubing, dome, or transducer	Insufficient pressure on IV bag Loose connections	Maintain 300 mm Hg pressure on IV bag. Use Luer-Lok stopcocks; tighten periodically.	Replace transducer. "Fast flush" through system. Tighten all connections.
Hemorrhage	Loose connections	Keep all connecting sites visible. Observe connecting sites frequently. Use built-in alarm system. Use Luer-Lok stopcocks.	Tighten all connections.
Emboli	Clot from catheter tip into bloodstream	Always aspirate and discard before flushing. Use continuous flush device. Use 1 unit heparin/1 ml IV fluid. Gently flush <2-4 ml.	Remove catheter.
Local infection	Forward movement of contaminated catheter Break in sterile technique Prolonged catheter use	Carefully suture catheter at insertion site. Always use aseptic technique. Remove catheter after 72-96 hr. Inspect and care for insertion site daily, including dressing change and antibiotic or iodophor ointment.	Remove catheter. Prescribe antibiotic.

Continued.

Table 7-2. Problems encountered with arterial catheters—cont'd

Problem	Cause	Prevention	Treatment
Sepsis	Break in sterile technique	Use percutaneous insertion.	Remove catheter.
		Always use aseptic technique.	Prescribe antibiotic.
	Prolonged catheter use	Remove catheter after 72-96 hr.	
	Bacterial growth in IV fluid	Change IV fluid bag, stopcocks, dome, and tubing every 24-48 hr.	
		Do not use IV fluid containing glucose.	
		Use sterile dead-ender caps on all ports of stopcocks.	
		Carefully flush remaining blood from stopcocks after bloodsampling.	

frequency to approximately 10 Hz (which is well within the frequency range of the arterial pressure wave), producing an inaccurate pressure reading.

Because of the complexity of the arterial pressure wave, optimal use of the dynamic response of the monitoring system is necessary to obtain useful hemodynamic data. Assessment of the system's dynamic response should be made at regular intervals, as well as at any time suspicion exists regarding the accuracy of the data or whenever changes have occurred with any components of the fluid-filled monitoring system. (See Chapter 3 for a detailed discussion of dynamic response assessment.) Tables 7-2 and 7-3 identify problems commonly encountered with measurement of intraarterial pressures and suggestions to optimize monitoring and minimize risks.

Maintenance of Catheter Patency

Maintaining catheter patency can be a greater problem with an arterial catheter than with a venous catheter because the arterial catheter is a high-pressure system.

An effective method of maintaining catheter patency is to use a pressure bag setup and continuous flush device, as shown in Fig. 7-25. The continuous flush device allows a flow of approximately 2 to 5 ml/hr of IV fluid into the arterial catheter; this amount of fluid is usually sufficient to maintain catheter patency while not altering the measured pressure. In addition, most continuous flush devices allow the rapid delivery of fluid (between 0.75 and 1.5 ml/sec) when the flush valve is completely open.

Thrombus formation almost invariably occurs, to at least a small degree, on the catheter tip, as well as on the entire catheter surface. Flushing of this material creates an embolus that can be carried distally and occlude a small critical artery (e.g., to a finger). To prevent this serious complication, the catheter should be aspirated before flushing, and the blood, which may contain a clot from the catheter tip, should be discarded. This should then be followed by gentle flushing of *small* volumes (2 to 4 ml) of flush solution to prevent embolization. If flushing is performed with the continuous flush device, the flush valve should be opened only for a few seconds. This precaution is based on Lowenstein, Little, and Lo's study showing that a vigorous flush of as little as 7 ml of fluid into a radial artery catheter could reach the aortic arch and possibly result in cerebral embolization.

The results of a very large clinical trial (the Thunder Project) confirm the benefits of using heparinized flush solution to improve arterial catheter patency. The addition of 0.25 to 2 units of heparin per milliliter of flush solution can increase catheter longevity and patency. Of course this practice applies only to patients who have no contraindications to heparin therapy.

It is very important that the cannulated extremity with the arterial line be left uncovered, so that it may be easily observed for bleeding caused by loose connections in the line. An alarm also should be built into the monitoring system to alert the nurse if the arterial line should become disconnected. An arterial line requires close and frequent observation because a loose connection could allow potentially fatal bleeding from the cannulated artery. The pulse distal to the arterial catheters should be checked every 2 hours for early signs of compromise or absence that may indicate thrombosis. Circulation and movement of the extremity distal to the arterial catheter also should be checked every 2 hours.

Prevention of Infection of Arterial Lines

Studies of the bacterial contamination of stopcocks connected to arterial lines have reported positive cultures in 15% to as high as 50% of patients with arterial lines. In many instances this high contamination rate most likely reflects nosocomial contamination during blood sampling. Cultures from arterial site catheters also have shown contamination at the tip of the catheter, although these studies have been of limited value because of the difficulty in determining whether contamination was present while the catheter was indwelling or at the time of withdrawal for study or replacement. The recommendations made for arterial sampling procedures outlined in the next section therefore should be followed.

Arterial Blood Sampling

Arterial blood gas measurements frequently are obtained in the critically ill patient to monitor and identify any dysfunctions of the metabolic, respiratory, or

Table 7-3. Guide for optimal arterial monitoring

Procedure	Reason
Label IV tubing of arterial line as "artery" or "arterial line."	Visual aid may help to avoid confusion with venous lines.
Keep pressure bag inflated to pressure greater than patient's arterial pressure.	Slow deflation of bag will result in blood flow back into tubing.
Maintain constant fluid flow with continuous flush device (2-4 ml/hr).	Constant fluid flow maintains patency and prevents clotting.
Check all connections.	Loose connections can introduce air or allow blood loss.
Immobilize extremity.	Extremity movement can result in needle or catheter displacement.
Keep all connectors and puncture sites visible.	Possible bleeding may be observed.
Frequently check pulse distal to puncture site.	Weakening or loss of pulse may indicate thrombosis.
Check circulation, movement, and sensation of extremity distal to puncture site.	Any changes in circulation, movement, or sensation may indicate hematoma formation.
Label date of catheter insertion on dressing.	Removal of catheter after 72-96 hr may reduce risk of infection.

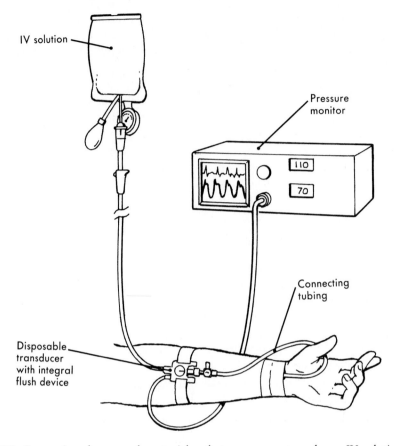

Fig. 7-25. Connections between the arterial catheter, pressure transducer, IV solution, and pressure monitor.

cardiovascular systems. An indwelling arterial catheter facilitates frequent evaluation of these parameters.

Several "in-line" blood sampling systems are now available that allow blood withdrawal without discarding any blood. Blood is withdrawn via and *up to* a self-sealing port located distal to the catheter hub. The amount of blood drawn back is equal to the dead space volume of the catheter and tubing. A syringe is placed on a second self-sealing port located proximal to the catheter hub, and the required blood sample volume is withdrawn. The blood remaining in the catheter and in-line sample tubing is then reinfused into the patient by flushing the infusion system. This method reduces the blood loss associated with blood sampling, provides a uniformly nondiluted blood sample, and minimizes the risk of infection by eliminating open stopcocks and reducing the number of entries into the system. For these reasons it is the preferred way of obtaining blood samples from an arterial line.

INDIRECT ARTERIAL PRESSURE MONITORING

Indirect, or noninvasive, arterial blood pressure measurement has been used for more than 100 years and provides valuable information in a number of clinical situations. However, it is important to remember that invasive — that is, direct arterial monitoring — measures pressure changes *directly,* whereas noninvasive techniques rely on changes in blood flow to *indirectly* reflect changes in pressure. Thus, differences in values obtained with these two different methods are common and likely are caused by changes in the relationship between the pressure pulse and blood flow. (See further discussion at the end of this section.) Although many consider the invasive arterial pressure measurement the "gold standard," its associated risks and complexity appropriately limit its clinical application.

Indirect arterial pressure can be measured noninvasively by the use of cuff occlusion (auscultation or oscillometry) or tonometry.

Cuff-Occlusion Method

The cuff-occlusion method utilizes inflation of a cuff to occlude blood flow through an artery. Slow deflation of the cuff permits a gradual increase in flow through the vessel. With the auscultatory method, as introduced by Korotkoff in 1905, the onset and cessation of sounds heard via a stethoscope over the artery distal to the cuff represent the systolic and diastolic arterial pressure, respectively. With the oscillometric method, which is most commonly used in automatic blood pressure devices, small oscillations that occur in the cuff pressure in response to increases in blood flow during cuff deflation are measured and analyzed. The maximum increase in oscillations represents the systolic pressure, whereas the maximum decrease in oscillations represents the diastolic pressure. The automatic device allows blood pressure measurements to be regularly and automatically obtained at set intervals. Studies comparing the auscultatory and oscillometric methods reveal conflicting and sometimes confusing results. Although MAP values have a fairly high correlation, the systolic and diastolic pressure measurements often correlate very poorly when auscultatory and oscillometry results are compared with direct arterial pressure measurements in hypotensive and hypertensive patients (see Frucht et al., Bruner et al., and Loubser references).

When using automatic blood pressure devices, clinicians need to pay special attention to the circulation of the arm used for measurement. Venous congestion, nerve damage, and petechial hemorrhages can occur as a result of faulty equipment or too-frequent cuff inflations, particularly in elderly patients, patients receiving nonsteroidal antiinflammatory drugs, steroids, anticoagulants, or thrombolytic agents, and patients with large arm circumferences. Frequent limb inspection beneath the cuff and application of a stockinette or soft cotton padding beneath the cuff can help reduce some of these complications.

Tonometry Method

Arterial tonometry is a noninvasive method that allows measurement of a peripheral artery pressure (systolic, diastolic, and mean), as well as continuous monitoring of the arterial pressure waveform. A special housing unit is aligned over a superficial artery (typically the radial artery) and strapped into place. A pneumatic system within the housing unit applies sufficient pressure to partially flatten the artery against the rigid bone beneath it (Fig. 7-26). Within the housing unit is an array of very small transducer sensors that rest on the skin surface over the flattened artery and that measure the transmitted arterial blood pressure. Periodic automatic calibrations enhance accuracy of measurements that correlate favorably with invasive arterial

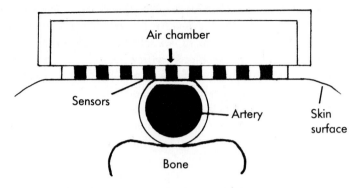

Fig. 7-26. Schematic illustration of arterial tonometry showing the tonometer sensor flattening the artery against the bone, allowing the transducer elements within the sensor to measure the arterial pressure.

blood pressure measurements. This method of arterial pressure monitoring provides all the information available through direct arterial monitoring but without the risks associated with invasive arterial monitoring. The reliability of this technique in critically ill patients has not been established, but clearly it offers promise.

Direct Versus Indirect Blood Pressure Measurement

Discrepancies frequently exist between noninvasive and directly measured arterial pressures. As mentioned earlier, this is a common finding and likely is due to the different methods of measurement (i.e., pressure vs. flow). Nonetheless, confusion regarding the "true" arterial pressure often exists when such discrepancies occur, particularly when one of the measured pressures falls within a range that would prompt treatment. When discrepancies exist, several methods are used clinically to determine the "true" or actual arterial pressure. First and foremost is determination and optimization by optimal use of the dynamic response of the direct arterial monitoring system (see discussion, Chapter 3).

An "occluded blood pressure" measurement sometimes is used to determine the actual systolic blood pressure. In this technique, a blood pressure cuff is placed over the brachial artery on the ipsilateral arm of the cannulated artery. While the examiner observes the arterial waveform on the oscilloscope, the cuff is inflated until the characteristic waveform is no longer present. The cuff is then slowly released until the arterial waveform reappears. The gauge reading noted when the waveform reappears represents the systolic arterial pressure.

Another method used to determine the actual arterial systolic pressure when a discrepancy exists between cuff and directly measured arterial pressures involves the use of the pulse oximeter. With the use of this technique, the blood pressure cuff, placed on the same arm as the pulse sensor, is inflated until the pulse oximeter ceases to sense pulsations. The gauge reading noted at this precise point is thought to reflect the actual systolic arterial pressure. A variation of this technique involves averaging the readings obtained at the disappearance and the appearance of the arterial signal on the pulse oximeter. Good agreement was obtained when this technique was compared with data based on Korotkoff sounds in normal healthy volunteers. However, this technique needs to be tried in a variety of critical care settings and on a larger number of patients before it can be recommended as a reliable method.

Significant differences also may exist between the digitally displayed arterial systolic pressure and that recorded on a paper writeout or strip chart. Some of these variations may be the result of large changes during portions of the respiratory cycle, but greater differences have been noted in the presence of hypertension, hypotension, or dysrhythmias. As with the PA and PAW pressures, measurement of arterial pressures should be obtained at end-expiration from a strip chart.

REFERENCES

American Association of Critical-Care Nurses: Evaluation of the effects of heparinized and nonheparinized flush solutions on the patency of arterial pressure monitoring lines: The AACN Thunder Project, *Am J Crit Care* 2:3-15, 1993.

Band JD, Maki DG: Infections caused by arterial catheters used for hemodynamic monitoring, *Am J Med* 67:735-741, 1979.

Bazaral MG et al: Radial artery pressures compared with subclavian artery pressure during coronary artery surgery, *Cleve Clin J Med* 55:448-457, 1988.

Bedford RF: Radial arterial function following percutaneous cannulation with 18- and 20-gauge catheters, *Anesthesiology* 47:37-39, 1977.

Bedford RF: *Invasive blood pressure monitoring.* In Blitt CD, editor: *Monitoring in anesthesia and critical care medicine,* ed 2, New York, 1990, Churchill Livingstone.

Bogliano CS et al: The effect of two concentrations of heparin on arterial catheter patency, *Crit Care Nurse* 10:47-56, 1990.

Bruner JMR et al: Comparison of direct and indirect methods of measuring arterial blood pressure, *Med Instrum* 15:11-21, 1981.

Centers for Disease Control: *Nosocomial bacteremia for intravascular pressure monitoring systems.* In National nosocomial infections study report, 1977 (6-month summaries), Atlanta, 1979, US Department of Health, Education, and Welfare.

Chawla R et al: Can pulse oximetry be used to measure systolic blood pressure? *Anesth Analg* 70:196, 1992.

Coyle JP et al: Respiratory variations in systemic arterial pressure as an indicator of volume status, *Anesthesiology* 58:A53, 1983.

Crossland SG, Neviaser RJ: Complications of radial artery catheterization, *Hand Clin* 9:287-290, 1977.

Curtiss EI et al: Pulsus paradoxus: definition and relation to the severity of cardiac tamponade, *Am Heart J* 115:391-398, 1988.

Davis FM: Radial artery cannulation: influence of catheter size and material on arterial occlusion, *Anaesth Intensive Care* 6:49-53, 1978.

Friedman HS, Sakura H, Lajam F: Pulsus paradoxus: a manifestation of a marked reduction of left ventricular end-diastolic volume in cardiac tamponade, *J Thorac Cardiovasc Surg* 79:74-82, 1980.

Frucht U et al: *How reliable are indirect blood pressure measurement devices in the intensive care unit (ICU)?* In Meyer-Sabellek W et al, editors: *Blood pressure measurements,* New York, 1990, Springer-Verlag.

Gardner RM: Direct blood pressure dynamic response requirements, *Anesthesiology* 54:227-236, 1981.

Gardner RM et al: Percutaneous indwelling radial artery catheters for monitoring cardiovascular function: prospective study of the risk of thrombosis and infection, *N Engl J Med* 290:1227-1231, 1974.

Gloyna DF et al: A comparison of blood pressure measurement techniques in the hypotensive patient, *Anesth Analg* 63:222, 1984.

Gravlee GP et al: Comparison of brachial, radial, and aortic arterial pressure monitoring during cardiac surgery, *Circulation VII* 61:A69, 1984.

Gravlee GP et al: A comparison of brachial, femoral and aortic intra-arterial pressures before and after cardiopulmonary bypass, *Anaesth Intensive Care* 17:305-322, 1989.

Jones RM et al: The effect of method of radial

artery cannulation on post cannulation blood flow and thrombus formation, *Anesthesiology* 55:76-78, 1981.

Kaye W: Catheter- and infusion-related sepsis: the nature of the problem and its prevention, *Heart Lung* 11:221-227, 1982.

Kaye W: Invasive monitoring techniques: arterial cannulation, bedside pulmonary artery catheterization, and arterial puncture, *Heart Lung* 12:395-428, 1983.

Kelly RP et al: Noninvasive registration of the arterial pressure pulse waveform using high-fidelity applanation tonometry, *J Vasc Med Biol* 1:142-149, 1989.

Kelly RP et al: Nitroglycerin has more favorable effects on left ventricular afterload than apparent from measurement of pressure in a peripheral artery, *Eur Heart J* 11:138-144, 1990.

Kemmotsu O et al: Blood pressure measurement by arterial tonometry in controlled hypotension, *Anesthesiology* 71:A406, 1989.

Kim JM, Arakawa K, Bliss J: Arterial cannulation: factors in the development of occlusion, *Anesth Analg* 54:836-841, 1975.

Korbon GA et al: Systolic blood pressure measurement: Doppler vs. pulse oximeter, *Anesthesiology* 67:A188, 1987.

Lantiegne KC, Civetta JM: A system for maintaining invasive pressure monitoring, *Heart Lung* 7:610-621, 1978.

Larrivee E, Joseph DH: Strategies for teaching decision making: discrepancies in cuff versus invasive blood pressures, *Dimens Crit Care Nurs* 11:278-285, 1992.

Laskey WK, Kussmaul WG: Arterial wave reflection in heart failure, *Circulation* 75:711-722, 1987.

Little JM, Clarke B, Shanks C: Effects of radial artery cannulation, *Med J Aust* 2:791-793, 1975.

Loubser PG: Comparison of intra-arterial and automated oscillometric blood pressure measurement in postoperative hypertensive patients, *Med Instrum* 20:255-259, 1986.

Lowenstein E, Little JW, Lo HH: Prevention of cerebral embolization from flushing radial-artery cannulas, *N Engl J Med* 285:1414-1415, 1971.

Maki DG, Hassemer CA: Endemic rate of fluid contamination and related septicemia in arterial pressure monitoring, *Am J Med* 70:733-738, 1981.

Maloy L, Gardner RM: Monitoring systemic arterial blood pressure: strip chart recording versus digital display, *Heart Lung* 15:627-635, 1986.

Mandel MA, Dauchot PJ: Radial artery cannulation in 1,000 patients: precautions and complications, *J Hand Surg* 2:482-485, 1977.

Molter N: Arterial blood gas analysis: a study of sampling techniques from indwelling arterial catheter systems, *Heart Lung* 12:428, 1983 (abstract).

Nystrom E et al: A comparison of automated indirect arterial blood pressure meters: with recordings from a radial arterial catheter in anesthetized surgical patients, *Anesthesiology* 62:526, 1985.

O'Rourke MF: Pressure and flow waves in systemic arteries and the anatomical design of the arterial system, *J Appl Physiol* 23:139-149, 1967.

O'Rourke MF: *Arterial function in health and disease,* Edinburgh, 1982, Churchill Livingstone.

O'Rourke MF, Kelly R, Avolio A: *The arterial pulse,* Philadelphia, 1992, Lea & Febiger.

Perel A, Pizov R, Cotev S: The systolic blood pressure variation is a sensitive indicator of hypovelemia in ventilated dogs subjected to graded hemorrhage, *Anesthesiology* 67:498-502, 1987.

Rothe CF, Kim KC: Measuring systolic arterial blood pressure. Possible errors from extension tubes or disposable transducer domes, *Crit Care Med* 8:683-689, 1980.

Shinozaki R et al: Bacterial contamination of arterial lines, *JAMA* 249:223-225, 1983.

Simkus GJ, Fitchett DH: Radial arterial pressure measurements may be a poor guide to the beneficial effects of nitroprusside on left ventricular systolic pressure in congestive heart failure, *Am J Cardiol* 66:323-326, 1990.

Singh S et al: Catheter colonization and bacteremia with pulmonary and arterial catheters, *Crit Care Med* 10:736-739, 1983.

Slogoff S, Keats AS, Arlund C: On the safety of radial artery cannulation, *Anesthesiology* 59:42-47, 1983.

Stamm WE et al: Indwelling arterial catheters as a source of nosocomial bacteremia, *N Engl J Med* 292:1099-1102, 1975.

Talke P, Nichols RJ Jr, Traber DL: Does measurement of systolic blood pressure with a pulse oximeter correlate with conventional methods? *J Clin Monit* 45:992-993, 1990.

Yang SS et al: *From cardiac catheterization data to hemodynamic parameters,* Philadelphia, 1972, FA Davis Co.

Chapter 8

Cardiac Output Measurements

Cardiac output is the amount of blood ejected by the heart per unit of time and is reported as liters per minute. Although there may be slight discrepancies, the cardiac output of both right and left ventricles is the same unless there is an intracardiac shunt. The importance of considering cardiac output in the evaluation of overall cardiac status and left ventricle (LV) performance, as well as its value in the determination of valve areas and resistances, has long been recognized. Even more important is the use of repeated cardiac output measurements to assess a patient's response to therapy.

Methods of determining cardiac output are the Fick method and the indicator-dilution method, which includes the thermodilution method. Although each method is sound and has particular advantages and disadvantages (Table 8-1), the simplicity of its performance makes the thermodilution method the most applicable to bedside use. Other methods currently under investigation include the pulse contour technique, and the noninvasive bioimpedance technique.

PHYSIOLOGIC REVIEW

The function and viability of all body tissues are dependent on an adequate supply of oxygen and nutrients from the circulating blood. This supply depends on the flow rate of blood and local tissue diffusion. The heart itself extracts the greatest amount of oxygen from the blood (approximately 70% of the oxygen present in every milliliter of blood). The brain is the next highest extractor of oxygen per milliliter of blood. Deprivation of oxygen supply to brain tissue for more than 2 to 4 minutes can result in severe, irreversible brain damage.

A demand for increased tissue oxygen can be met in two ways: (1) by an increase in flow rate (cardiac output) or (2) by an increase in oxygen extraction from the blood.

Cardiac output is the product of heart rate and stroke volume (CO = HR × SV). Stroke volume is the volume of blood ejected with each heartbeat and is the difference between the volume of the left ventricle at end-diastole (the end of the filling period) and the volume remaining in the ventricle at end-systole (the end of ejection). Most ventricular filling occurs rapidly early in diastole and is affected by the filling pressure

Table 8-1. Advantages and disadvantages of Fick and thermodilution methods for determining cardiac output

Advantages	Disadvantages
FICK	
Gives accurate results even in presence of low cardiac output states, valvular insufficiencies, and shunts.	Requires constant or steady state hemodynamic and respiratory conditions.
Gives an indication of patient's pulmonary status.	Requires simultaneous withdrawal of both arterial and mixed venous blood samples (10-20 ml).
Considered "gold standard" because of accuracy.	Requires patient cooperation in collecting expired air.
	Requires at least two persons for simultaneous collection of expired air and blood samples.
	Requires more time in analyzing samples.
	Oxygen administration affects results.
	Changes in pulmonary volume affect results.
THERMODILUTION	
Requires only one catheter.	Presents possible electrical hazard if there are damaged thermistor wires in catheter.
Catheter can be inserted at bedside.	
Does not require blood withdrawal.	Indwelling pulmonary artery catheter can be a hazard.
Rapidly performed.	
Good reproducibility.	Requires proper recording device and computer for calculations.
Minimally affected by recirculation.	
Requires only one person.	Not accurate in presence of shunts.
Not affected by oxygen administration.	Specific heat and gravity of blood changes with hematocrit changes.

of the left atrium and the distensibility of the ventricular wall. Systolic ejection occurs during contraction of the ventricle and is partly dependent on the degree of muscle fiber shortening attained by the ventricle. Starling and his associates found a direct correlation between the diastolic volume (increasing volume causing lengthening of muscle fibers) and the energy released in the following systole (the shortening of muscle fibers). Therefore one way the heart can increase stroke volume is by increasing the diastolic volume and length of muscle fibers, which will result in a greater ejection fraction and stroke volume. This is one of the primary compensatory mechanisms the heart inherently uses to increase cardiac output.

Actual measurements of LV volume are difficult to obtain because of the nonsymmetric shape of the left ventricle and its constantly changing volume during the cardiac cycle. However, a mean stroke volume can be calculated by dividing the cardiac output by the ventricular rate during that period. The normal range of stroke volume is 60 to 130 ml.

Unlike a mechanical pump, whereby a specific amount of fluid is ejected regardless of any change in rate, the heart adapts itself to changes in heart rate. For example, the increased time of diastole that occurs with a slow heart rate allows greater ventricular filling with resultant greater lengthening of the muscle fibers. According to the Frank-Starling law, the result is increased muscle shortening, an increased ejection fraction, and increased stroke volume. Therefore a decrease in heart rate is compensated for by an increase in stroke volume, maintaining a constant average blood flow, or normal cardiac output. Tachycardia, on the other hand, decreases the duration of diastole with minimal effect on the systolic time period. If the tachycardia is excessive, it prevents sufficient time for adequate filling of the LV to occur. This decrease in LV filling results in a reduced stroke volume and a reduced cardiac output in spite of the rapid heart rate. Tachycardia and cardiac dysrhythmias can significantly reduce stroke volume and cardiac output by preventing adequate time for LV filling. A failing heart also increases in size (dilates) to try to compensate for a lower efficiency by increasing diastolic volume to effect increased muscle shortening and to improve stroke volume.

Cardiac output is affected not only by the factors within the heart but by resistance to ejection of the blood from the ventricle (afterload). The higher the systolic blood pressure, the higher is the resistance to ejection of an adequate stroke volume. This factor is particularly serious in a patient with a failing heart and an already low stroke volume. Reducing peripheral resistance (afterload reduction) can increase stroke volume sufficiently so that little or no reduction in blood pressure occurs. This is particularly clear when the formula $BP = CO \times SVR$ is reviewed. If the resistance is decreased and the cardiac output is increased, the blood pressure remains nearly the same.

Normal resting cardiac output is 4 to 8 L/min. These values, however, do not take into account individual needs of tissues according to body size. Whereas a cardiac output of 4 L/min might be adequate for a person of small stature, it would not be adequate for a larger person. A more specific measurement is the cardiac index, which is the cardiac output per square meter (m^2) of body surface area (BSA). The body surface area can be calculated from Dubois's height-weight formula (Appendix C). A normal resting cardiac index is 2.5 to 4 L/min/m^2.

EXAMPLE: A 77-kg man has a cardiac output of 6.7 L/min. He is 180 cm tall and according to the Dubois body surface chart has a BSA of 1.96 m^2. His cardiac index (CI) is therefore 3.4 L/min/m^2.

$$CI = \frac{6.7}{1.96} = 3.4 \text{ L/min/m}^2$$

A low cardiac output may be the result of poor filling of the ventricle or poor forward emptying of the ventricle (Table 8-2). A common cause of low resting cardiac output is diminished myocardial function resulting from myocardial infarction.

Some other factors that affect the cardiac output include age, body temperature, environmental temperature, anxiety, and changes in body position. Cardiac output decreases approximately 10% from supine to sitting position and nearly 20% from the supine to standing position.

FICK METHOD
Principle

The Fick method of cardiac output determination (Fig. 8-1) is based on Adolph Fick's principle, which states that the difference between the arterial and mixed

Table 8-2. Factors causing low cardiac output

Inadequate LV filling	Inadequate LV ejection
Tachycardia	Coronary artery diseases causing LV ischemia or infarction
Rhythm disturbance	
Hypovolemia	Primary myocardial disorders such as myocarditis, cardiomyopathy
Mitral or tricuspid stenosis	
Pulmonic stenosis	Increased afterload
Pulmonary embolus	Aortic stenosis
↑ Pulmonary vascular resistance	Hypertension
Constrictive pericarditis or tamponade	Mitral regurgitation
Restrictive cardiomyopathy	Drugs with negative inotropic effect
	Metabolic disorders
	Ventricular septal defect

venous oxygen concentration reflects oxygen uptake per unit of blood as it flows through the lungs.

The amount of oxygen removed from inspired air over a given time period reflects the oxygen consumption of the tissues. If the oxygen saturations of mixed venous blood (flowing into the lungs) and arterial blood (leaving the lungs) are measured, the amount of blood flowing through the lungs can be calculated. The following formula is used to calculate cardiac output:

$$\text{CO (ml/min)} = \frac{O_2 \text{ consumption (ml/min)}}{\text{Arterial } O_2 \text{ content (vol \%)} - \text{Venous } O_2 \text{ content (vol \%)}}$$

(Vol % = ml O_2/100 ml blood)

EXAMPLE: O_2 consumption = 250 ml/min
Arterial O_2 content = 20 vol %
Mixed venous O_2 content = 15 vol %
Arteriovenous O_2 difference = 5 vol % (20 vol % − 15 vol %)

On the basis of this formula, the calculation for cardiac output would be as follows:

$$\text{CO} = \frac{250 \text{ ml/min}}{20 \text{ vol \%} - 15 \text{ vol \%}} = \frac{250 \text{ ml/min}}{5 \text{ vol \%}} = \frac{250}{0.05} = 5000 \text{ ml/min} = 5 \text{ L/min}$$

Because accurate calculation of the cardiac output with the direct Fick method requires collection of expired air and P_{O_2} and P_{CO_2} measurements, this method rarely is used for bedside monitoring. Rather, it is the standard against which other methods are validated.

Various instruments, including pulse oximeters and fiberoptic catheters, are available for measuring the oxygen saturation of blood. Because most of these instruments provide a reading in direct percentage of saturation, it is necessary to convert the data to volume percent saturation (oxygen saturation per 100 ml blood) or oxygen content for use in the Fick formula of cardiac output determination. Some instruments that measure oxygen saturation also measure hemoglobin in grams per 100 ml blood. Each gram of hemoglobin is able to carry 1.34 ml of oxygen. This

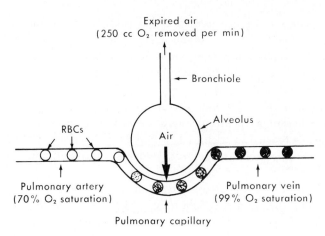

Fig. 8-1. Uptake of oxygen from the alveolus by red blood cells *(RBCs)* in the pulmonary capillary in a person with an oxygen consumption of 250 ml/min. The oxygen taken up is measured in the collected expired air and represents the body's oxygen consumption.

represents the total amount of oxygen that can combine with each gram of hemoglobin. If the oxygen saturation and hemoglobin concentration of the patient's blood are known, the following formula can be used to calculate volume percent oxygen content:

Hemoglobin (g/100 ml) $\times$ 1.34 $\times$ O_2 saturation = vol % O_2 content

> **EXAMPLE:** A patient's venous oxygen saturation is 75%, and the hemoglobin concentration is 15 g/100 ml.
>
> 15 g/100 ml $\times$ 1.34 $\times$ 0.75 = 15.06 vol % O_2 content

Some oxygen also combines with the plasma portion of blood and is referred to as *dissolved oxygen.* (See discussion, p. 218.) However, the contribution of dissolved oxygen to the cardiac output calculation is minimal and for the purpose of bedside hemodynamic monitoring is usually not included.

The arteriovenous oxygen difference (a-vD_{O_2}) is obtained by subtracting the volume percent saturation of mixed venous blood from the volume percent saturation of arterial blood. The normal range of the a-vD_{O_2} is 3 to 5.5 vol %.

> **EXAMPLE:** A patient's arterial blood oxygen saturation is 95%, the mixed venous oxygen saturation is 75%, and the hemoglobin concentration is 15 g/100 ml.
>
> 15 g/100 ml $\times$ 1.34 $\times$ 0.95 = 19.10 vol % *arterial* O_2 content
> 15 g/100 ml $\times$ 1.34 $\times$ 0.75 = 15.06 vol % *venous* O_2 content
> Arterial O_2 content $-$ Venous O_2 content = a-vD_{O_2}
> 19.10 vol % $-$ 15.06 vol % = 4.04 vol % a-vD_{O_2}

Estimated Calculation of Fick Cardiac Output

At times, an estimation of the cardiac output according to the Fick method (indirect Fick) is obtained by use of an expected or "normal" value for oxygen consumption and a measured arteriovenous oxygen difference (a-vD_{O_2}).

The a-vD_{O_2} varies inversely with the cardiac output; that is, the greater the blood flow, the less oxygen is removed per unit of blood and the smaller the arteriovenous oxygen difference. As blood flow decreases, tissue oxygen extraction increases and venous blood returning to the heart is less saturated with oxygen; thus a wide arteriovenous oxygen difference (> 5.5 vol %) usually reflects a low cardiac output.

Oxygen consumption, the other factor in this estimated calculation of cardiac output, is presumed to be relatively constant and within the normal range of 110 to 150 ml/min/m^2 (average 125 ml/min/m^2). However, oxygen consumption can vary with changes in body temperature, external work, pain, anxiety, and restlessness. (See Table 10-5.)

The following steps are taken to *estimate* the cardiac output by the Fick method.

1. Use the patient's height and weight to calculate BSA according to Dubois's chart (Appendix C). For example, a man weighing 80 kg who is 180 cm tall has a BSA of 2.00 m^2.
2. Multiply the BSA times 125 ml oxygen/min/m^2:

$$2.00 \times 125 = 250 \text{ ml } O_2/\text{min} = \text{Estimated } O_2 \text{ consumption}$$

3. Calculate arterial and venous oxygen contents and hemoglobin (see preceding example for steps in calculation).
4. Divide the estimated oxygen consumption by the arteriovenous oxygen difference.

$$\frac{250}{4.04} = 61.88 \times 100 = 6188 \text{ ml/min} = 6.19 \text{ L/min CO}$$

THERMODILUTION METHOD
Principle

Fegler described the measurement of cardiac output by thermodilution as early as 1954. This method applies the indicator-dilution principle, whereby a solution (indicator) having a known temperature is injected into the bloodstream and the resulting temperature change is detected downstream. The detected temperature change is equal to the flow rate (CO) and the change in indicator temperature over time. The resultant determination is averaged for an entire minute, giving the average rate of flow in liters per minute (L/min). The thermodilution method did not gain popular acceptance until Swan and Ganz introduced a flow-directed, thermal-sensitive catheter, which resulted in a simple, safe, and accurate measurement of cardiac output that could be easily used in the clinical setting. Its results compare favorably with both the Fick and indicator-dilution methods of measuring blood flow. Because of its rapidity and minimal recirculation, measurements can be made as frequently as every 60 seconds, and reproducibility is good.

The *accuracy* of the thermodilution technique has been evaluated, both in vivo and in vitro, by comparing its results with those obtained from other measurements of known flow rates. Under strictly controlled in vitro conditions, differences of 3% to 13% have been reported. Thus, in the clinical setting where conditions are often less than optimal, it is prudent to consider that the error in the accuracy of thermodilution cardiac output values may exceed this range.

The *reproducibility* of the thermodilution method, a clinically relevant factor, also

Table 8-3 Reproducibility of thermodilution*

Number of injections	± 10%	± 5%
2	70%	49%
3	89%	70%
4	96%	81%
5	98%	87%
6		92%
7		95%
8		96%

Modified from Hoel BL: *Scand J Clin Lab Invest* 38:383, 1978.
*The percent probability that the cardiac output based on n thermodilution curves will lie within ± 10% or ± 5% of cardiac output based on an infinite number of thermodilution curves.

has been studied both in vivo and in vitro. The reproducibility, or the variability of thermodilution cardiac output, determines how many determinations must be made to obtain an accurate value. With the use of probability calculus, Hoel calculated that to reach a 95% probability of obtaining a true (within 5%) cardiac output value it would be necessary to perform seven injections (Table 8-3). With use of three injections, which is the most common practice, there would be an 89% probability of obtaining a true cardiac output measurement that is within 10%! To assess reproducibility, Stetz and colleagues analyzed 14 publications on the clinical use of thermodilution. They concluded that a *minimal* difference of 12% to 15% (average 13%) among cardiac output values (when averaging three measurements) is required to suggest clinical significance. Thus clinicians, as well as researchers, should seriously consider the basis of their practice of eliminating cardiac output determinations that are not within 10% of the mean values.

An injection of solution, either cold or at room temperature, can be used as the indicator. The use of room-temperature solution results in less temperature change and requires greater amplification of the temperature-time curve. Numerous studies have satisfactorily correlated cardiac output determinations using room temperature and cold temperature injectate with other methods of measurement. Although these studies have been performed in a variety of patient populations, the clinician should be aware that certain individual patients may exhibit wide variations in cardiac output readings and require the use of iced injectate to maximize the physiologic signal and reduce background interference. In most instances, however, use of room-temperature injectate is satisfactory and clinically easier.

Technique

A bolus of cold or room-temperature fluid is injected into the right atrium through the proximal lumen of a thermodilution catheter; the resulting temperature change is detected by the thermistor on the catheter tip in the pulmonary artery and is recorded as a temperature-time curve by the cardiac output computer (Fig. 8-2).

The formula used in calculating the blood flow or cardiac output is based on the premise that the heat gain recorded when the injectate is mixed with the blood equals

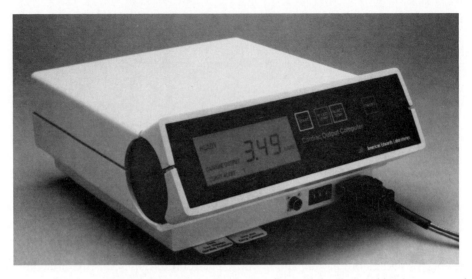

Fig. 8-2. Cardiac output computer for immediate analysis of the thermodilution curve and calculation of the cardiac output.

Courtesy American Edwards Laboratories, Santa Ana, Calif.

the heat lost by the blood. A certain amount of heat is naturally lost through handling of the syringe and through the catheter itself before entry into the right atrium. Although the cardiac output computer adds a constant factor to the calculations to offset this heat loss, the actual amount of heat lost is not constant and may be responsible for some of the error encountered with the thermodilution method of cardiac output determination. Details of the formula and calculations are not discussed here. They can, however, be found in the article by Forrester and co-workers listed at the end of this chapter.

Equipment

The following equipment is used:
1. Flow-directed thermodilution catheter
2. Closed injectate system (optional if room temperature injectate used)
3. Sterile plastic 10- or 5-ml syringe for injection of solution
4. Thermodilution cardiac output computer (COC) with connecting cable
5. Sterile IV solution (normal saline or D5W) at room temperature or at 0° to 4° C
6. Injectate temperature probe
7. IV tubing
8. Ice (if iced injectate used)

All thermodilution catheters are precalibrated. Immediately before the catheter is inserted, however, its electrical continuity should be tested by connecting the thermistor connector cable to the appropriate catheter hub and depressing the *self-test* button of the COC. If there is some fault with the catheter or the connection, the computer will signal "faulty catheter." A new catheter should then be used. The balloon of the catheter also should be tested by filling it with the designated amount of air and immersing it in sterile water. The appearance of any air bubbles in the water indicates a leak in the balloon, and it should not be used.

Procedure

The following procedure is used.

1. Insert the spiked end of the IV tubing into the solution bag and hang it from an IV pole.
2. If iced injectate solution is used, run the tubing through the prepared closed injectate system (Fig. 8-3).
3. Attach a 10-ml syringe to the stopcock of the injectate system.
4. Attach the in-line temperature probe to the distal end of the tubing.
5. Attach the distal end of the temperature probe cable to the COC.
6. Completely fill the tubing and ports with IV fluid.
7. Attach the injectate system to the proximal port of the pulmonary artery (PA) catheter via a three-way Luer-Lok stopcock.
8. Attach the thermistor connector cable from the COC to the thermistor hub of the catheter.
9. Turn on the power of the COC. (A "ready" signal should be displayed after approximately 2 seconds indicating that the computer is ready.)
10. Depress the *self-test* button to check the patency of the system (once each day).
11. Check the PA blood temperature and the injectate temperature by depressing the appropriate button on the COC. Cardiac output determinations should not be performed if the injectate temperature is unstable. To obtain accurate readings it is necessary to wait for the injectate temperature to stabilize. This may take up to 45 to 60 minutes when using iced injectate that has not been prechilled.
12. Enter the appropriate computation constant on the side panel of the computer. The correct computation constant (CC) is included in the package insert of each catheter. Most institutions tape one of these inserts to the top of each cardiac output computer. If the wrong computation constant has been entered, the data may still be used according to the formula listed in Table 8-4.
13. Depress the *cardiac output* button on the COC and wait for a *ready* signal to appear.
14. Check the pressure waveform from the distal lumen of the PA catheter to verify a PA waveform.
15. Start the strip chart recorder, if used.
16. Slowly withdraw the plunger of the syringe and fill it with exactly 10 ml (or 5 ml) of injectate.
17. Turn the stopcock closed to the IV solution and open from the injectate syringe to the proximal lumen of the catheter.
18. Press the *start* button, and rapidly and evenly inject the solution in the syringe through the proximal lumen of the catheter. To enhance accuracy, this must be done smoothly in less than 4 seconds.
19. Check the CO curve on the paper writeout or on the monitor display, and observe for the presence of a smooth, rapid upstroke indicating a rapid, even injection (Fig. 8-4).
20. Repeat steps 13 through 18 for repeated CO measurements. Usually at least three cardiac output determinations are performed to obtain an average reading. If these readings vary significantly, up to five or six determinations may be necessary to obtain a more accurate mean value. It is best to wait at least 1 minute between CO determinations to reflect the mean flow rate over a longer period.

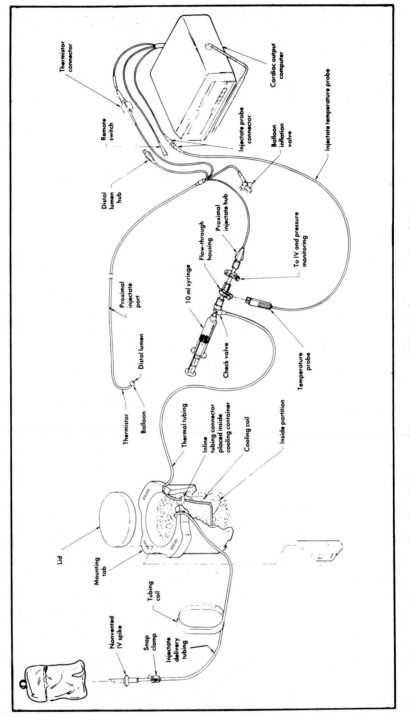
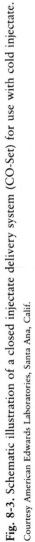

Fig. 8-3. Schematic illustration of a closed injectate delivery system (CO-Set) for use with cold injectate.

Courtesy American Edwards Laboratories, Santa Ana, Calif.

Table 8-4. Troubleshooting problems with thermodilution cardiac output measurements

Problem	Cause	Action
Cardiac output values lower than expected	Injectate volume greater than designated amount	Inject exact volume to correspond to computation constant used. Discontinue rapid infusion through proximal or distal port.
	Catheter tip in RV or RA	Verify PA waveform from distal lumen. Reposition catheter.
	Incorrect computation constant (CC)	Reset computation constant. Correct prior CO values: $$\text{Incorrect CO value} \times \frac{\text{Correct CC}}{\text{Wrong CC}}$$
	Left-to-right shunt (VSD)	Check RA and PA oxygen saturations. Use alternative CO measurement technique.
	Catheter kinked or thermistor partially obstructed with clot	Check for kinks at insertion site; straighten catheter; aspirate and flush catheter.
	Faulty catheter (communication between proximal and distal lumens)	Replace catheter.
Cardiac output values higher than expected	Injectate volume less than designated amount	Inject exact volume to correspond to computation constant. Carefully remove all air bubbles from syringe.
	Catheter too distal (PAW)	Verify PA waveform from distal lumen. Pull catheter back.
	RA port lies within sheath	Advance catheter.
	Thermistor against wall of PA	Reposition patient. Rotate catheter to turn thermistor away from wall. Reposition catheter.
	Fibrin covering thermistor	Check a-vDo$_2$; change catheter.
	Incorrect computation constant (CC)	Correct prior CO values (see formula above). Reset computation constant.
	Right-to-left shunt (VSD) Severe tricuspid regurgitation	Use alternative CO measurement technique.
	Incorrect injectate temperature	Use closed injectate system with in-line temperature probe. Handle syringe minimally. Do not turn stopcock to reestablish IV infusion through proximal port between injections; reduce or discontinue IV flow through VIP port.
	Magnetic interference producing numerous spikes in CO curve	Try to determine cause of interference. Wipe CO computer with damp cloth.
	Long lag time between injection and upstroke of curve	Press *start* button *after* injection completed to delay computer sampling time..

RV, Right ventricle; *RA,* right atrium; *CO,* cardiac output; *VSD,* ventricular septal defect; *PA,* pulmonary artery; *PAW,* pulmonary artery wedge; *a-vDo$_2$,* arteriovenous oxygen content difference; *PVCs,* premature ventricular contractions; *AF,* atrial fibrillation.

Continued.

Table 8-4. Troubleshooting problems with thermodilution cardiac output measurements—cont'd

Problem	Cause	Action
Irregular upslope of CO curve	Uneven injection technique	Inject smoothly and quickly (10 ml in ≤4 sec).
	RA port partially occluded with clot	Always check catheter patency by withdrawing, then flushing proximal port before CO determinations.
	Catheter partially kinked	Check for kinks, particularly at insertion site; straighten catheter; reposition patient
Irregular downslope of CO curve	Cardiac dysrhythmias (PVCs, AF, etc).	Note ECG during CO determinations. Try to inject during a stable period. Increase the number of CO determinations.
	Marked movement of catheter tip	Obtain x-ray film to determine position of tip. Advance catheter tip away from pulmonic valve.
	Marked variation in PA baseline temperature	Use iced temperature injectate to increase signal/noise ratio. Increase the number of CO determinations. Inject at various times during respiratory cycle.
	Curve prematurely terminated	Press *start* button *after* injection completed to delay computer sampling time.
	Right-to-left shunt	Use alternative CO measurement technique.

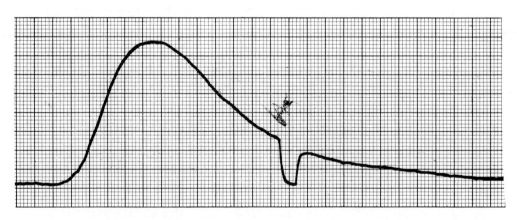

Fig. 8-4. Normal thermodilution cardiac output curve demonstrating a smooth, rapid upstroke and even downslope. (Dip on the downslope indicates end of the computer sampling period.)

The obvious advantage of the closed system is that it eliminates the need for frequent interruption of the system, with the inherent risks of contamination that accompany each entry. The primary disadvantage is the increased bulk on or near the patient, because the entire system must remain attached to the catheter. This arrangement can potentially interfere with patient movement and can be inadvertently loosened or dislodged, resulting in bleedback, introduction of air, and/or contamination. Special care is required to prevent these complications.

Sources of Error

In addition to the previously discussed issues affecting the accuracy of thermodilution cardiac output, it must be emphasized that this technique provides information over a very brief "window" of time, that is, only over several seconds of actual measurement. This value, then, is used as a reflection of the patient's flow rate per minute of time, and depending on how frequently measurements are performed, it is assumed to reflect the patient's cardiac output over the ensuing hours. Obviously, these assumptions frequently can be erroneous. The shorter the time of measurement, the larger the sampling error. In addition to the patient's changing condition, the technique itself can introduce errors that further compound the problem.

Technical considerations

Injectate temperature. Because thermodilution cardiac output measurement is calculated from a resultant change in blood temperature, it is paramount that the temperature of *both* the blood and the injectate solution be accurate and stable. Improvements in cardiac output equipment—specifically a closed injectate system with an in-line thermistor that measures the injectate's temperature as it leaves the syringe (see Fig. 8-3)—have reduced, but certainly not eliminated, this source of error. Heat from the injectate, whether iced or room temperature, is transferred during handling of the injectate syringe and throughout the shaft of the catheter. This transfer is relatively greater with the use of iced temperature injectate than with room temperature injectate. A warm environment or the use of heat lamps can appreciably alter the injectate temperature. Some ways to minimize injectate heat transfer or loss include the following:

1. Use a closed-injectate system with an in-line temperature probe. This reduces exposure to environmental influences and minimizes the amount of hand contact with the injectate. (Every 1° increase in injectate temperature results in an approximate 3% overestimation of the cardiac output.) In addition, the in-line temperature probe measures the temperature of the injectate *after* it leaves the syringe.

2. Use room-temperature rather than iced-temperature injectate. Numerous studies have demonstrated similar results between room-temperature and ice-temperature cardiac output determinations in a number of patient populations. In addition, room-temperature injectate is less likely to cause a slowing of the heart rate, as can occur with cold injectate. However, to ensure a minimum temperature difference of *12°* between the blood temperature and the injectate temperature, it may be necessary to use iced injectate in patients who are very hypothermic.

3. Keep injectate solution and tubing, as well as the catheter, away from direct sunlight or heat lamps.

Because the thermodilution measurement of cardiac output integrates a change in blood temperature produced by a bolus of fluid of different temperature, it is essential that the injectate be administered rapidly (10 ml in 4 seconds or less) and evenly as a bolus injection. Slow or uneven injection techniques will produce inaccurate data and frequently are responsible for discrepancies between serial cardiac output readings. Faulty injection techniques are visually apparent on the cardiac output curve, revealing a slow or uneven upstroke similar to that seen in Fig. 8-5. When such a cardiac output curve is produced, the data should be discarded from calculations of cardiac output. Accurate thermodilution cardiac output determinations require careful inspection of each cardiac output curve to assess technical adequacy. This requires a display or paper printout of each curve. Figs. 8-6 and 8-7 depict other errors apparent in the cardiac output curves resulting in erroneous measurements. If reliance

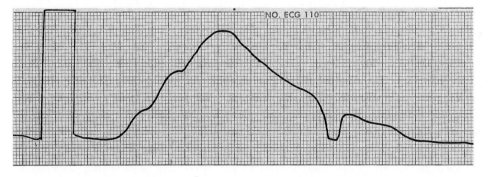

Fig. 8-5. Irregular thermodilution cardiac output curve demonstrating an uneven upslope as a result of poor injection technique.

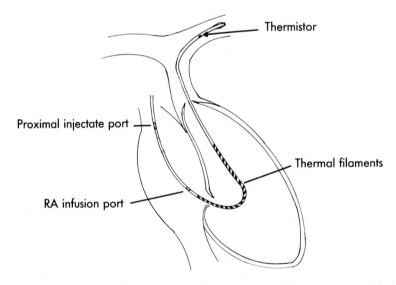

Fig. 8-6. Continuous cardiac output thermodilution catheter in proper position, with the right atrium (RA) infusion port just above the tricuspid valve, the thermal filaments in the right ventricle (RV), and the thermistor in the pulmonary artery (PA).

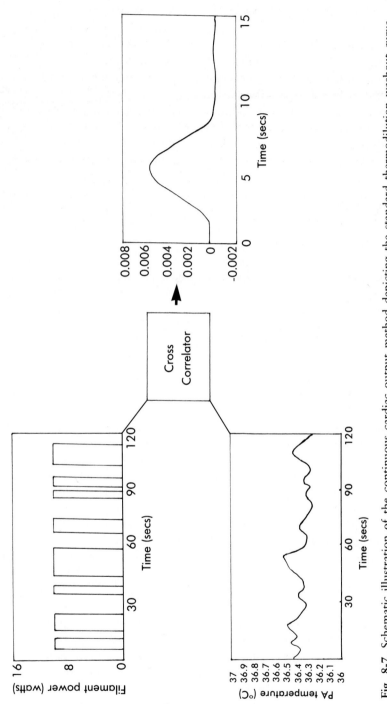

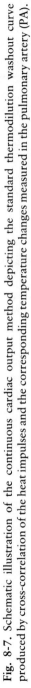

Fig. 8-7. Schematic illustration of the continuous cardiac output method depicting the standard thermodilution washout curve produced by cross-correlation of the heat impulses and the corresponding temperature changes measured in the pulmonary artery (PA).

is placed solely on the digitally displayed value, no assessment of technical accuracy can be made. This would be like monitoring the numerical value of the PA or pulmonary artery wedge (PAW) pressure without assessing the corresponding waveform!

While the upslope of the cardiac output curve indicates the injection technique, the downslope, as well as the area under the curve, relates to the rate of blood flow through the right side of the heart. A slow, prolonged downslope producing a large area beneath the curve is associated with a low flow rate, or cardiac output (Fig. 8-8). This is in contrast to the rapid downslope and smaller area seen in patients with high cardiac outputs in whom the temperature change is sensed very quickly (Fig. 8-9). If the digital display on the cardiac output computer does not correlate with this curve depiction, troubleshooting steps should be initiated to determine the cause of error (see Table 8-4). In this way analysis of the cardiac output curve, including the upslope, downslope, and area beneath the curve, is used to assess the accuracy of cardiac output determinations.

All cardiac output computers measure temperature changes over a specific limited amount, or window, of time. This measurement begins when the *start* button is initiated and continues until the slope returns to 30% of baseline, or until some specific time period has elapsed. Usually the *start* button is depressed at the beginning of each injection, signaling the computer to begin analysis. However, in patients with very low stroke volumes in whom blood moves very slowly from the right atrium (RA) to the pulmonary artery (PA), the cardiac output computer may complete its period of analysis before the maximum temperature difference has been sensed in the PA. The result would be a cardiac output curve with a small area producing an erroneously high cardiac output value. This problem can be eliminated by delaying the cardiac output computer's period of analysis until *after* injection is completed and the *start* button is not depressed until after the injectate is fully administered. Once again, careful analysis of the cardiac output curve is necessary to ensure that accurate measurements are obtained.

The formula used by the COC to measure cardiac output is based, among other factors, on the specific properties of 5% dextrose in water. To avoid the possible bacterial growth that can occur with dextrose solutions, it is not uncommon to substitute a saline solution for the injectate. However, the specific properties, including the density, of saline differ from dextrose and can introduce a small error (probably less than 2%) in the cardiac output determinations.

Errors in measurement of cardiac output via a thermodilution catheter inserted through a percutaneous sidearm sheath have been reported. As the length of the sidearm sheath is 15 cm, it is possible for the RA port of the catheter to open within the sheath rather than in the RA. This is particularly likely with catheters introduced percutaneously into small persons via the subclavian or internal jugular veins, in whom the in vivo catheter length is shorter. Indications of this occurrence include erroneously high cardiac output values and the appearance of a retrograde surge of blood-tinged fluid through the sidearm of the sheath during injection into the RA port. Correction of this problem consists of proper placement of the proximal port of the catheter within the RA and temporarily turning off the sidearm IV infusion during cardiac output measurements.

Several studies have evaluated the feasibility of obtaining thermodilution cardiac

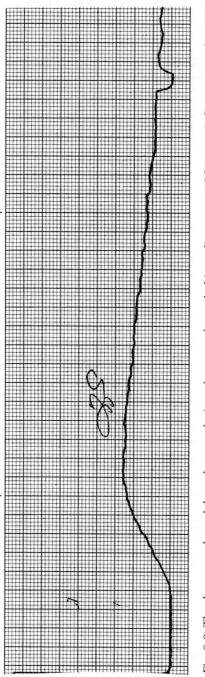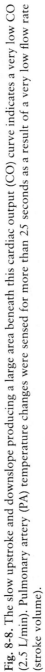

Fig. 8-8. The slow upstroke and downslope producing a large area beneath this cardiac output (CO) curve indicates a very low CO (2.5 L/min). Pulmonary artery (PA) temperature changes were sensed for more than 25 seconds as a result of a very low flow rate (stroke volume).

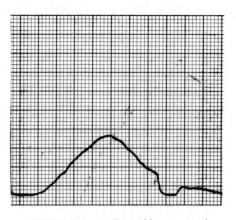

Fig. 8-9. High cardiac output (7.3 L/min) as indicated by a normal, smooth upstroke and rapid downslope producing a small area beneath the curve.

output measurements by means of injection of iced or room-temperature solution into other catheter ports (Lee and Stevens reference and Pesola references). The acceptable correlations reported permit the use of a second RA port, a right ventricle (RV) port, or even the side port of the introducer catheter in situations in which the standard proximal RA port becomes dysfunctional. Although increased variability in cardiac output values may be encountered, increasing the number of samples averaged (at least three or four determinations) minimizes this effect while providing the opportunity of continuing trend monitoring of the cardiac output.

Positional variations

Patient position can affect a number of the determinants of flow rate and thus cardiac output measurements. Changing from a flat to an elevated position produces an expected decrease in preload that may result in lower cardiac output readings. Reported differences in cardiac output values obtained from supine and lateral positioning, although statistically significant, are clinically minor (Doering and Dracup and Whitman et al.). Yet, to evaluate significant differences (>15%) in mean cardiac output values obtained from one sampling time to the next, it is important to make sure that both sampling technique and conditions are the same. For example, if a patient's average cardiac output determination is 3.1 L/min at one time and changes to a mean of 4.1 L/min several hours later, does this really represent an improvement in flow, or does it reflect a change in measurement technique because of a change in the patient's position? With so many variables affecting the measurement of cardiac output, it is important to try to achieve as constant a state as possible.

PHYSIOLOGIC CONSIDERATIONS
Respiratory Variations

Marked variations in serial cardiac output values (>10%) can result from certain physiologic changes. During the ventilatory cycle the temperature of the PA blood

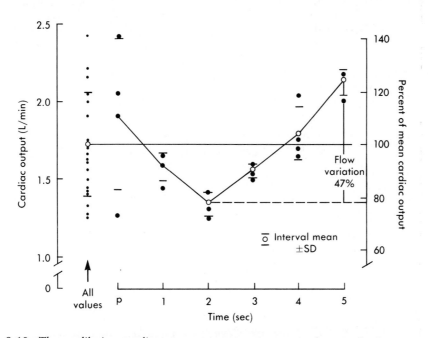

Fig. 8-10. Thermodilution cardiac output measurements at each second of a 6-second ventilation cycle. All measurements are plotted on the left, and the same points are grouped by time of the cycle on the right. (*P*, Peak inspiration.)

From Snyder JV, Powner DJ: *Crit Care Med* 10:677-682, 1982.

varies. This effect can be exaggerated during mechanical ventilation or other irregularities in the ventilatory cycle. These changes in baseline PA temperature, from which the cardiac output is calculated, introduce error in thermodilution cardiac output measurements. Again, visualization of the baseline on a paper writeout or observation of the displayed PA temperature should reveal such changes (see Fig. 8-7). When the PA temperature appears to be fluctuating, it might be necessary to use iced injectate (to increase the signal-to-noise ratio), as well as to increase the number of cardiac output determinations to five or six for averaging. Timing of indicator injections relative to the ventilatory phase also can be responsible for wide discrepancies between serial cardiac output measurements. Fig. 8-10 demonstrates the corresponding changes in cardiac output when measurements are made at different times in the respiratory cycle. However, inasmuch as temperature change and cardiac output are measured at some later time (depending on the rate of flow) after injection, no one particular moment of the ventilatory cycle will yield more *accurate* data. Injections timed to occur at one particular phase of the respiratory cycle will certainly yield more *reproducible* data but not actually reflect the average or mean flow rate per minute of time. A more accurate and clinically meaningful cardiac output measurement would reflect the average of the changes in flow that occur during both inspiration and expiration. Therefore, indicator injections should be timed to occur at various phases of the respiratory cycle. Again, if marked variation occurs, the number of determinations can be increased to five or six, or more.

Heart Rate Variations

Changes in stroke volume resulting from dysrhythmias or changing heart rates also can produce wide variations in serial cardiac output readings. The patient's heart rate and rhythm should be monitored during each cardiac output measurement. When possible, determinations should be made during a stable, dysrhythmia-free period. Because this is often difficult to do, it is again necessary to increase the number of cardiac output determinations in patients with irregular or varying heart rates.

Spurious cardiac output readings often can be checked by obtaining a mixed venous oxygen saturation or by continuously monitoring venous oxygen saturation (Svo_2) if an oximeter PA catheter is in place. If low cardiac output readings are obtained in the face of a normal Svo_2, troubleshooting steps should be initiated to determine the cause of error (see Table 8-4). Likewise, high cardiac output readings with low Svo_2 values also indicate an erroneous cardiac output measurement (except in patients with sepsis and inadequate oxygen utilization).

CONTINUOUS CARDIAC OUTPUT MEASUREMENTS

Modification of the PA catheter with the attachment of a specialized filament that provides heat as the indicator has resulted in the ability to continuously monitor cardiac output by means of thermodilution principles. As with standard thermodilution catheter positioning, the thermistor at the distal portion of the catheter rests in the PA while the thermal or heating filament lies within the right ventricle (see Fig. 8-6). The catheter is attached by means of a cable to a computer that sequentially drives the delivery of bursts of heat (approximately 15 W) to the filament, measures the corresponding temperature changes distally in the PA, and—by means of cross-correlation—yields an indicator washout curve (see Fig. 8-7) from which flow is computed. The cardiac output readout, which is updated every 30 seconds, reflects the average of the data collected within the previous 3 to 6 minutes.

Heating of the filament—and thus the catheter and surrounding blood—is intermittent and brief (1 to 4 seconds). An absolute temperature limitation of 44° C is an important safety feature that prevents rheologic changes as a result of the heating of blood.

Limited data (Yelderman et al.) on the clinical utility of this technique demonstrate an excellent correlation (r = 0.94) compared with standard bolus thermodilution cardiac output determinations of patients in intensive care units (ICUs). The theoretic advantages of this technique include the maintenance of a closed system that reduces the risk of infection, the reduced delivery of fluid volume, the reduced amount of nursing time to perform cardiac output determinations, the elimination of effects of injection technique, and the ability to continuously monitor changes in blood flow. Further clinical research is necessary to determine the realization of these potential benefits, as well as to evaluate the risks, including the cost, of this new technique.

REFERENCES

Barcelona M et al: Cardiac output determination by the thermodilution method: comparison of ice-temperature injectate versus room-temperature injectate contained in prefilled syringes or a closed injectate delivery system, *Heart Lung* 14:232-235, 1985.

Bazaral M, Petre J, Novoa R: Errors in thermodilution cardiac output measurements caused by rapid pulmonary artery temperature decreases after cardiopulmonary bypass, *Anesthesiology* 77:31-37, 1992.

Bearss MG et al: A complication with thermodilution cardiac outputs in centrally-placed pulmonary artery catheters, *Chest* 81:527, 1982 (correspondence).

Carpenter JP, Sreedhar N, Staw I: Cardiac output determination: thermodilution versus a new computerized Fick method, *Crit Care Med* 13:576-579, 1985.

Daily EK, Mersch J: Comparison of Fick method of cardiac output with thermodilution method using two indicators, *Heart Lung* 16:294-300, 1987.

Doering L, Dracup K: Comparisons of cardiac output in supine and lateral positions, *Nurs Res* 37:114-118, 1988.

Ehlers KC et al: Cardiac output measurements. A review of current techniques and research, *Ann Biomed Engin* 14:219-239, 1986.

Elkayan U et al: Cardiac output by thermodilution technique: effect of injectate volume and temperature on accuracy and reproducibility in the critically ill patient, *Chest* 84:418-422, 1983.

Fegler G: Measurement of cardiac output in anesthetized animal by a thermodilution method, *Q J Exp Physiol* 39:153-164, 1954.

Forrester JS et al: Thermodilution cardiac output determination with a single flow-directed catheter, *Am Heart J* 83:306-311, 1972.

Gardner PE, Woods SL: Accuracy of the closed injectate delivery system in measuring thermodilution cardiac output, *Heart Lung* 16:552-561, 1987.

Gillman PH: Continuous measurement of cardiac output: a milestone in hemodynamic monitoring, *Focus Crit Care* 19:155-158, 1992.

Grose BL, Woods SL, Laurent DJ: Effect of backrest position on cardiac output measured by the thermodilution method in acutely ill patients, *Heart Lung* 10:661-665, 1981.

Hainsworth R: Mixed venous oxygen content and its meaning, *Intensive Care Med* 7:153-155, 1981.

Haites NE et al: How far is the cardiac output? *Lancet* 3:1025-1027, 1984.

Hankeln KB et al: Continuous, on-line, real-time measurement of cardiac output and derived cardiorespiratory variables in the critically ill, *Crit Care Med* 13:1071, 1985.

Hoel BL: Some aspects of the clinical use of thermodilution in measuring cardiac output, *Scand J Clin Lab Invest* 38:383, 1978.

Hunn D et al: Thermodilution cardiac output values obtained by using a centrally placed introducer sheath and right atrial port of a pulmonary artery catheter, *Crit Care Med* 18:438-439, 1990.

Jansen JRC, Schreuder JJ, Verspille A: Reliability of cardiac output measurements by the thermodilution method. In Vincent JL, editor: *Update in intensive care and emergency medicine,* Berlin, 1990, Springer-Verlag.

Jewkes C et al: Non-invasive measurement of cardiac output by thoracic electrical bioimpedance: a study of reproducibility and comparison with thermodilution, *Br J Anaesth* 67:788-794, 1991.

Kashtan HI et al: Effects of tricuspid regurgitation on thermodilution cardiac output: studies in an animal model, *Can J Anaesth* 34:246-251, 1987.

Lee DW, Stevens GH: Comparison of thermodilution cardiac output measurements by injection of the proximal lumen versus side port of the Swan-Ganz catheter, *Heart Lung* 14:126-127, 1985.

Mintz R et al: Comparison of cardiac outputs determined by impedance cardiography and thermodilution in cardiac transplant patients, *Anesthesiology* 67:A213, 1987.

Moxham J, Armstrong RF: Continuous monitoring of right atrial oxygen tension in patients with myocardial infarction, *Intensive Care Med* 7:157-164, 1981.

Nelson LD, Anderson HB: Patient selection for iced versus room-temperature injectate for thermodilution cardiac output determinations, *Crit Care Med* 13:182-184, 1985.

Nishikawa T, Nimiki A: Mechanism for slowing of heart rate and associated changes in pulmonary circulation elicited by cold injectate during thermodilution cardiac output determination in dogs, *Anesthesiology* 68:221-225, 1988.

Paulsen AW, Valek TR: Artifactually low cardiac outputs resulting from a communication between the proximal and distal lumens of an Edwards pacing thermodilution catheter, *Anesthesiology* 68:308-309, 1988.

Pesola GR, Carlon GC: Thermodilution cardiac output: proximal lumen versus right ventricular port, *Crit Care Med* 19:563-565, 1991.

Pesola GR, Rostata HP, Carlon GC: Room-temperature thermodilution cardiac output: central venous vs right ventricular port, *Am J Crit Care* 1:76-80, 1992.

Pitt B, Strauss HW: Evaluation of ventricular function by radioisotopic technics, *N Engl J Med* 296:1097-1099, 1977.

Raffin TA: Technique of thermodilution cardiac output measurements, *J Crit Illness* 2:73-79, 1987.

Runciman WB, Ilsly AH, Roberts JG: Thermodilution cardiac output—a systematic error, *Anaesth Intensive Care* 9:135, 1981.

Sanmarco ME et al: Measurement of cardiac output by thermal dilution, *Am J Cardiol* 28:54-58, 1971.

Sedlock S: Cardiac output: physiologic variables and therapeutic interventions, *Crit Care Nurse* 1:14-22, 1981.

Shellock FG, Riedinger MS: Reproducibility and accuracy of using room-temperature vs. ice-temperature injectate for thermodilution cardiac output determination, *Heart Lung* 12:175-176, 1983.

Shellock FG et al: Thermodilution cardiac output determination in hypothermic post cardiac surgical patients: room- vs. ice-temperature injectate, *Crit Care Med* 11:668-670, 1983.

Siegel LC et al: Comparison of simultaneous intraoperative measurements of cardiac output by thermodilution, esophageal Doppler and electrical impedance in anesthetized patients, *Anesthesiology* 67:A181, 1987.

Slonim NB, Bell B, Christensen S: *Cardiopulmonary laboratory basic methods and calculations,* Springfield, Ill, 1972, Charles C Thomas.

Snyder JV, Powner DJ: Effects of mechanical ventilation on the measurement of cardiac output by thermodilution, *Crit Care Med* 10:677-682, 1982.

Spahn DR et al: Noninvasive versus invasive assessment of cardiac output after cardiac surgery: clinical validation, *J Cardiothorac Anesth* 4:46-59, 1990.

Steele PP et al: Simple and safe bedside method for serial measurement of left ventricular ejection fraction, cardiac output, and pulmonary blood volume, *Br Heart J* 36:122-131, 1974.

Stetz CW et al: Reliability of the thermodilution method in the determination of cardiac output in clinical practice, *Am Rev Respir Dis* 126:1001-1004, 1982.

Stevens JH et al: Thermodilution cardiac output measurement—effects of the respiratory cycle on its reproducibility, *JAMA* 253:2240-2242, 1985.

Tahvanainen J, Meretoja O, Nikki P: Can central venous blood replace mixed venous blood samples? *Crit Care Med* 10:758-761, 1982.

Thys DM: Cardiac output, *Anesth Clin North Am,* 6:803-823, 1988.

Van Grondelle A et al: Thermodilution method overestimates low cardiac output in humans, *Am J Physiol* 245:H690-692, 1983.

Vaughn S, Puri VK: Cardiac output changes and continuous mixed venous oxygen saturation measurement in the critically ill, *Crit Care Med* 16:495-498, 1988.

Vennix CV, Nelson DH, Pierpont GL: Thermodilution cardiac output in critically ill patients: comparison of room temperature and iced injectate, *Heart Lung* 13:574-578, 1984.

Vicar M, Ogle V: Comparison of measurements of cardiac output from the side port versus the proximal lumen of the Swan-Ganz catheter: follow-up study, *Heart Lung* 16:379, 1987.

Weisel RD et al: Clinical application of thermodilution cardiac output determination, *Am J Surg* 129:449-454, 1975.

Wetzel RC, Larson TW: Major errors in thermodilution cardiac output measurement during rapid volume infusion, *Anesthesiology* 62:684-687, 1985.

Whitman G, Howaniak D, Verga T: *Comparison of cardiac output measurements in 20° right and left lateral recumbent positions.* Proceedings of the Ninth Annual National Teaching Institute of the American Association of Critical-Care Nurses, Irvine, Calif, 1982.

Woog RH, McWilliam DB: A comparison of methods of cardiac output measurement, *Anaesth Intensive Care* 11:141-146, 1983.

Yang SS et al: *From cardiac catheterization to hemodynamic parameters,* Philadelphia, 1972, FA Davis Co.

Yelderman ML et al: Continuous thermodilution cardiac output measurement in intensive care unit patients, *J Cardiothoracic Vasc Anesth* 6:270-274, 1992.

Zaret BL, Cohen LS: Evaluation of cardiac performance, *Mod Concepts Cardiovasc Dis* 46(7):33-36, 1977.

Zaret BL, Cohen LS: Evaluation of perfusion and viability, *Mod Concepts Cardiovasc Dis* 46(8):37-42, 1977.

Chapter 9

Right Ventricular Volume Measurements

The evaluation of cardiac performance and, specifically, ventricular function traditionally has been directed at the left ventricle, with the right ventricle considered little more than a passive conduit transporting blood to the left heart pump. This concept was supported by studies performed on animals in the 1940s and 1950s in which extensive damage to the right ventricular free wall had very little impact on hemodynamic parameters. However, these studies were performed in animals with an open pericardium, which would be expected to evoke a different hemodynamic response than would occur with an intact pericardium. Nonetheless, an incidental role for the right ventricle was erroneously propagated. However, the performance of the right ventricle has been restudied, and its role in maintaining circulation, as well as the impact of right ventricular dysfunction on hemodynamics, has become recognized. This is due, in large part, to the development of more sophisticated assessment and imaging technologies. Among these new technologies is the ability to obtain volumetric measurements of the right ventricle (RV) as part of on-line hemodynamic monitoring.

PHYSIOLOGIC REVIEW
Normal RV Function

Although it performs the same basic function—that is, delivery of the same stroke volume—the RV differs from the left ventricle (LV) in several important ways (Table 9-1). The thin-walled, more compliant RV is architecturally and structurally designed to handle large volumes of blood with little myocardial fiber shortening or pressure development. In contrast, the thick-walled and muscular LV is designed to generate high pressures but is much less capable of handling large volumes. These inherent differences in structure and design underlie the distinct responses of each ventricle to various pathologic conditions.

Table 9-1. RV and LV structural and functional differences

Right ventricle (RV)	Left ventricle (LV)
Thin, compliant walls	Thick, muscular walls
Surface area large relative to volume	Surface area small relative to volume
Little myocardial fiber shortening	Significant myocardial fiber shortening
Unable to generate high pressures (to handle increased afterload)	Able to generate high pressures (can handle increased afterload)
Well-suited to handle large volumes	Not well-suited to handle large volumes
Coronary perfusion during systole and diastole	Coronary perfusion mainly in diastole

These dissimilarities aside, the function of both ventricles is determined by the same factors—preload, afterload, and contractility.

According to the Frank-Starling mechanism, increases in myocardial fiber stretch, or the filling volume (*preload*) of the ventricle, result in increases in stroke volume. This mechanism is operative in the RV as well as the LV. Because of the difficulty in measuring ventricular volume, the intraventricular *pressure* indirectly measured at the end of filling (end-diastole) is used clinically as a measurement of preload. The nonlinear relationship between pressure and volume, however, limits the applicability of pressure measurements as a reflection of preload, or filling volume. In addition, the usual pressure-volume relationship is altered by changes in ventricular compliance so that a decrease in compliance causes a marked increase in filling pressure for the same filling volume. The inherent difference in the compliance of the RV versus the LV also affects this relationship. As depicted in Fig. 9-1, the more distensible and compliant RV permits the accommodation of greater volume with less increase in pressure than does the less compliant LV. Thus, to interpret the patient's *preload*, or volume status, on the basis of pressure measurements is potentially misleading.

In recognition of this unpredictable relationship, it is common practice to administer volume to patients with low cardiac output even when their filling pressures—right atrial (RA) or pulmonary artery wedge (PAW)—are elevated. In this situation, careful assessment of cardiac output follows each bolus of fluid administered in an effort to ascertain the response to therapy and evaluate the patient's volume status. If both the filling pressures and cardiac output increase after the administration of a fluid bolus, it is assumed that a state of relative hypovolemia likely existed and that the fluid therapy increased the preload and, according to the Frank-Starling mechanism, appropriately increased cardiac output. If the cardiac output increases but the filling pressure remains unchanged, a state of continuing hypovolemia is assumed and further volume is given. If, however, the filling pressures increase but the cardiac output remains the same or falls, it is presumed that the elevated filling pressures reflect a decrease in ventricular compliance and that the volume status, or preload, was optimal. Clearly, the evaluation of pressures as a reflection of volume may lead to erroneous interpretation and therapies inasmuch as increasing *preload* can increase wall tension and myocardial oxygen consumption ($M\dot{V}_{O_2}$), resulting in a decrease in LV compliance and collateral coronary blood flow.

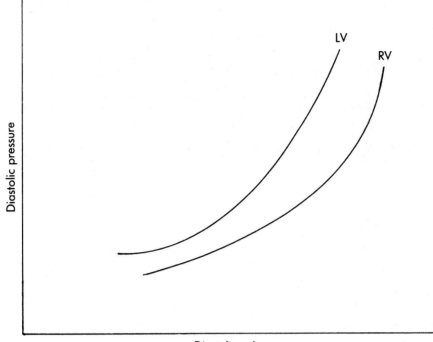

Fig. 9-1. Pressure-volume curves for the right and left ventricles. Note that for the same diastolic volume, the right ventricle *(RV)* generates less pressure than does the left ventricle *(LV)*.

The *afterload* of the ventricle refers to the load the ventricle must move during ejection. Although afterload is determined by a number of factors, a primary determinant is the vascular resistance. For the LV, this is the systemic vascular resistance (SVR), whereas for the RV, it is the pulmonary vascular resistance (PVR). Normally the resistance to flow from the RV is low, about one tenth the resistance met by the LV for the same stroke volume. For either ventricle, an increase in afterload may result in a decrease in stroke volume, as well as an increase in $M\dot{V}O_2$. The structural differences between the RV and LV, however, impose a different magnitude of response to increases in afterload, with the thicker-walled LV usually able to sustain ejection even in the face of increased afterload or pressure load. This is not the case with the thin-walled RV, which is twice as sensitive as the LV to changes in afterload. Even in the normal RV, an increase in afterload results in reduced ejection fraction. Clinical studies indicate that the maximal afterload the normal RV can adapt to, without failing, is represented by a mean pulmonary artery (PA) pressure of approximately 40 mm Hg. This afterload-dependency characteristic of the RV becomes even more exaggerated under pathologic conditions. As the RV increases in size (dilation) as a compensatory mechanism to maintain stroke volume, afterload and $M\dot{V}O_2$ are increased further, and a vicious cycle ensues.

Contractility, the degree of myocardial fiber shortening achieved by either ventricle independent of both preload and afterload, is determined by sympathetic

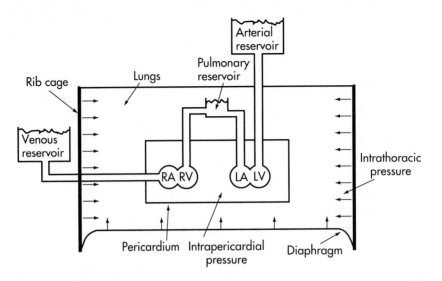

Fig. 9-2. A schematic illustration representing the thorax and its components. Intrathoracic pressure surrounds the right and left heart and lungs, whereas intrapericardial pressure is applied solely to the right and left heart.

From Weber KT et al: *Crit Care Med* 11:323-328, 1983.

stimulation and the amount of effective muscle mass. Although the RV is able to increase its contractility to a certain extent, it is more limited in this ability than is the LV as a result of its reduced muscle mass and reduced coronary blood flow to the RV free wall.

Intrathoracic Influences

The cardiopulmonary unit, which consists of the filling chambers (the RA and the LA), the two pumps (the RV and the LV), and the lungs, is surrounded by changing *intrathoracic pressure* (Fig. 9-2). However, the two systemic reservoirs—the venous and arterial vascular spaces—are located outside the thorax. As the flow of blood is proportional to pressure differences, the amount of blood returning to the right heart from the venous reservoir is determined by the difference between intrathoracic and extrathoracic pressure. This is not the case for the left heart, whose filling reservoir, the pulmonary venous reservoir, resides within the thorax and therefore is not affected by the intrathoracic/extrathoracic pressure gradient. Therefore, increases in intrathoracic pressure, whether intrinsic or extrinsic from positive pressure ventilation, reduce the intrathoracic/extrathoracic pressure gradient and decrease venous return to the right heart, reducing RV filling (preload). In addition, positive end-expiratory pressure (PEEP) ventilation at moderate levels produces an increase in RV afterload that cannot be compensated for by an inherent increase in preload.

Ventricular Interdependence

The two pumps, the RV and the LV, are coupled by the intraventricular septum (IVS), which plays an important role in the systolic and diastolic function of both ventricles. It is the transseptal ventricular pressure gradient that defines the shape and the position of the IVS. The relative dominance of the LV during systole causes the

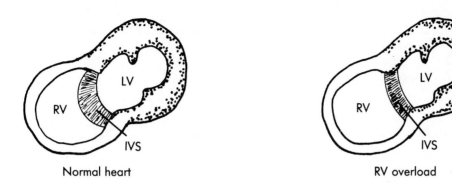

Fig. 9-3. Diagrammatic representation of ventricular interdependence. Note that during RV overload the septum flattens and moves toward the LV, reducing LV capacity. (*RV,* Right ventricle; *LV,* left ventricle; *IVS,* intraventricular septum.)

IVS to bow into the RV in the normal heart (Fig. 9-3). With elevations in RV systolic pressure (to near systemic levels), the transseptal pressure gradient is reduced and septal motion becomes abnormal.

When RV diastolic pressure becomes elevated (either from an increase in volume or a decrease in compliance), the IVS shifts to the left, toward the LV. This, in turn, distorts the LV and decreases its compliance, as well as its distensibility and filling, and stroke volume falls. An opposite effect occurs when LV volume and diastolic pressure increase, causing the IVS to shift to the right and to result in increased RV end-diastolic pressure. Thus the distensibility of either ventricle, which can be altered via the IVS, is affected by the diastolic filling of the opposite ventricle.

Ventricular interaction during diastole is further affected by the pericardium, the membranous sac that surrounds both ventricles. As pericardial pressure increases as a result of effusion or constriction, or because of an abrupt increase in RV size, the distensibility of the ventricles is impeded and the *volume* filling the ventricles declines, even though measured end-diastolic *pressures* rise. Because of its thinner wall and greater distensibility, the RV experiences greater restraint from the pericardium than does the thicker-walled LV. Thus the compensatory mechanism of RV dilation, although initially able to maintain filling, is severely limited by increases in pericardial pressure.

Acute RV Failure

Failure of the right ventricle can be considered to occur when adaptive mechanisms fail to compensate, and its systolic performance no longer can supply adequate delivery to the left heart to maintain systemic circulation. This may occur as the result of excessive RV volume or pressure loads or decreased RV contractility (Table 9-2). Clinically, abnormalities of both preload (volume) and afterload (pressure) frequently coexist and conjointly contribute to the development of acute RV failure.

Increased RV volume load

Both acute and chronic increases in RV volume usually are well-tolerated by the distensible RV and result in minimal hemodynamic consequences. However, the pathophysiologic conditions responsible for the increased volume often negatively

Table 9-2. Clinical causes of acute RV failure

Dysfunction	Clinical condition
↑ Volume load	RV ischemia/infarction
	Atrial septal defect
	Ventricular septal defect
	Pulmonic insufficiency
	Tricuspid insufficiency
↑ Pressure load	Pulmonary venous hypertension
	Mitral valve disease
	Left ventricular failure
	Primary pulmonary hypertension
	Pulmonary disease
	Pulmonary embolism
	Adult respiratory distress syndrome (ARDS)
	Pulmonic stenosis
	Positive pressure ventilation/PEEP
↓ Contractility	Ischemia
	RCA occlusion
	Decreased coronary perfusion pressure
	Right ventricular contusion
	Beta adrenergic-blockers
	Calcium channel blockers

RV, Right ventricle; *PEEP*, positive end-expiratory pressure; *RCA*, right coronary artery.

affect the afterload or contractility, or both, which intensifies the negative effects on RV function. With excessive volume, the RV dilates, which often causes the development of functional tricuspid regurgitation with decreased forward stroke volume and cardiac output. Increased RV volume also causes a leftward shift of the IVS with consequent decreases in LV chamber size, filling volume, and, hence, stroke volume. In addition, RV volume overload increases wall stress and $M\dot{V}_{O_2}$, which can result in myocardial ischemia and decreased RV contractility. Clinical conditions associated with excessive RV volume include atrial or ventricular septal defects, as well as pulmonic insufficiency. Most commonly, however, excessive RV volume occurs secondary to decreased RV ejection, either as a result of an increase in RV afterload or decreased RV contractility.

Increased RV pressure load

Increases in RV afterload, or pulmonary vascular resistance (PVR), evoke a deleterious response of the RV that is proportional to the magnitude of the PVR and accompanying pulmonary hypertension. The RV responds to an increase in pressure load by dilation and hypertrophy. Although this compensatory response initially can provide increased volume and contractility, it eventually leads to RV failure. The time course required for the development of RV failure depends on the acute or chronic nature of the pulmonary hypertension.

A major impact of increased RV pressure load is an increase in RV work and $M\dot{V}_{O_2}$. With mild-to-moderate increases in RV pressure load (mean PA pressures < 30

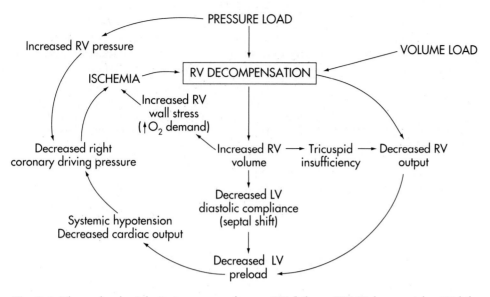

Fig. 9-4. The pathophysiologic responses of acute RV failure. (*RV,* Right ventricle; *LV,* left ventricle.)

From Wiedemann HP, Matthay RA: *Crit Care Clin* 1:631-661, 1985.

mm Hg), RV end-diastolic volume increases. Although this increase in preload may result in an adequate stroke volume from the RV to the LV according to the Frank-Starling mechanism, the associated increase in RV work and $M\dot{V}o_2$ are intensified.

As the pressure load increases, RV systolic pressure rises, and ejection fraction, which is highly dependent on afterload, declines. The higher the PA pressure, the lower the ejection fraction. Although normal coronary blood flow to the RV occurs during both systole and diastole, elevations in RV systolic pressure reduce the coronary pressure gradient and may restrict coronary flow to the period of diastole. This reduction in coronary blood flow occurring at a time of increased myocardial oxygen demand results in myocardial ischemia, particularly of the hypertrophied free walls, and decreased contractility. Even with normal coronary arteries, high PA pressures are associated with diminished coronary vascular reserve.

The negative impact of increased pressure load on RV function is exacerbated in the presence of other pathophysiologic conditions that increase preload or decrease contractility. Conditions responsible for an acute increase in RV pressure load are listed in Table 9-2.

Decreased contractility

Decreased RV contractility most commonly results from ischemia or infarction of the RV because of occlusion of the right coronary artery or decreased coronary perfusion pressure, or both. As contractility declines, ejection fraction decreases, and both RV end-diastolic and end-systolic volumes increase. Without some intervention, the RV becomes unable to supply adequate stroke volume to the LV to allow it to maintain sufficient circulation.

In summary, RV pressure or volume overload, or decreased contractility, may result in RV decompensation and initiate a vicious cycle of pathophysiologic responses that result in circulatory collapse (Fig. 9-4). The spectrum of these responses depends on the degree of dysfunction and the presence of other co-morbid conditions. In addition, certain therapeutic interventions, such as PEEP or beta-adrenergic blockade, can evoke responses that contribute to acute RV failure.

ASSESSMENT OF RV PERFORMANCE

The increased recognition of the importance of RV function to the maintenance of circulation underscores the need to accurately assess RV systolic and diastolic performance in some patients. One simple expression of RV function is the ejection fraction (the percentage of RV volume ejected each beat), which is sensitive to changes in RV preload, afterload, and contractility. Assessment of the RV may be performed by measurement of hemodynamic pressures, by echocardiography, by radionuclide angiography, and by thermodilution RV ejection fraction with volumetric measurements.

Hemodynamic Pressure Measurements

Indirect measurement of both RV end-diastolic and systolic pressures can be obtained with the PA catheter. The mean RA pressure, obtained from the proximal port of the PA catheter, represents the RV filling pressure, or end-diastolic pressure. Normal filling pressure of the RV is ≤5 mm Hg. Volume overload of the RV results in elevations of the mean RA pressure and, when tricuspid regurgitation develops, a dominant and elevated RA *v* wave (Fig. 9-5). RV pressure overload, likewise, results in an elevated RA pressure, usually with a dominant *a* wave. As previously discussed, the difficulty in interpreting elevations in the RA pressure relate to the nonlinear relationship of pressure to volume, which can be exaggerated by certain disease states, drugs, increased intrapleural pressure, or any conditions that increase RV afterload (see Fig. 9-1). In patients with RV ischemia or infarction, the degree of RA pressure elevation is related directly to the extent of RV dysfunction.

In the absence of pulmonic stenosis, the PA systolic pressure equals the RV systolic pressure and is used clinically to evaluate the RV pressure load (Fig. 9-6). Normal RV (and PA) systolic pressure is <25 mm Hg. As PVR increases, RV and PA pressures rise. However, the structural design of the RV prevents it from acutely generating pressures >60 to 80 mm Hg. Much higher pressures can be achieved with chronic pressure overload. The reduced ejection fraction and stroke volume associated with increases in RV afterload are evidenced by a narrow PA pulse pressure. Occasionally, pulsus alternans may be evident in the PA pressure waveform, indicating severe RV failure (Fig. 7-13).

Echocardiography

Both M-mode and two-dimensional echocardiographic assessment of the RV can be used to determine RV dimensions and to evaluate RV performance. The recent development of transesophageal probes for use with two-dimensional echocardiography has expanded the monitoring capability of this technique. In addition to problems associated with the RV shape, however, technical considerations limit its ability to quantitatively and qualitatively assess RV function.

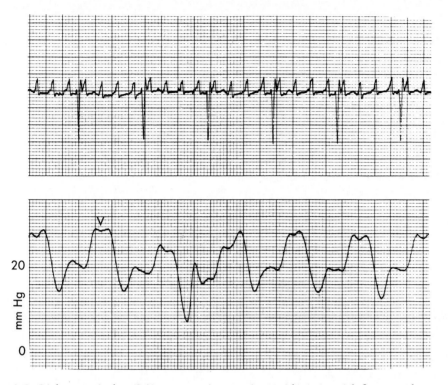

Fig. 9-5. Right ventricular (RA) pressure in a patient with 4:1 atrial flutter and severe cardiomyopathy with biventricular failure. Note the "ventricularized" appearance of this atrial waveform as a result of the elevated, dominant v wave (approximately 28 mm Hg) produced by marked tricuspid regurgitation.

Radionuclide Angiography

Two radionuclide techniques, the "first-pass" technique and the equilibrium-gated pool scan, are used to evaluate RV function by determining ejection fraction, systolic ejection time, peak filling rates, and rate of contractility. The first-pass technique measures these parameters during one cycle, whereas the gated pool scan uses repeated measurements obtained over approximately 5 minutes. Although useful for diagnostic evaluation, the technicalities associated with both these techniques preclude their use as a monitoring method.

Thermodilution Measurement of RV Ejection Fraction and Volumes
Principle

Recent modification of the standard PA catheter has resulted in a thermodilution technique that allows bedside assessment of systolic and diastolic volume measurements of the right ventricle. In addition to the standard monitoring capabilities (RA, PA, and PAW pressures and cardiac output) via proximal (RA) and distal (PA) ports, this catheter is equipped with two intracardiac electrodes and a rapid response thermistor (Fig. 9-7). The proximal and distal electrodes, located 16 cm and 6 cm from the tip of the catheter, respectively, sense the R-wave activity that is necessary for computation of beat-to-beat volume data. The thermistor, located 4 cm from the

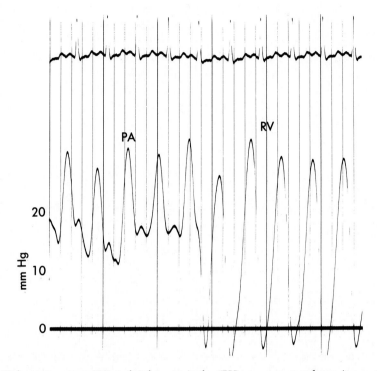

Fig. 9-6. Pulmonary artery *(PA)* and right ventricular *(RV)* pressure waveforms in a patient with left ventricular *(LV)* failure. Note the similarity of the PA and RV systolic pressures (approximately 30 mm Hg).

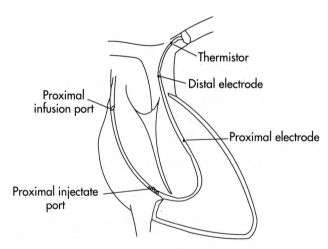
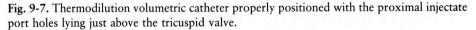

Fig. 9-7. Thermodilution volumetric catheter properly positioned with the proximal injectate port holes lying just above the tricuspid valve.

catheter tip, is a very sensitive, rapid response thermistor that detects small temperature changes in the PA.

Equipment

To determine thermodilution volumetric measurements of the right ventricle, the following equipment is required:
1. PA thermodilution ejection fraction/volumetric catheter
2. Ejection fraction/cardiac output computer (Fig. 9-8)
3. Catheter connecting cable
4. ECG reference lead connector
5. Injectate temperature probe
6. Closed cardiac output injectate system or chilled, prefilled syringes
7. Ice bucket with ice
8. Chilled (0° to 4° C) injectate solution (5% dextrose in water or normal saline)
9. 10-ml syringe(s)
10. Paper recorder (optional)

Catheter placement

Insertion of the thermodilution ejection fraction/volumetric PA catheter is performed following standard procedure. The precision required for volume measurements, however, requires optimal catheter positioning so that the injectate port (which consists of several closely approximated openings) lies just above the tricuspid valve (see Fig. 9-7). This position is best achieved by monitoring both the proximal and distal pressure waveforms during passage of the catheter. When an RV waveform is obtained via the proximal port, the catheter should be withdrawn slightly (a few centimeters) just until the RV pressure waveform changes to that of an RA waveform (Fig. 9-9). Of course, a PA waveform should be obtained from the distal

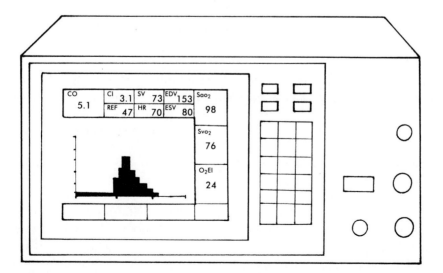

Fig. 9-8. Diagrammatic representation of the ejection fraction/cardiac output computer combined with continuous venous oximetry.

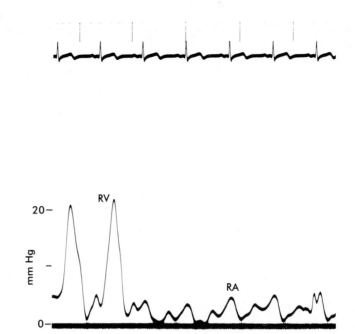

Fig. 9-9. Normal right ventricular *(RV)* waveform (first two waveforms) that changes to a right atrial *(RA)* waveform as the thermodilution ejection fraction/volumetric pulmonary artery (PA) catheter is withdrawn slightly. This change in waveform indicates that the injectate port (site of pressure measurements) lies just above the tricuspid valve — an optimal location for obtaining accurate RV volumetric data.

From Daily EK, Schroeder JS: *Hemodynamic waveforms: exercises in identification and analysis,* ed 2, St Louis, 1990, Mosby–Year Book.

port of the catheter. Verification of this position, which is accomplished by observing an RA waveform and a PA waveform from the proximal and distal ports, respectively, also should take place before each volumetric determination.

Procedure

The technique of measuring thermodilution cardiac output (CO) and ventricular volumes is the same as for standard thermodilution CO measurements. The quantified nature of the measurement, however, requires that the signal be enhanced. This necessitates use of iced rather than room-temperature injectate for volumetric measurements.

The technique described in this section refers to use of the REF-1 system of Baxter Edwards Laboratories (Irvine, Calif.).

Setup

1. Plug the ejection fraction/CO computer into an electrical outlet; turn on the rear power switch and depress the *on* switch on the front panel of the computer. The digital display will appear on the screen, and a short power-up test will be performed.

2. Insert the proximal and distal electrode connectors into the flat end of the catheter's connecting cable, and plug the other end of the connecting cable into the appropriate slot in the front of the computer.

3. Insert the ECG reference lead into the flat end (middle port) of the connecting cable, and attach the clip-end of the reference lead to an ECG electrode placed on the patient's upper torso. Assess correct R-wave sensing by observing the timing of the flashing R-wave trigger light on the front of the computer and comparing it with the patient's heart rate.

4. Connect the thermistor connection of the connecting cable to the thermistor port of the catheter.

5. Enter the patient's height and weight, and verify the correct computation constant using the control keys.

6. Prepare the iced injectate using the closed injectate system or prefilled syringes. Attach to the proximal injectate port of the catheter via a three-way stopcock. Turn the stopcock to fill the injectate syringe with exactly 10 ml of iced injectate.

Technique

1. Verify the appearance of an RA waveform from the proximal injectate lumen and a PA waveform from the distal lumen of the catheter (see Fig. 9-9). (If fluid is being rapidly infused into either the proximal or distal catheter lumens, it should be slowed or stopped during measurements.)

2. Depress the *start* button of the CO computer.

3. Turn the stopcock open between the proximal injectate lumen and the syringe, and rapidly (within 4 seconds) inject the iced bolus. (To enhance reproducibility, perform each injection at the same time in the respiratory cycle, preferably at end-expiration.)

4. The display will indicate that a CO measurement is in progress. The temperature of the patient (within the PA) and the injectate solution, as well as the patient's heart rate and the computation constant, also will be displayed. Observe these variables for accuracy. In addition, observe the CO curve to assess technical accuracy and the corresponding R-wave signals to assess the heart rate and rhythm during the determination.

5. When the sampling period is finished, the computer automatically performs the necessary volumetric computations, and the display indicates that such computations are in progress. The calculated CO and ejection fraction values will appear on the digital display.

6. Additional derived parameters, such as end-systolic volume (ESV), end-systolic volume index (ESVI), end-diastolic volume (EDV), end-diastolic volume index (EDVI), stroke volume (SV), and stroke volume index (SVI) can be observed by depressing the *more* control key.

7. Repeat steps 2 and 3 at least two more times for the determination of average flow rate and ejection volume. Repeat determinations can be made when the display changes from *in progress* to *ready* (usually about 45 seconds) after each determination.

8. Depress the *print* control key to obtain a hard copy of the CO curve as well as the calculated volumetric data.

9. Turn the stopcock on the proximal injectate port to reestablish continuous infusion. If infusion rates have been altered during the determinations, resume their previous rates.

Volumetric parameters

In addition to the CO measurement, both the ejection fraction and volume measurements of the right ventricle can be calculated from the thermodilution curve. The rapid response thermistor of the REF-1 catheter senses the total temperature change over time, as well as with each beat (R wave) during a determined period of measurement. By selecting two reference measurement points on the downslope of the thermodilution CO curve—one between 80% and 95% of the maximum temperature change and the other between 15% and 30% of the maximum temperature change—the exponential slope of the curve can be divided by the number of RR intervals during that period to yield the percent of blood ejected each beat, or the *ejection fraction (EF)*. As can be seen in Fig. 9-10, this method results in a stepwise decline in the CO curve, in contrast to the smooth downslope associated with standard thermodilution CO curves. Normal right ventricular ejection fraction, as determined by the thermodilution technique, is approximately 40%, which is slightly lower than normal values reported with the use of other techniques. Changes in EF may be due to changes in RV preload or contractility, but the EF is most sensitive to changes in afterload.

Inasmuch as the RR interval and thus the heart rate is measured during the cardiac output measurement, the calculation of *stroke volume*—the volume ejected with each heartbeat—is readily determined and calculated by the computer. Normal stroke volume is 60 to 100 ml per beat. By entering the patient's height and weight during the initial setup, the computer is able to index all parameters to the patient's body size. Normal stroke volume index is 33 to 47 ml/beat/m^2.

The volume of blood in the right ventricle at end-diastole represents the true preload of the right heart. This measurement, end-diastolic volume (EDV), also is calculated by the computer by dividing the volume ejected each beat (stroke volume) by the percentage of total volume ejected each beat (ejection fraction). Normal RV EDV is 100 to 160 ml. Changes in this measurement may be due to changes in preload, afterload, or contractility.

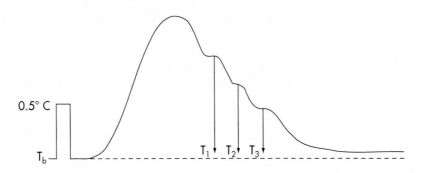

Fig. 9-10. Schematic drawing of thermodilution cardiac output curve and method of measuring right ventricular (RV) ejection fraction. (T_b, Baseline temperature; T_1, T_2 and T_3 represent the temperature differences from baseline.) Each plateau on the downslope of the curve represents the diastolic phase of the cardiac cycle, during which there is little temperature change. The mean residual fraction (RF) for each of these phases is determined by the ratio of T_2/T_1, and T_3/T_2. From this, the average ejection fraction is determined by subtracting the mean residual fraction from 1.00.

The final volume parameter calculated by the thermodilution volumetric technique is the volume of blood remaining in the right ventricle at the end of systole, the end-systolic volume (ESV). Normal right ventricular ESV is 50 to 100 ml. Changes in this measurement primarily reflect changes in RV afterload and contractility.

Validation

Numerous studies—both past and current—deal with assessing the accuracy and applicability of the thermodilution RV volumetric technique. Use of this technique in an in vitro pulsatile flow model study demonstrated a very good comparison between the CO, SV, and EF values (Ferris and Konno). Greater variation was observed in thermodilution ESV and EDV measurements. Good correlation has been demonstrated in comparing RV EF measurements obtained by use of thermodilution technique, ventricular angiography, gated and first-pass radionuclide angiography, and 2-D echocardiography (Spinale et al., Starling et al., and Vitolo et al.).

Clinical application

The occurrence of RV dysfunction has been observed in a number of illnesses and conditions, including chronic obstructive pulmonary disease (COPD), adult respiratory distress syndrome (ARDS), primary and secondary pulmonary hypertension, arterial hypertension, pulmonary embolus, postcardiac surgery and transplantation, septic shock, trauma, and burns. However, the observation made by Paul Dudley White in 1936—that the most common cause of RV failure is LV failure—remains true today.

Any condition that causes an increase in pulmonary vascular resistance (right heart afterload) increases the work of the right ventricle and impedes right ventricular ejection. If the RV ejects less completely, the stroke volume decreases and greater volume remains in the ventricle at the end of systole (end-systolic volume). During the following diastolic period, the ventricle fills with more volume, resulting in an even greater volume at the end of diastole (end-diastolic volume). Under such conditions, both the calculated ESV and EDV are elevated and RV EF is reduced. Therapeutic interventions should be directed toward reducing both the EDV and ESV and increasing the EF. This can be achieved by administration of a vasodilator with both venous and arterial dilatory properties (such as nitroprusside) to reduce preload and afterload, which may result in an increased EF. If necessary, further increases in the EF can be obtained with administration of positive inotropic agents, such as dobutamine or dopamine.

Increases in intrathoracic pressure with positive pressure ventilation and PEEP also increase RV afterload. Although the effect of PEEP on RV preload may vary, the associated increased intrathoracic pressure definitely limits any preload recruitment ability. Volumetric measurements and evaluation of EF can aid in the assessment of the impact of this therapy and direct changes in, or additions to, this intervention.

Although measurement of the patient's EF, defined as the stroke volume divided by the end-diastolic volume, provides a valuable global assessment of RV systolic performance, the assessment of RV volumes provides more specific information on the conditions that influence RV performance. For example, the EF of a patient with a stroke volume of 60 ml per beat, and an end-diastolic volume of 150 ml, is 40%. If the patient's condition changes and a tachycardia develops, stroke volume might fall to 40 ml per beat. However, as tachycardia limits diastolic filling, the RV end-diastolic volume might be reduced to 100 ml, yielding the same EF of 40%. In addition to limiting diastolic filling, tachycardia increases the $M\dot{V}o_2$. Consequently, although the EF may remain essentially unchanged, clinically significant changes in the volume conditions of the RV may occur, which can negatively affect RV performance.

The increased morbidity and mortality associated with acute RV failure from a variety of causes may be modified by the measurement of RV volumes and ejection in response to therapeutic interventions. Several studies have demonstrated the usefulness of thermodilution volumetric measurements in certain patient populations.

The measurement of RV EF in patients undergoing coronary artery bypass surgery was found to be an early and sensitive indicator of RV dysfunction secondary to RV ischemia (Hines and Barash). Although in another study of patients undergoing coronary bypass surgery, thermodilution RV EF demonstrated high variability (16%), it was still considered to be of value in the management of patients undergoing cardiopulmonary bypass (Dorman et al.). Right ventricular performance indexes, particularly the RV EF, also were found to facilitate an earlier diagnosis of postoperative cardiac tamponade when compared with standard hemodynamic pressure measurements (Jones et al.).

The measurement of RV volumes in critically ill patients has been demonstrated to be a better indicator of preload than corresponding hemodynamic pressure measurements. In two studies the RV end-diastolic volume was found to be a useful guide to fluid challenge therapy in that patients with an RV end-diastolic volume index (RVEDVI) < 140 ml/m^2 demonstrated a favorable hemodynamic response to fluid challenges (Reuse et al. and Diebel et al.).

Conditions in which RV volumetric measurements are not valid include any conditions that prevent homogeneous mixing of the thermal bolus. These include tricuspid regurgitation, pulmonic insufficiency, atrial septal defect, ventricular septal defect, and cardiac dysrhythmias such as atrial fibrillation.

Although the cost-benefit ratio of this new technology remains to be determined, it may be very helpful in the management of certain critically ill patients.

Patient Example

A 72-year-old man was admitted to the surgical ICU after coronary artery bypass grafting of the right coronary artery and the left anterior descending coronary artery. The patient was receiving an infusion of nitroglycerin at 2 μg/kg/min. The following hemodynamic data were obtained 2 hours after the patient's admission to the ICU:

HR (beats/min)	85
MAP (mm Hg)	76
PA systole/diastole (mm Hg)	28/14
PAW mean (mm Hg)	13
RA mean (mm Hg)	8
CO/CI (L/min; L/min/m^2)	3.9/2.0
SVR (dynes/sec/cm^{-5})	1395
PVR (dynes/sec/cm^{-5})	123
Urine output (ml/hr)	20

RV volumetric measurements

RV EF	0.30
RV stroke volume (ml/beat)	46
RV end-diastolic volume (ml)	153
RV end-systolic volume (ml)	107

The low CO/CI and urine output and the relatively low PAW pressure, along with the condition of rewarming, prompted the decision to administer volume in an attempt to increase stroke volume and CO (the Starling mechanism). The following hemodynamic parameters were obtained after the administration of 250 ml albumin:

HR (beats/min)	90
MAP (mm Hg)	71
PA systole/diastole (mm Hg)	32/15
PAW mean (mm Hg)	13
RA mean (mm Hg)	10
CO/CI (L/min; L/min/m^2)	4.1/2.1
SVR (dynes/sec/cm^{-5})	1190
PVR (dynes/sec/cm^{-5})	156
Urine output (ml/hr)	16

RV volumetric measurements

RV EF	0.26
RV stroke volume (ml/beat)	46
RV end-diastolic volume (ml)	176
RV end-systolic volume (ml)	130

The hemodynamic parameters change very little after volume administration, although the urine output is further decreased despite a somewhat improved CO. However, when the additional RV volumetric data are reviewed, it is clear that, although the RV EF is depressed (0.30) before the volume administration, it is not a result of low RV preload inasmuch as the end-diastolic volume is in the high normal range (153 ml). Likely, the RV EF is low as a result of increased afterload (PVR 123 dynes/sec/cm^{-5}) and decreased contractility.

Although the administration of 250 ml albumin resulted in a slightly higher CO, the stroke volume remained the same because the heart rate also increased somewhat. Volume administration, predictably, increased the end-diastolic volume, but the RV EF fell even further, indicating the RV was unable to increase its ejection despite increased preload. This likely was due to the even higher RV afterload (PVR 156 dynes/sec/cm^{-5}) and depressed RV contractility after cardiac surgery. Evaluation of the RV volumetric data in conjunction with the hemodynamic data points to the potential benefit of a positive inotropic agent to improve RV contractility. The following hemodynamic data were obtained after initiating an infusion of dobutamine 5 µg/kg/min:

HR (beats/min)	81
MAP (mm Hg)	81
PA systole/diastole (mm Hg)	24/11
PAW mean (mm Hg)	11
RA mean (mm Hg)	7
CO/CI (L/min; L/min/m^2)	4.7/2.4
SVR (dynes/sec/cm^{-5})	1259
PVR (dynes/sec/cm^{-5})	68
Urine output (ml/hr)	58

RV volumetric measurements

RV EF	0.37
RV stroke volume (ml/beat)	58
RV end-diastolic volume (ml)	156
RV end-systolic volume (ml)	98

The administration of a positive inotropic agent (dobutamine) resulted in an improved CO and stroke volume, as well as enhanced RV performance as indicated by the increased EF (37%) and improved RV volume measurements. In this instance of RV dysfunction after coronary artery bypass grafting, the hemodynamic pressure measurements are not accurate indicators of true preload.

Patient Example

A 45-year-old woman with no significant past medical history was transferred from a community hospital to the medical ICU with the diagnoses of streptococcal pneumonia, septic shock, and ARDS. She was receiving 20 cm H_2O PEEP, 1 : 1 I : E ratio with inspiratory plateau to maintain the Pao_2 in the 60s and the fractional inspired oxygen concentration (Fio_2) at 0.60.

On arrival her blood pressure was 56/43 mm Hg; dopamine and phenylephrine infusions were started and increased to maintain a systolic blood pressure of 90 to 100 mm Hg. An RV volumetric catheter was inserted into the PA, and the following hemodynamic parameters were obtained:

HR (beats/min)	123
MAP (mm Hg)	66
PA systole/diastole (mm Hg)	42/25
PAW mean (mm Hg)	16
RA mean (mm Hg)	8
CO/CI (L/min; L/min/m^2)	3.3/2.0
SVR (dynes/sec/cm^{-5})	1406
PVR (dynes/sec/cm^{-5})	364
Urine output (ml/hr)	18

RV volumetric measurements

RV EF	0.46
RV stroke volume (ml/beat)	28
RV end-diastolic volume (ml)	61
RV end-systolic volume (ml)	33

The hemodynamic measurements were improved with the dopamine and phenylephrine infusions; however, the patient's CO remained extremely low. Evaluation of the *pressure* measurements of preload indicated adequate filling pressures in this patient. However, the volumetric measurement of preload revealed a very low and inadequate filling volume of 61 ml, resulting in an extremely low stroke volume (28 ml/beat). As the contractility of the RV was normal (EF 46%), the decision was made to administer volume in an attempt to increase preload and thus cardiac output. The patient subsequently was given approximately 5 L of fluid (2 units of blood, plus crystalloid solution). The following hemodynamic parameters were obtained after this treatment:

HR (beats/min)	112
MAP (mm Hg)	70
PA systole/diastole (mm Hg)	44/24

PAW mean (mm Hg)	19
RA mean (mm Hg)	14
CO/CI (L/min; L/min/m^2)	5.9/3.5
SVR (dynes/sec/cm^{-5})	759
PVR (dynes/sec/cm^{-5})	149
Urine output (ml/hr)	28
RV volumetric measurements	
RV EF	0.42
RV stroke volume (ml/beat)	53
RV end-diastolic volume (ml)	126
RV end-systolic volume (ml)	73

The increased volume resulted in an improved stroke volume and cardiac output, as well as overall improved hemodynamics. The volumetric measurements combined with the hemodynamic measurements were used to titrate therapy carefully to obtain optimal perfusion over the next 72 hours.

REFERENCES

Anardi DM: Assessment of right heart function, *J Cardiovasc Nurs* 6:12-32, 1991.

Badke FR: Left ventricular dimensions and function during right ventricular pressure overload, *Am J Physiol* 11:H611, 1982.

Biondi JW et al: The effect of PEEP on right ventricular function, *Am Rev Resp Dis* 133:303-307, 1986.

Brinker J et al: Leftward septal displacement during right ventricular loading in man, *Circulation* 61:626, 1980.

Dhainaut JF, Brunet F: Right ventricular performance in adult respiratory distress syndrome, *Eur Resp Jnl* 11:490s-495s, 1990.

Diebel LN et al: End-diastolic volume: a better indicator of preload in the critically ill, *Arch Surg* 127:817-822, 1992.

Dorman BH et al: Use of a combined right ventricular ejection-oximetry catheter system for coronary bypass surgery, *Crit Care Med* 20:1650-1655, 1992.

Eddy AC, Rice CL, Anardi DM: Right ventricular dysfunction in multiple trauma victims, *Am J Surg* 155:712-715, 1988.

Ferris SE, Konno M: In vitro validation of a thermodilution right ventricular ejection fraction method, *J Clin Monit* 8:74-80, 1992.

Headley JM, Diethorn ML: Right ventricular volumetric monitoring. In Osguthorpe S, editor: *AACN Clinical Issues in Critical Care Nursing*, Philadelphia, 1993, JB Lippincott.

Hines R: Monitoring right ventricular function, *Anesth Clin North Am* 6:851-863, 1988.

Hines R, Barash PG: Intraoperative right ventricular dysfunction detection with a right ventricular ejection fraction catheter, *J Clin Monit* 2:206-208, 1986.

Jones JW et al: Usefulness of right ventricular indices in early diagnosis of cardiac tamponade, *Ann Thorac Surg* 54:44-49, 1992.

Klinger JR, Hill NS: Right ventricular dysfunction in chronic obstructive pulmonary disease: evaluation and management, *Chest* 99:715-723, 1991.

Martyn JA et al: Right ventricular dysfunction in acute thermal injury, *Ann Surg* 191:330-335, 1980.

McIntyre KM, Sasahara AA: The hemodynamic response to pulmonary embolism in patients without prior cardiopulmonary disease, *Am J Cardiol* 28:288-294, 1971.

McIntyre K, Sasahara AA: Determinants of right ventricular function and hemodynamics after pulmonary embolism, *Chest* 65:534-543, 1974.

Mitsuo T, Shimazaki S, Matsuda H: Right ventricular dysfunction in septic patients, *Crit Care Med* 20:630-634, 1992.

Neubaur R, Schwartzkopff B, Strauer BE: Right ventricular performance in hypertension, *Eur Heart J* 13(suppl D):33-38, 1992.

Reuse C, Vincent JL, Pinsky MR: Measurements of right ventricular volumes during fluid challenge, *Chest* 98:1450-1454, 1990.

Schulman DS, Matthay RA: The right ventricle in pulmonary disease, *Cardiol Clin* 10:111-135, 1992.

Schulman DS et al: Effect of positive end-expiratory pressure on right ventricular performance: importance of baseline right ventricular function, *Am J Med* 84:57-67, 1988.

Sibbald W, Driedger A: Right ventricular function

in acute disease states: pathophysiological considerations, *Crit Care Med* 11(5):339-345, 1983.

Skowronski EW et al: Right and left ventricular function after cardiac transplantation: changes during and after rejection, *Circulation* 84:2409-2417, 1991.

Spinale FG et al: Right ventricular function computed by thermodilution and ventriculography, *J Thorac Cardiovasc Surg* 99:141-152, 1990.

Starling RC et al: Thermodilution measures of right ventricular ejection fraction and volumes in heart transplant recipients: a comparison with radionuclide angiography, *J Heart Lung Transplant* 11:1140-1146, 1992.

Stojnic BB et al: Left ventricular filling characteristics in pulmonary hypertension: a new mode of ventricular interaction, *Br Heart J* 68:16-20, 1992.

Thompson EP, White PD: The commonest cause of hypertrophy of the right ventricle: left ventricular strain and failure, *Am Heart J* 12:641, 1936.

Vitolo E et al: Two-dimensional echocardiographic evaluation of right ventricular ejection fraction: comparison between three different methods, *Acta Cardiol* 43:469-480, 1988.

Vlahakes GJ, Turley K, Hoffman JIE: The pathophysiology of failure in acute ventricular hypertension: hemodynamic and biochemical correlates, *Circulation* 63:87-95, 1981.

Weber KT et al: Contractile mechanics and interaction of the right and left ventricles, *Am J Cardiol* 47:685, 1981.

Weber KT et al: The right ventricle: physiologic and pathophysiologic considerations, *Crit Care Med* 11:323-328, 1983.

Weyman AE: *Right ventricle.* In Weyman AE, editor: *Cross-sectional echocardiography,* Philadelphia, 1982, Lea & Febiger.

Chapter 10

Monitoring of Oxygenation

The function and viability of all mammalian cells depend on a continuing supply of oxygen in amounts equal to or greater than their needs. When oxygen delivery becomes inadequate, cellular metabolism continues anaerobically at the price of critical biochemical changes within the cell. Some of these changes result in increased lactic acid accumulation, which further inhibits normal mitochondrial metabolism, and a vicious cycle ensues. For this reason, assessment and monitoring of the adequacy of oxygenation are of primary importance in the care and management of all critically ill patients. Technology now permits continuous bedside monitoring of both arterial and mixed venous oxygen saturation, tissue oxygen tension, and continuous or intermittent cardiac output determinations to closely assess overall tissue oxygenation. From these measurements, calculations of the amount of oxygen consumed ($\dot{V}o_2$) by the tissues can be determined, and interventions aimed at optimizing oxygenation can be made.

OXYGEN DELIVERY ($\dot{D}o_2$)

Oxygen delivery ($\dot{D}o_2$), the amount of oxygen delivered to the tissues each minute, is one of the primary functions of the cardiopulmonary system. The delivery of oxygen from the lungs to the tissues depends on the blood flow (cardiac output), as well as the content of oxygen in the blood. The oxygen content, in turn, is determined by the hemoglobin concentration and the oxygen saturation of the hemoglobin (Fig. 10-1), which is expressed by the formula:

$$\dot{D}o_2 = CO \times Cao_2 \times 10$$

where:

$\dot{D}o_2$ = Oxygen delivery (ml/min)
CO = Cardiac output (L/min)
Cao_2 = Oxygen content of arterial blood (ml/dl)
10 = Conversion factoring dl to L

215

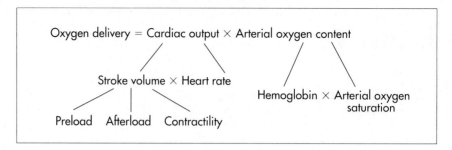

Fig. 10-1. Oxygen delivery—in milliliters per minute (ml/min)—is a product of the cardiac output and the oxygen content of arterial blood. In turn, cardiac output is a product of stroke volume and heart rate. The stroke volume is subsequently determined by the preload, afterload, and contractility. The arterial oxygen content is a product of the patient's hemoglobin and oxygen saturation of arterial blood. Alterations in oxygen delivery can be achieved by manipulation of any of these parameters.

Cardiac Output

Cardiac output, the rate of blood flow from the heart to the lungs and systemic circulation per minute, is a major determinant of oxygen delivery. In general, the rate of blood flow is regulated on a moment-to-moment basis by the metabolic needs of each organ system. However, when cardiac output falls, oxygen delivery also falls. The role of cardiac output in maintaining the balance between oxygen delivery and oxygen demand is discussed in more detail in Chapter 8.

Arterial Oxygen Content (Cao_2)

The content, or total amount of oxygen, carried in arterial blood is the sum of the oxygen bound to the hemoglobin and the oxygen that is dissolved in plasma. The amount of oxygen carried by hemoglobin is determined by the total concentration of hemoglobin in blood and the percentage of total hemoglobin that combines with oxygen (arterial oxygen saturation). The content of oxygen can be measured directly or calculated as follows:

$$Cao_2 = \text{Hemoglobin} \times 1.34 \times Sao_2 + Pao_2 \times 0.003$$

where:

Cao_2 = Arterial oxygen content *(ml O_2/dl blood)*
1.34 = ml oxygen carried by each gram hemoglobin
Sao_2 = Arterial oxygen saturation (%)
Pao_2 = Partial pressure of oxygen in arterial blood (mm Hg)
0.003 = ml oxygen/mm Hg Pao_2

Normal arterial oxygen content is 18 to 20 ml/dl blood. The content of oxygen in venous blood is normally 14 to 16 ml/dl blood. The difference between these two oxygen content values is termed the arteriovenous oxygen difference (a-vDo_2) and often is used clinically as a gross indicator of perfusion. Normal a-vDo_2 difference ranges from 3 to 5.5 ml/dl. However, more important than the absolute value is the directional trend of changes in the a-vDo_2. If the a-vDo_2 increases (i.e., the venous oxygen content falls), it is often the result of decreased cardiac output. However, it also could be the result of decreased hemoglobin (caused by hemorrhage or hemodilution) or an increase in oxygen consumption.

Hemoglobin

As blood passes through the lungs, oxygen is taken up by both the hemoglobin and the plasma portion of the blood. Each heme molecule of hemoglobin can chemically and reversibly combine with four oxygen molecules. (If every heme molecule combines fully with oxygen, the hemoglobin is said to be *fully saturated* or 100% saturated with oxygen). This corresponds to a mean volume of approximately 1.34 ml of oxygen bound to every gram of hemoglobin. (Some confusion exists about the actual oxygen-combining capacity of hemoglobin, with reported values ranging from 1.34 ml/g to 1.39 ml/g. Throughout this text the original value of 1.34 ml O_2/g hemoglobin/dl blood will be used.) Thus a patient with a normal hemoglobin of 15 g/dl could carry 20 ml O_2/dl blood) via hemoglobin, if every heme molecule were fully saturated with oxygen (100% saturation).

The inverse relationship of hemoglobin concentration to blood flow constitutes an important consideration in terms of oxygen delivery. As hemoglobin concentration falls, blood viscosity and, hence, arterial resistance are reduced. This reduction in resistance (afterload) results in improved flow (cardiac output) at decreased myocardial work. This concept forms the basis of isovolemic hemodilution therapy.

Consequently, although a fall in hemoglobin implies a reduction in the oxygen-carrying capacity of blood, the associated rise in cardiac output may maintain overall $\dot{D}o_2$.

> **EXAMPLE:** ($\dot{D}o_2$)   750 ml/min = 14 g/dl × 1.34 × 1.00 × 4.0 × 10
> ($\dot{D}o_2$)   750 ml/min = 8 g/dl × 1.34 × 1.00 × 7.0 × 10

Arterial oxygen saturation (Sao_2)

The percentage of the total hemoglobin that combines or becomes saturated with oxygen is known as the oxygen saturation of blood. This is referred to as *functional* oxygen saturation of arterial blood, in that it considers only those hemoglobin molecules that are capable of binding with and transporting oxygen. The presence of other abnormal or *dysfunctional* hemoglobin, such as methemoglobin or carboxyhemoglobin, reduces the oxygen-carrying capacity of the hemoglobin molecules either by preventing oxygen from binding to hemoglobin or by interfering with the release of oxygen from hemoglobin. Methemoglobin is formed when the iron ion in the hemoglobin molecule is oxidized from the ferrous (Fe^{++}) to the ferric (Fe^{+++}) form. This may occur in the presence of certain toxic substances such as potassium chlorate, certain intravascular dyes, and nitroprusside, as well as in patients with familial methemoglobinemia. Carboxyhemoglobin is formed when carbon monoxide preferentially binds with hemoglobin, displacing oxygen from the hemoglobin molecule. This can occur in patients who are heavy smokers or patients suffering from smoke inhalation or carbon monoxide poisoning. (Increased levels of carboxyhemoglobin also can be seen in persons who are exposed to extended periods of heavy freeway traffic.) The oxygen saturation of hemoglobin can be measured directly by means of a spectrophotometer or oximeter, or it can be calculated from the measured Pa_{O_2} with use of a nomogram or oxyhemoglobin dissociation curve. Normal arterial oxygen saturation is 95% to 100%.

Oxygen also is carried in the plasma, where it is physically dissolved. The solubility coefficient of oxygen in human plasma is 0.003 ml/mm Hg partial pressure of arterial blood, if the patient is breathing room air. This amounts to approximately 0.25 ml O_2/dl at a normal Pa_{O_2}. Because this amount is so small, it is generally clinically ignored, particularly with the use of trend monitoring. (If oxygen were carried only in plasma, maintenance of normal oxygen delivery would require a flow rate in excess of 100 L/min!)

Oxyhemoglobin Dissociation Curve

Both the uptake and the release of oxygen by the hemoglobin molecules are represented visually by the oxyhemoglobin dissociation curve (Fig. 10-2), which relates the partial pressure of oxygen (P_{O_2}) in blood to the saturation of hemoglobin. The S-shape of the curve is a result of the increased affinity of hemoglobin for oxygen as more oxygen molecules combine with it, despite large alveolar P_{O_2} changes (the flat, upper portion of the curve) and the rapid unloading of oxygen from hemoglobin, with small changes in P_{O_2} (the steep, lower portion of the curve). In this way, the oxygen tension gradient necessary for the diffusion of oxygen from blood into the mitochondria is maintained. A normal uptake and release of oxygen by hemoglobin is characterized by a hemoglobin saturation of 50% when the P_{O_2} is 26.5 mm Hg. This is known as the P_{50} (see Fig. 10-2). Certain conditions can change this relationship, resulting in a shift of the oxyhemoglobin curve to the right or to the left, which thus changes the ability of the hemoglobin to either combine with or release oxygen. Changes in the P_{O_2} associated with a hemoglobin saturation of 50% have become a

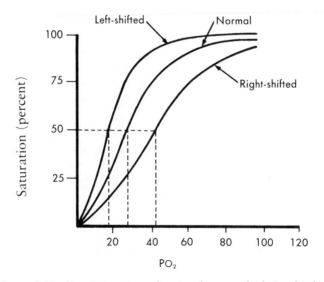

Fig. 10-2. Oxyhemoglobin dissociation curve showing the normal relationship between the P_{O_2} and oxygen saturation, as well as a left and right shift of the curve as defined by either a decreased or an increased P_{50}, respectively.

convenient way to express directional shifts in the dissociation curve. A right shift is defined by a hemoglobin saturation of 50% at a Pa_{O_2} higher than 26.5 mm Hg, inasmuch as less tightly bound oxygen is more easily released (see Fig. 10-2). A left shift, conversely, describes the hemoglobin saturation of 50% at a Pa_{O_2} less than 26 mm Hg, a low pressure gradient of oxygen that prevents diffusion and, thus, tissue oxygenation. These shifts, or changes in affinity, are affected by changes in body temperature, the pH of blood, and the level of 2,3-diphosphoglycerate (2,3-DPG) in blood. Table 10-1 lists factors that produce these changes or shifts in the oxyhemoglobin dissociation curve.

Normal Values of Oxygen Delivery ($\dot{D}_{O_2}$)

The amount of oxygen delivered to all the body tissues ($\dot{D}_{O_2}$) each minute can be calculated when the values for cardiac output, hemoglobin, and arterial saturation are known.

$$
\begin{aligned}
\textbf{EXAMPLE:} \quad & CO = 5 \text{ L/min} \\
& Hgb = 15 g/dl \\
& Sa_{O_2} = 99\% \\
10 \text{ dl/L} = & \text{ Conversion factor} \\
& \dot{D}_{O_2} = 5 \text{ L/min} \times 15 g/dl \times .99 \times 1.34 \times 10 \\
& \dot{D}_{O_2} = 5 \times 15 \times .99 \times 1.34 \times 10 \\
& \dot{D}_{O_2} = 995 \text{ ml/min}
\end{aligned}
$$

The quantity of oxygen delivered to the tissues each minute ($\dot{D}_{O_2}$) is a commonly used index of the performance of the cardiopulmonary transport system. However, it does not indicate the adequacy of oxygen in relation to tissue oxygen demands. Although low oxygen delivery values usually are associated with tissue hypoxia, normal or even high values do not necessarily ensure that oxygen delivery is adequate.

Diffusion

Oxygenation of tissues depends not only on the bulk transport of oxygen but also on the diffusion of oxygen from the capillaries to the mitochondria of the cell, where 80% to 90% of oxygen uptake occurs. This movement of oxygen occurs through passive diffusion and is determined primarily by the pressure gradient between the oxygen tension (P_{O_2}) in the capillaries and the tissues. Initially, capillary P_{O_2} nearly

Table 10-1. Factors affecting the position of the oxyhemoglobin dissociation curve

Left shift (increased affinity)	Right shift (decreased affinity)
Alkalosis ($\uparrow$ pH)	Acidosis ($\downarrow$ pH)
Hypocapnia ($\downarrow$ Pa_{CO_2})	Hypercapnia ($\uparrow$ Pa_{CO_2})
Decreased temperature	Increased temperature
Decreased 2,3-DPG	Increased 2,3-DPG
Hypophosphatemia	
Carbon monoxide	
Sepsis	

Pa$_{CO_2}$, Arterial oxygen pressure; *2,3-DPG*, 2,3-diphosphoglycerate.

equals arterial P_{O_2}, but it falls as oxygen is extracted by the tissues. Mitochondrial P_{O_2} values in vivo are unknown but are considered to be quite low.

Other determinants of oxygen diffusion include capillary surface areas, the distance between the capillary and the mitochondria, and the oxygen consumption of the tissues. Oxygen diffusion is impaired when Pa_{O_2} is low or when interstitial edema or inflammation increases the distance between the capillary and the cell.

OXYGEN DEMAND

The amount or quantity of oxygen needed or demanded by the tissues to maintain aerobic metabolism is determined primarily by their metabolic rate. This, in turn, is determined by the rate of cellular activity. Normally, changes in oxygen needs or demands are regulated, in an automatic fashion, by changes in blood flow. Under normal resting conditions, global $\dot{D}_{O_2}$ is more than adequate to meet tissue oxygen demands for aerobic metabolism (Table 10-2).

Oxygen Consumption ($\dot{V}_{O_2}$)

Whole body oxygen consumption ($\dot{V}_{O_2}$) is simply the amount of oxygen actually used by the tissues per minute of time. Normally, at rest, the tissues consume approximately 25% of the available oxygen. Therefore, if oxygen delivery is normally about 1000 ml/min, oxygen consumption at rest is approximately 25% of this, or 250 cc/min. During exercise or other forms of stress, oxygen consumption may increase about threefold, using about 75% of the available oxygen.

Oxygen consumption is increased by numerous conditions, as well as interventions, therapeutic procedures, and various other stresses imposed on hospitalized patients. Oxygen consumption may increase from 25% to 100% in critically ill patients. Increased work of breathing can increase $\dot{V}_{O_2}$ by 25%; severe infections increase $\dot{V}_{O_2} \geq 60\%$; and shivering can increase $\dot{V}_{O_2} > 100\%$. (See Table 10-4 for various interventions that also increase $\dot{V}_{O_2}$ in critically ill patients.) In fact, failure of $\dot{V}_{O_2}$ to increase in the face of increasing oxygen demands, or a persistent decline in $\dot{V}_{O_2}$ not associated with a decrease in metabolic rate, is associated with a poor prognosis.

$\dot{V}_{O_2}/\dot{D}_{O_2}$ Relationships

The magnitude of the normal relationship between $\dot{D}_{O_2}$ and $\dot{V}_{O_2}$ (about $4:1$) provides sufficient reserve to maintain $\dot{V}_{O_2}$ *independent* of $\dot{D}_{O_2}$ over a wide range of

Table 10-2. Oxygen consumption, blood flow, and percentage of total flow to various organs

Organ	Flow (ml/min)	$\dot{V}_{O_2}$ (ml/min)	Cardiac output (%)
Heart	210	26	10
Brain	750-800	50-60	15
Kidney	1200-1300	15-20	20
Muscle	750-800	50	15
Liver	500	65-75	10

delivery values. This is illustrated in Fig. 10-3, which depicts a relatively constant $\dot{V}_{O_2}$ (plateau) despite decreases in oxygen delivery. However, further decreases in $\dot{D}_{O_2}$, below some critical level, eventually result in a linear fall in $\dot{V}_{O_2}$. This area of $\dot{V}_{O_2}$ decline is termed *supply-dependent* $\dot{V}_{O_2}$ because the amount of oxygen used is limited by the amount of oxygen delivered.

The point at which $\dot{V}_{O_2}$ abruptly falls and becomes limited by the amount of oxygen delivered is termed the *critical level* of oxygen delivery ($\dot{D}_{O_2\ crit}$). It represents maximal oxygen extraction and typically is associated with anaerobic metabolism and lactic acidosis. This critical level of $\dot{D}_{O_2}$ varies among individuals and depends somewhat on the cause of the fall in $\dot{D}_{O_2}$. A decline in $\dot{D}_{O_2}$ as a result of anemia or low cardiac output is tolerated better than a similar decline as a result of hypoxemia, and it may be associated with a lower $\dot{D}_{O_2\ crit}$.

Most studies of $\dot{D}_{O_2\ crit}$ have been performed in animals, and little data exist regarding critical $\dot{D}_{O_2}$ levels in human beings. Shibutani and colleagues reported a critical $\dot{D}_{O_2}$ of 330 ml/min/m^2 in relatively healthy anesthetized humans before cardiac bypass surgery. Other clinical studies have reported $\dot{D}_{O_2\ crit}$ levels ranging from 7 to 15 ml/kg/min. Such differences in values likely reflect variations in metabolic rates and oxygen extraction abilities. It can be assumed, however, that the $\dot{D}_{O_2\ crit}$ of critically ill patients is significantly higher than normal.

Some critically ill patients may exhibit a pathologic *supply-dependent* $\dot{V}_{O_2}$ in which $\dot{V}_{O_2}$ is *dependent* on $\dot{D}_{O_2}$ over a wide range of $\dot{D}_{O_2}$ values and does not become *independent* of $\dot{D}_{O_2}$ except at very high levels of oxygen delivery, if at all. This concept is depicted in Fig. 10-3 as a very shallow slope of the supply-dependent line. This pathologic response is due to the fixed oxygen extraction ratio (O_2ER) present in many critically ill patients.

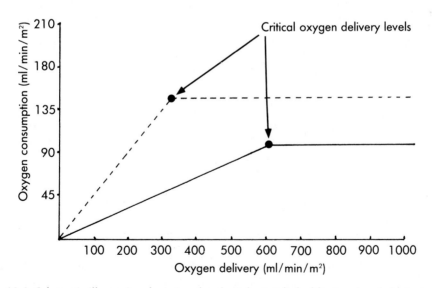

Fig. 10-3. Schematic illustration depicting the physiologic *(slashed line)* and pathologic *(solid line)* relationships between oxygen consumption ($\dot{V}_{O_2}$) and oxygen delivery ($\dot{D}_{O_2}$). The critical level of oxygen delivery ($\dot{D}_{O_2\ crit}$) defines that level of $\dot{D}_{O_2}$ at which $\dot{V}_{O_2}$ abruptly falls and $\dot{V}_{O_2}$ becomes dependent on $\dot{D}_{O_2}$. This critical level is substantially higher in certain pathologic states in which oxygen extraction is fixed.

MAINTAINING OXYGEN SUPPLY AND DEMAND BALANCE

As previously mentioned, increases in oxygen demand by the tissues normally are met by increases in oxygen supply or delivery ($\dot{D}o_2$). Remembering the three components of oxygen delivery: cardiac output, hemoglobin concentration, and arterial oxygen saturation — it is apparent that there are several ways in which oxygen supply can be increased to meet increased oxygen demands.

Cardiac Output

As tissue demands for oxygen increase, cardiac output automatically increases, primarily via vasoregulatory mechanisms. Normally, blood flow can increase by a factor of at least three (and even higher in exercise). This ability represents the primary compensatory mechanism involved in maintaining the balance between oxygen supply and demand. Clearly, increasing cardiac output up to 15 L/min (three times normal) can maintain very high levels of oxygen delivery, if necessary. Many critically ill patients, however, are without such cardiac reserve or already are functioning at maximum cardiac performance.

Hemoglobin

Compensatory increases in hemoglobin can occur over time (e.g., in persons living at high altitudes) to maintain adequate oxygen delivery, but because this adjustment cannot occur quickly in response to acute increases in oxygen demand, it is not applicable to the critically ill patient.

Arterial Oxygen Saturation

Normally, arterial blood becomes fully or almost fully saturated with oxygen (97% to 100%) as it passes through the lungs. If this does not occur, hypoxemia results. Inherent compensatory mechanisms such as increased depth and frequency of respiration, can improve arterial oxygen saturation, but in general, this mechanism is limited, particularly in acutely ill patients.

Oxygen Extraction Ratio (O_2ER)

If increased oxygen demands are not met with adequate increases in oxygen supply, by means of increased cardiac output, the tissues extract more oxygen from the circulating hemoglobin. The average amount of oxygen extracted by the tissues is normally about 25% (22% to 32%). This ratio is determined by either of the following formulae:

$$O_2ER = \frac{(\dot{V}o_2)}{(\dot{D}o_2)}$$

where:

O_2ER = Oxygen extraction ratio
$\dot{V}o_2$ = Oxygen consumption
$\dot{D}o_2$ = Oxygen delivery

or

$$O_2ER = \frac{Cao_2 - Cvo_2}{Cao_2}$$

where:

    Cao_2 = Arterial oxygen content
    Cvo_2 = Venous oxygen content

As a compensatory mechanism, O_2ER increases to maintain effective tissue oxygenation. The maximum O_2ER that can be obtained by critically ill patients is unknown and depends on numerous factors, but it is not likely to exceed 45% and may be as low as 25%. An increasing level of O_2ER, or a value $>32\%$, indicates that the tissues are extracting more oxygen per unit of blood flow as a result of an imbalance in oxygen supply and demand. This imbalance may be caused by an increase in $\dot{V}o_2$ at the same or reduced $\dot{D}o_2$, or a decrease in $\dot{D}o_2$ with no change in the $\dot{V}o_2$.

A decreased O_2ER ($<22\%$) also may be due to an imbalance, with the $\dot{D}o_2$ substantially exceeding $\dot{V}o_2$. This may occur with conditions that reduce oxygen demands, such as anesthesia or hypothermia. However, it also may represent a pathologic condition in which the O_2ER becomes fixed despite increasing oxygen demands. This may occur in patients with sepsis, adult respiratory distress syndrome (ARDS), or multiple organ failure secondary to a maldistribution of systemic or microcirculatory blood flow.

When the O_2ER is maximal, or unable to increase appropriately, $\dot{V}o_2$ falls. As previously discussed, this point identifies the critical $\dot{D}o_2$ level and pathologic supply-dependency $\dot{V}o_2$. However, some controversy exists regarding the validity of this concept inasmuch as not all studies support such a finding. One major criticism of this concept of a linear relationship between $\dot{D}o_2$ and $\dot{V}o_2$ concerns the mathematic coupling error that results from using similar variables to calculate both parameters. In fact, the only variable that differs in the equations for calculating $\dot{V}o_2$ and $\dot{D}o_2$ is the venous oxygen saturation! Direct measurement of $\dot{V}o_2$ by calorimetry avoids this error but can incorporate other technical errors. Studies in which both methods of measuring $\dot{V}o_2$ were compared have reported conflicting results.

In reviewing the components of the formula for O_2ER, it is apparent that venous oxygen saturation (Svo_2) is directly related to the O_2ER in an inverse fashion. As O_2ER increases above a normal value of approximately 25%, Svo_2 likewise decreases below its normal value of 75%.

When the partial pressure of oxygen in blood reaches approximately 20 mm Hg, the diffusion gradient between the cell and capillary blood may be insufficient for appropriate transfer of oxygen out of the capillary and into the tissue. In reviewing a normal oxyhemoglobin dissociation curve (see Fig. 10-2), it is apparent that a partial pressure of venous oxygen (Pvo_2) of 20 mm Hg corresponds to a venous oxygen saturation of 30%. Therefore, oxygen extraction by the tissues can increase until the oxygen saturation of blood is approximately 30%, after which point further extraction is limited.

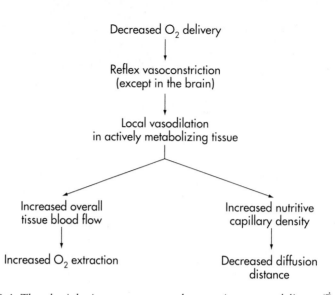

Fig. 10-4. The physiologic responses to a decrease in oxygen delivery ($\dot{D}o_2$).
From Dantzker DR, Gutierrez G: *Respir Care* 30:456-461, 1985.

Vasoregulatory Response

In addition to systemic mechanisms, local vasoregulatory reflexes are capable of maintaining blood flow and, therefore, oxygenation to critical tissues (Fig. 10-4). As $\dot{D}o_2$ falls, arterial chemoreceptors stimulate reflex vasoconstriction, which maintains systemic blood pressure and diverts flow from less demanding tissues. At a local level, arteriolar vessels in actively metabolizing tissues dilate, providing increased flow and oxygen. Arteriolar vasodilation also results in the recruitment of more capillary reserve, increasing capillary density, and decreasing diffusion distances.

Summary

The first compensatory mechanism called upon to maintain a balance between oxygen demand and supply is an increase in cardiac output. If this does not supply adequate oxygen delivery relative to demands, *or* if cardiac dysfunction prevents such an increase in cardiac output, the second compensatory mechanism is evoked. This mechanism is increased oxygen extraction by the tissues, resulting in decreased saturation of venous blood returning to the heart. Healthy tissues can extract nearly three times more oxygen than usual, until Po_2 falls to approximately 20 mm Hg. However, this mechanism is ineffective in several pathologic conditions in which oxygen extraction is fixed and limited.

TISSUE HYPOXIA

Tissue hypoxia occurs when oxygen is delivered either in insufficient quantity to meet the tissues' demands or at an insufficient pressure for diffusion to occur. Insufficient oxygen uptake by the tissues limits the conversion of adenosine diphosphate (ADP) to adenosine triphosphate (ATP), the essential energy source for

Table 10-3. Causes and associated conditions of tissue hypoxia

Type of hypoxia	Cause	Conditions
Hypoxic	↓ Sao_2	Pulmonary disease Pulmonary edema ↓ Fio_2 Carbon monoxide poisoning
Anemic	↓ Hemoglobin	Hemorrhage Anemia Dysfunctional hemoglobins
Stagnant	↓ CO	Cardiac disease Dysrhythmias Drugs ↑ SVR
Dysoxic	↓ O_2ER a-v shunting	Sepsis ARDS MOF
Histotoxic	Cell poisoning	Cyanide poisoning

Sao_2, Arterial oxygen saturation; Fio_2, fractional inspired oxygen concentration; *CO*, cardiac output; *SVR*, systemic vascular resistance; O_2ER, oxygen extraction ratio; *a-v*, arteriovenous; *ARDS*, adult respiratory distress syndrome; *MOF*, multiple organ failure.

metabolic processes. Anaerobic metabolism is initiated and glucose is metabolized to pyruvate in the cytoplasm. Pyruvate subsequently is reduced to lactate, which spills over into the blood. Although lactate can provide a small amount of energy, it is insufficient for high energy demands, and an energy debt develops. In addition, lactic acid results in intracellular acidosis, which impairs cellular integrity and leads to tissue and organ dysfunction and eventual failure.

Causes of tissue hypoxia are listed in Table 10-3, along with commonly associated clinical conditions.

Indicators of Tissue Hypoxia

Lactate

The time-honored method of assessing the adequacy or inadequacy of tissue oxygenation is the measurement of the concentration of lactate in blood. Normal arterial lactate level is < 1 mmol. Lactate levels > 1.5 mmol indicate inadequate $\dot{D}o_2$, and levels > 2.0 mmol are associated with increased mortality. However, lactate concentrations can be elevated in other conditions, such as respiratory alkalosis and liver disease. In addition, lactate accumulation is a fairly late marker of tissue hypoxia and may not be elevated even when some organs, are hypoxic because of insufficient blood flow.

Gastric intramucosal pH

Some clinicians assess tissue oxygenation by measuring the pH level of the gastric mucosa with a nasogastrically placed tonometer. As gastrointestinal hypoperfusion

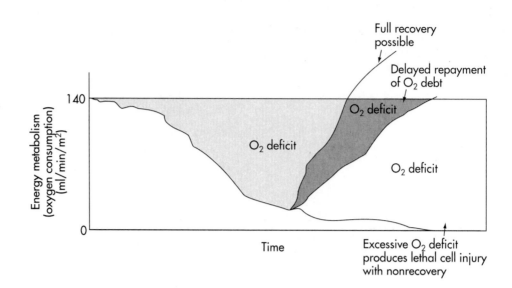

Fig. 10-5. Diagrammatic representation of the concept of oxygen (O_2) debt that occurs as oxygen consumption ($\dot{V}o_2$) falls below the patient's oxygen requirements over a period of time. If this deficit is corrected rapidly with interventions that increase $\dot{V}o_2$ to levels *above* baseline requirements, full recovery is possible. (See overshoot.) If the O_2 debt continues or increases over a longer period of time, significant organ damage occurs. If the O_2 debt remains uncorrected for a prolonged period, lethal cell injury prevents patient recovery.

From Siegel JA: *Trauma: emergency surgery and critical care,* New York, 1992, Churchill Livingstone.

and hypoxia develop, the pH of the gastric mucosa falls. Gastric mucosal pH levels <7.32 have been correlated with decreased regional oxygen delivery.

Venous oxygen saturation (Svo_2)

As oxygen delivery falls, O_2ER, if not impaired by underlying disease processes, increases. As a result, the saturation in blood returning to the heart via the venous circulation is reduced. When the arterial oxygen saturation (Sao_2) is maintained close to 100%, Svo_2 provides information on the patient's O_2ER. An Svo_2 <50% probably denotes significant potential tissue hypoxia.

Oxygen Debt

An oxygen debt develops when inadequate oxygen uptake relative to oxygen demand occurs over a period of time (Fig. 10-5). As the duration of oxygen deficiency increases, the chances for survival decrease.

The oxygen debt in critically ill patients is determined by subtracting the patient's actual $\dot{V}o_2$ (calculated or measured) from the patient's predicted $\dot{V}o_2$ (Table 10-4). Whereas normal resting $\dot{V}o_2$ is 250 ml/min (140 ml/min/m²), this value is much higher in critically ill patients. Although exact $\dot{V}o_2$ values for each critical condition are unknown, numerous studies of $\dot{V}o_2$ measurements in critically ill patients have provided valuable information regarding expected $\dot{V}o_2$ changes. For example, $\dot{V}o_2$ increases 10% to 13% for each degree of centigrade temperature elevation above normal. Thus the expected $\dot{V}o_2$ of a patient with a temperature of 39°C would be *at least* 168 ml/min/m² ([.10 × 2° C × 140 ml/min/m²] + 140 ml/min/m²). Typically,

Table 10-4. Increases in energy expenditure ($\dot{V}o_2$) related to various ICU interventions

Activity	% ↑ Increase of energy expenditure ($\dot{V}o_2$ and $\dot{V}co_2$)
Bed scale weights	36 (± 12)
Repositioning	31 (± 11)
Portable chest x-ray	22 (± 16)
Bed bath	19 (± 11)
Visitors	18 (± 18)
Agitation/restlessness	18 (± 8)
Nursing assessments	11 (± 7)
Chest physiotherapy	10 (± 10)
Dressing change	10 (± 9)

Modified from Swinamer DL et al: *Crit Care Med* 15:637-643, 1987.

multiple conditions are simultaneously present in the critically ill patient to increase $\dot{V}o_2$ far above that observed in healthy resting adults. All possible factors should be considered in calculating the patient's expected $\dot{V}o_2$.

The patient's oxygen debt (the difference between the actual and predicted $\dot{V}o_2$) must be identified and corrected rapidly to achieve full recovery. This is accomplished by manipulating the parameters of oxygen delivery to increase $\dot{D}o_2$ and thereby increase $\dot{V}o_2$ to values that exceed the patient's expected $\dot{V}o_2$ value (Table 10-5). According to Siegel (see Siegel reference), a supranormal period is necessary to "repay the debt" that developed during the ischemic period.

THERAPEUTIC INTERVENTIONS

The maintenance of a balanced oxygen supply/demand ratio frequently necessitates therapeutic interventions aimed at either increasing one of the three components of oxygen delivery or decreasing oxygen demands.

Table 10-5 lists some of the therapeutic ways these determinants are manipulated.

Oxygen Challenge Test

In patients suspected of having insufficient oxygen uptake or experiencing supply-dependent $\dot{V}o_2$, an oxygen challenge test should be considered. This intervention consists of deliberately increasing $\dot{D}o_2$ and observing the $\dot{V}o_2$ response. If $\dot{V}o_2$ increases >10 to 20 ml/min/m^2 in response to an increase in $\dot{D}o_2$ of >50 ml/min/m$_2$, $\dot{V}o_2$ is considered to be supply-dependent and further interventions are necessary to maximize $\dot{D}o_2$ until $\dot{V}o_2$ plateaus or increases <10 ml/min/m^2. This is especially important in patients with hyperlactemia.

Interventions that increase $\dot{D}o_2$ should, ideally, be targeted at the determinant of $\dot{D}o_2$ (cardiac output, hemoglobin, or Sao_2) that is inadequate. For example, in a patient with inadequate preload, a fluid challenge consisting of rapid administration of either 100-ml albumin (25%), 500-ml albumin (5%), 500-ml hetastarch (6%), or 2000-ml crystalloids is appropriate to increase cardiac output and therefore oxygen delivery.

Table 10-5. Therapeutic manipulations to increase oxygen delivery

Determinant	Therapeutic intervention
Cardiac output	↑ Preload (volume) ↓ Afterload (arterial vasodilators, calcium channel blockers, ACE inhibitors, counterpulsation) ↑ Contractility (positive inotropic agents, calcium) Maintain heart rate 50-100 beats/min (beta blockers, calcium channel blockers, pacemaker, atropine)
Arterial oxygen saturation (Sao_2)	Airway control ↑ Fio_2 Mechanical ventilation, CPAP, PEEP Hyperbarism ECMO
Hemoglobin	Blood or blood products Hemoglobin solutions
Oxygen demands	↓ Work of breathing (sedation, mechanical ventilation, paralysis) ↓ Fever Prevent/treat shivering Minimize/treat pain and anxiety Space necessary activities Eliminate unnecessary activities Relaxation therapy Music

ACE, Angiotensin-converting enzyme; *Fio₂*, fractional inspired oxygen concentration; *CPAP*, continuous positive airway pressure; *PEEP*, positive end-expiratory pressure; *ECMO*, extracorporeal membrane oxygenation.

One commonly used method to rapidly increase $\dot{D}o_2$ in an oxygen challenge test is the administration of dobutamine 5 µg/kg/min. However, the thermogenic effects of catecholamines directly affect $\dot{V}o_2$ as well as $\dot{D}o_2$ and may confound the issue of dependency.

Therapeutic Goals

Traditional therapeutic goals, which consist of normal values of physiologic parameters, have been shown to be inadequate in critically ill patients who have increased metabolic requirements associated with the inflammatory response, tissue repair, temperature elevations, and possible prior oxygen debt. Table 10-6 lists "supranormal" values identified by Shoemaker to be associated with improved survival in high-risk surgical patients. Other studies have confirmed the benefit of using "supranormal" values of physiologic parameters as therapeutic goals.

MONITORING TECHNIQUES
Oxygen Consumption ($\dot{V}o_2$)

Oxygen consumption can be measured directly by analyzing the amount and composition of the patient's inspired and expired air over a known period of time.

Table 10-6. Therapeutic goals of physiologic parameters of oxygen delivery in critically ill patients

Parameter	Goal
Cardiac index (CI)	>4.5 L/min/m^2
Oxygen delivery ($\dot{D}o_2$)	>600 ml/min/m^2
Oxygen consumption ($\dot{V}o_2$)	>170 ml/min/m^2
Total blood volume	>3.2 L/m^2 (males)
	>2.8 L/m^2 (females)

From Shoemaker WC: *Am J Crit Care* 1:38-53, 1992.

Other techniques have been developed to directly measure oxygen consumption in patients receiving ventilation. However, because of the technical difficulties involved in directly measuring oxygen consumption in critically ill patients, indirect calculation of $\dot{V}o_2$ with the Fick formula frequently is used in the critical care setting. The Fick formula is based on Adolf Fick's equation for cardiac output determination, whereby the difference between the oxygen content of arterial and venous blood in the pulmonary circulation reflects oxygen uptake per unit of blood as it flows through the lungs. This can be expressed as follows:

$$CO(L/min) = \frac{O_2 \text{ consumption (ml/min)}}{(\text{Arterial } O_2 \text{ content} - \text{Venous } O_2 \text{ content})}$$

Rearrangement of this formula is used to calculate oxygen consumption when cardiac output and arterial and venous oxygen contents are determined.

$$\dot{V}o_2 = CO \times \text{Arterial } O_2 \text{ content} - \text{Venous } O_2 \text{ content} \times 10$$

EXAMPLE: CO = 5 L/min
Arterial O_2 content = 20 ml/dl
Venous O_2 content = 15 ml/dl
$$\therefore \dot{V}o_2 = 5 \times (20 - 15) \times 10$$
or
$$\dot{V}o_2 = 250 \text{ ml/min}$$

This estimate of $\dot{V}o_2$ requires simultaneous and precise measurement of cardiac output and hemoglobin, as well as arterial and venous oxygen saturations. Obviously, this is not always possible in the critical care setting, resulting in estimations of $\dot{V}o_2$ that can vary by as much as 25% or more from direct measurement.

Pulse Oximetry (Sao$_2$)
Principle

The normal loading of oxygen into the arterial blood occurs as blood circulates through the lungs and is exposed to high concentrations of oxygen in the alveoli. The pressure difference between oxygen in the alveoli and the oxygen in the precapillary blood causes oxygen to diffuse into the blood where it combines with the hemoglobin molecules. Hypoxemia—inadequate loading of oxygen—results in a reduction in the oxygen saturation of the hemoglobin (less than 95%). Assessment of arterial oxygenation can be done by blood gas analysis, which requires removal of 5 to 10 ml of blood for each analysis. More important, analyzed results often are not available for 20 to 30 minutes, at which time appropriate therapy may no longer be appropriate or may be harmfully delayed. Continuous noninvasive monitoring of the oxygen saturation percentage of arterial blood (Sao_2) provides early and immediate detection of decreases in oxygen saturation and impending hypoxemia.

Technique

Noninvasive continuous measurement of the oxygen saturation of arterial blood can be accomplished with the use of a pulse oximeter that senses the light absorption differences between nonsaturated and saturated hemoglobin. A special sensor (Fig. 10-6) that contains two light-emitting diodes (LEDs) and a light detector is positioned so that the light emitter and light detector are directly across from one another on opposite sides of an arteriolar bed. (For adults, this is either on the thumb, one of the fingers, on the bridge of the nose, or on the ear; for infants, a finger, toe, foot, tongue, or central portion of the cheek can be used.) The LEDs emit a red light (approximately 660 nm) and an infrared light (approximately 910 nm). The light detector continuously measures the amount of each type of light that passes through the tissue. Saturated or oxyhemoglobin absorbs more infrared light, whereas unsaturated or deoxyhemoglobin absorbs more red light. When pulsatile blood is not present, the amount of light that is absorbed by tissue, bone, and venous blood remains constant and serves as a baseline for the increase in light absorbency that occurs as a pulse of arterial blood flows to the tissue. The light-absorbence differences between the oxyhemoglobin (saturated) and deoxyhemoglobin (unsaturated) are then described quantitatively according to Beer's law, resulting in a determination of the percent saturation of arterial hemoglobin (Sao_2). In addition, the oximeter automatically measures the pulse rate.

Equipment. Fig. 10-6 illustrates the various sensing devices used to measure Sao_2 by means of pulse oximetry. The sensor is connected directly to a pulse oximeter (Fig. 10-7) that provides visual and auditory data regarding the Sao_2 and the pulse rate. A beep accompanies each heartbeat. A change in the tone of the beep occurs when Sao_2 falls. This alerts the clinician to impending hypoxemia even when out of view of the monitor.

Preparation. No calibration of equipment is required inasmuch as the diodes are precalibrated and coded during the manufacturing process. In addition, frequent and automatic calibration checks are performed internally. Skin preparation for place-ment of the sensor is not necessary although the skin should be dry; wiping the skin with an alcohol wipe is usually sufficient. Skin pigmentation or clear or light-colored (nonfrosted) nail polish does not interfere with accurate oximetric measurement of the arterial pulse. Sensors are best placed on an extremity without an arterial catheter or blood pressure cuff that would either continuously or intermittently reduce arterial flow distally. Faster response times, with earlier detection of desaturation, have been noted when sensors are placed on the thumb or ear in adults or on the tongue or cheek in children. (See Young et al. and Reynolds et al. references.)

Table 10-7 lists some of the problems, as well as causes and recommended actions,

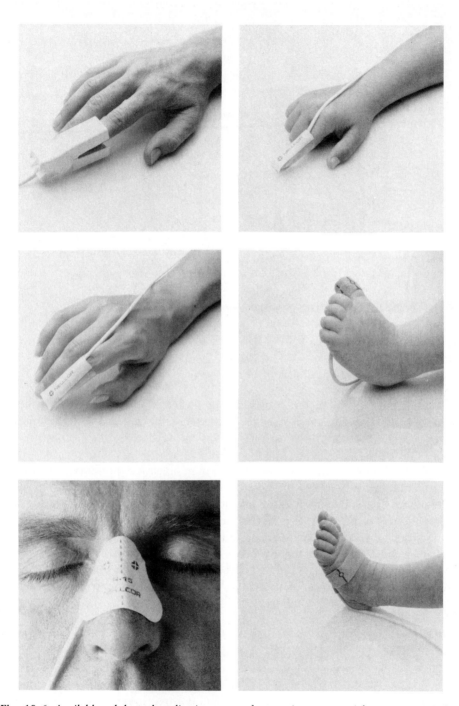

Fig. 10-6. Available adult and pediatric sensors for continuous arterial oxygen saturation monitoring with use of pulse oximetry.

Courtesy Nellcor, Inc., Hayward, Calif.

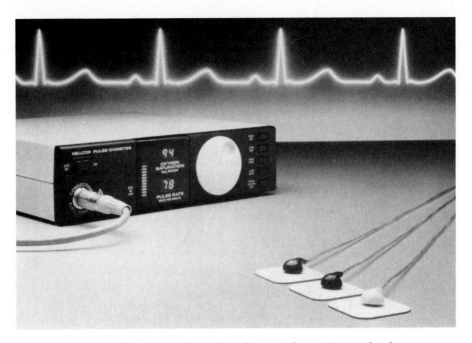

Fig. 10-7. A pulse oximeter displaying the arterial saturation and pulse rate.
Courtesy Nellcor, Inc., Hayward, Calif.

associated with pulse oximetry. To avoid finger necrosis, a spring-clip sensor should be moved every 2 hours and a standard finger sensor moved every 4 to 6 hours.

Clinical application

The use of continuous pulse oximetry for noninvasive monitoring of arterial oxygen saturation is an important monitoring tool in the care of all critically ill adults and children. It is widely used in the operating room, postanesthesia care units, and intensive care units, where patients are likely to experience anticipated or unanticipated periods of hypoxia. Continuous Sao_2 monitoring can provide immediate and early warning of impending hypoxemia. It is also useful in assessment of ventilatory management and the effects of other therapeutic interventions. Reductions in arterial saturation to 95% or less should prompt immediate assessment of the patient as well as the adequacy of oxygen delivery.

Continuous Venous Oximetry (Svo_2)
Principle

The amount of oxygen remaining in the venous blood reflects the oxygen used by the tissues. With a normal oxygen delivery of 1000 ml and a normal extraction of about 25%, mixed venous blood remains approximately 75% saturated with oxygen. When mixed venous blood remains 60% to 80% saturated with oxygen, it generally is assumed that oxygen delivery is adequate for the tissue's needs. However, in critically ill patients with oxygen-extraction impairment (such as sepsis or ARDS) this assumption is incorrect, making interpretation of this parameter difficult.

SVO$_2$ levels below 60% occur because of increased oxygen extraction by the tissues. When SVO$_2$ continues to fall to 50% or less, lactic acidosis can occur as a result of anaerobic metabolism. The precise SVO$_2$ level at which anaerobic metabolism and lactic acidosis begin varies, but an SVO$_2$ of less than 40% likely represents the limits of compensation and impending lactic acidosis. Generally, an SVO$_2$ of less than 30%

Table 10-7. Troubleshooting the pulse oximeter

Problem	Possible cause	Recommended action
? Inaccurate Sao$_2$	Excessive patient movement	Quiet patient, if possible. Check security of sensor; replace if necessary. Move sensor to different site. Use an adhesive sensor. Immobilize monitoring site. Use ECG signal synchronization. Select a longer (10-15 sec) averaging time, if possible.
	High carboxyhemoglobin or methemoglobin levels	Measure dysfunctional hemoglobin levels. Measure arterial blood gas.
	Reduced arterial blood flow	Do not place sensor on same side as indwelling arterial catheter or blood pressure cuff. Ensure sensor is not too tight.
	Electrocautery interference	Move sensor as far as possible from cautery cable; change sites if necessary. Check sensor; replace if damp. Place oximeter plug into a different circuit than cautery unit.
	Excessive ambient light (surgical lamps, heating lamps, bilirubin lights, bright fluorescent lights, direct sunlight)	Cover sensor with opaque material.
	Fungal infection of nail of finger	Move sensor to a different site.
Loss of pulse signal	Constriction by sensor	Check sensor; move to a different site or change type of sensor used.
	Reduced arterial blood flow	Same as above.
	Excessive ambient light	Same as above.
	Severe anemia	Check patient's hemoglobin.
	Hypothermia	Warm monitoring site and replace sensor.
	Shock (hypotension, vasoconstriction)	Check patient's condition, including vital signs.
Inaccurate pulse rate	Excessive patient motion	Same as above.
	Pronounced dicrotic notch on arterial waveform	Move sensor to a different site.
	Poor-quality ECG signal	Check ECG leads; replace if necessary.
	Electrocautery interference	Same as above.

(20 mm Hg) indicates insufficient oxygen availability to the tissues. Clinically, this degree of tissue hypoxia usually is accompanied by coma.

The oxygen saturation of venous blood varies, depending on the organ system it serves. Venous blood returning from high flow areas, such as the kidney or skin, have higher concentrations of oxygen than does venous blood from other areas (e.g., from the heart). Complete mixing of these varying oxygen saturations occurs in the right ventricle, making the pulmonary artery (PA) blood reflective of true *mixed* venous oxygen saturation. The oxygen saturation of PA blood is a flow-weighted average of all the different end-capillary oxygen saturations. Thus a normal mixed Svo_2 could be obtained despite tissue hypoxia of an individual organ.

Technique

The combination of fiberoptic technology with a modified 7.5- or 8-Fr thermodilution pulmonary artery catheter was first introduced in 1981. In addition to the standard features, this catheter has a lumen containing optical fibers that transmit light to and from the bloodstream. The light source consists of two or three diodes that emit alternating pulses of wavelengths of red light through one of the

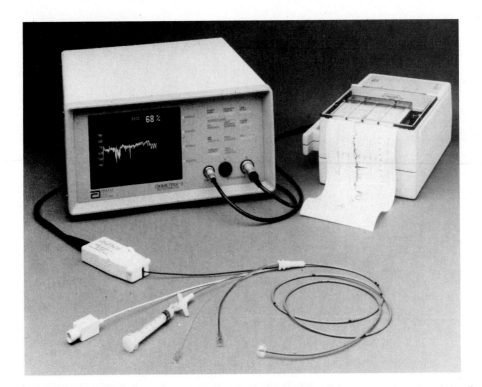

Fig. 10-8. A venous oxygen saturation (Svo_2) catheter showing the usual proximal and distal ports, as well as thermistor wires and a lumen for balloon inflation. The catheter is connected to an Svo_2 monitor with a digital readout of the current Svo_2 plus a graphic display of the frequently updated Svo_2. A small paper recorder attached to the monitor provides a hard copy of the graphic readings.

Courtesy Abbott Critical Care, Mountain View, Calif.

optical fibers. This light is absorbed, refracted by the hemoglobin constituents of the blood, and reflected back through the second optical fiber to the light detector. It is then converted to an electrical signal and transmitted to a remote data processor. The computed oxyhemoglobin saturation is averaged over a 5-second interval, updated every 1 to 2 seconds, and displayed digitally and graphically on a monitor, as well as on a slow-speed paper recorder. The recorded output also indicates the light intensity at the tip of the catheter. Changes in the light intensity signify a change in catheter position (i.e., against the wall of the vessel or spontaneous wedging), inadequate blood flow (thrombus at the tip of the catheter), or damage to the fiberoptic fibers. This light intensity indicator is valuable in troubleshooting problems with either oxygen saturation readings or PA pressure readings.

Equipment. A fiberoptic thermodilution PA catheter and a microprocessor with a strip chart recorder or data display and storage system are needed for this procedure (Fig. 10-8).

Preparation. The manufacturer's recommendations for preparation should be followed before the fiberoptic catheter is inserted in the patient. The catheter should be handled gently, avoiding any sharp bending of the catheter to prevent damage to the optical fibers. The balloon and thermostat wires of the catheter also should be checked, as discussed on p. 180. Although the fiberoptic PA catheter is somewhat stiffer than the standard PA catheter, it compares favorably in both ease of insertion and complication rates.

Table 10-8. Various causes of alterations in venous oxygen saturation (Svo_2)

	Svo_2 reading (%)	Physiologic alteration	Clinical causes
High	80-95	↓ O_2 consumption	Hypothermia
			Anesthesia
			Induced muscular paralysis
			Sepsis/ARDS
		↑ O_2 delivery	Hyperoxia
		Mechanical interference	Catheter wedged
			Left-to-right shunt
Normal	60-80	O_2 supply = O_2 demand	Adequate perfusion
		↓ O_2 Extraction	Sepsis/ARDS
Low	<60	↑ O_2 consumption	Shivering
			Pain
			Seizures
			Activity/exercise
			Hyperthermia
			Anxiety
			Suctioning
		↓ O_2 delivery	Hypoperfusion
			Anemia
			Hypoxemia

ARDS, Adult respiratory distress syndrome.

Calibration of the oximeter with a blood sample of known oxygen saturation is recommended on a daily basis or whenever there are doubts regarding the displayed Svo_2 reading. Calibration with a known saturation should be carried out at a time when the patient's saturation values are relatively stable, following the specific manufacturer's instructions.

Clinical application

Continuous monitoring of Svo_2 with a fiberoptic catheter can provide immediate "real-time" information on changes in cardiopulmonary function and the balance between oxygen demand and supply. A decrease in any of the determinants of oxygen supply (cardiac output, hemoglobin, or arterial saturation) usually is associated with a decrease in Svo_2. On the other hand, any change in oxygen consumption is associated with an inverse change in Svo_2. However, a "normal" mixed venous oxygen saturation does not ensure adequate oxygen delivery to any one specific organ system but rather reflects an overall picture of tissue oxygenation. In addition, a "normal" Svo_2 may reflect a pathologic inability to increase oxygen extraction despite increasing oxygen demands.

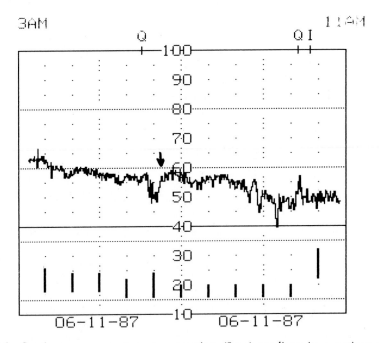

Fig. 10-9. Continuous venous oxygen saturation (Svo_2) readings in a patient who had undergone a mitral and aortic valve replacement. On a postoperative dopamine regimen, the patient showed hemodynamic stability, with a cardiac index (CI) of 2.6 L/min/m$_2$ and an Svo_2 of approximately 62%. At 3AM, her Svo_2 began to decline. A drop to 50%, which was associated with hypotension and a CI of 1.7 L/min/m$_2$, prompted administration of an epinephrine infusion, which resulted in an improved Svo_2 of approximately 58% (see *arrow*). However, over the next few hours the Svo_2 further declined despite blood and fluid administration. The patient was subsequently returned to the OR for relief of cardiac tamponade, with removal of approximately 400 ml blood.

Normal saturation of mixed venous blood ranges from 65% to 77%. Table 10-8 lists the probable causes and clinical states associated with high and low Svo_2 readings. A fall in Svo_2 below 60% lasting for 5 minutes or longer indicates a compromise in at least one of the determinants of oxygen transport (cardiac output, hemoglobin, or arterial oxygen saturation) relative to oxygen demands.

Changes in Svo_2 may, and often do, precede hemodynamic changes and events, providing an early warning that should prompt reassessment of the components of oxygenation. Sudden sustained (>3 to 5 minutes) falls in Svo_2 levels (no matter what the value) require immediate assessment to determine the possible cause. (Brief, minor changes in Svo_2 (5% or less) are clinically insignificant and are likely to be caused by some type of interference rather than changes in cardiac output.) The patient should be clinically evaluated to determine whether any sudden increases in oxygen demand (and therefore oxygen consumption) have occurred. Patient movement or agitation, pain, shivering, seizure activity, or increased body temperature will increase oxygen demand. If no apparent increase in oxygen consumption is noted, the determinants of oxygen delivery must then be assessed. A reduction in hemoglobin, unless associated with massive bleeding, is usually a slowly changing determinant and is less

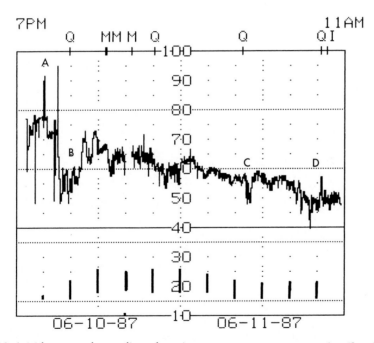

Fig. 10-10. A 16-hour trend recording of continuous venous oxygen saturation (Svo_2) readings in a victim of acute trauma. The initial high Svo_2 *(A)* is artifactual and represents distal migration and wedging of the tip of the Svo_2 catheter. This is confirmed by the marked decrease in the light-intensity indication at the bottom of the strip. A drop in Svo_2 *(B)* was associated with increased activity of the patient, which was effectively controlled with appropriate sedation. A decline in Svo_2 *(C)* occurred during turning of the patient, which reverted somewhat but remained $<60\%$. The Svo_2 continued to decline over the next 4 hours *(D)*. The measured cardiac output (CO) was 9.2 L/min. However, the patient's measured hemoglobin level had dropped to 7.5 g/dl, which severely reduced oxygen delivery and tissue oxygenation.

frequently responsible for sudden decreases in Svo_2. Hypoxemia, with a low Sao_2 can be evaluated by arterial blood gas determination or by continuous monitoring of Sao_2 with pulse oximetry. Although Sao_2 rarely changes more than 10% in most clinical situations, a decrease from 80% to 70% could represent a 30% drop in cardiac output.

Hypoperfusion resulting in decreased $\dot{D}o_2$ is by far the most common cause of a falling Svo_2. To confirm this, cardiac output determination should be performed. In this way cardiac output measurements are made when they are hemodynamically indicated, rather than at some routine or preset time. Use of continuous Svo_2 monitoring also has reduced the need for *routine* arterial blood gas analysis.

Continuous Svo_2 monitoring is also helpful in the immediate assessment of the effectiveness of therapeutic interventions directed at improving oxygen supply or decreasing oxygen demand. Frequently this results in initiation and/or titration of therapy in a more expedient manner (Figs. 10-9 to 10-11). Svo_2 monitoring is also a valuable adjunct to nursing care because the effects of nursing activities on the patient's oxygen balance can be immediately assessed.

Studies assessing the correlation between Svo_2 and any one of the individual determinants of oxygen delivery or of oxygen consumption have shown a rather poor

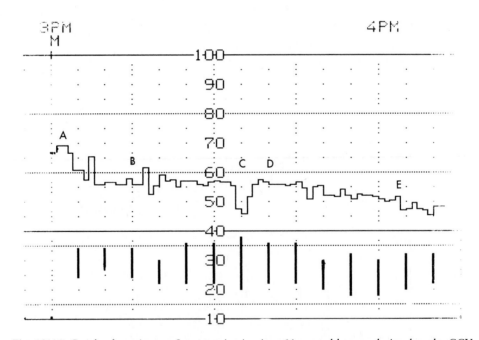

Fig. 10-11. Graph of continuous Svo_2 monitoring in a 64-year-old man admitted to the CCU with severe chest pain associated with dyspnea. Initial Svo_2 readings *(A)* were obtained after administration of oxygen and furosemide (Lasix), as well as a nitroglycerin infusion. The patient's chest pain waxed and waned over the next 6 to 8 hours *(B)* despite increases in nitroglycerin administration. Episodes of nonsustained ventricular tachycardia were associated with a drop of Svo_2 to <50% *(C)*. Lidocaine infusion was begun, which resulted in dysrhythmia suppression and improved Svo_2 *(D)*. However, the patient's cardiac output and Svo_2 continued to decline despite positive inotropic support *(E)*. An intraaortic balloon pump (IABP) subsequently was inserted in this patient in an attempt to improve myocardial and global tissue oxygenation.

relationship. However, correlation of Svo_2 and all the determinants (oxygen extraction or oxygen utilization) is inversely high. This suggests that changes in Svo_2 occur not because of alterations in any one single determinant of oxygen supply/demand balance but rather reflect an overall imbalance. In this way continuous Svo_2 monitoring is used as a "barometer" to reflect overall tissue oxygenation.

Dual Oximetry

Continuous dual oximetry combines pulse and venous oximetry to provide real-time information about oxygen utilization. The cables from both standard monitoring devices (pulse oximetry sensor and Svo_2 catheter) are connected to a single oximeter/computer that simultaneously displays both arterial and venous oxygen saturations. In addition, the computer calculates and displays the oxygen extraction ratio index (O_2ERI) as well as the shunt fraction (Qs/Qt). Continuous dual oximetry can provide rapid bedside evaluation of peripheral oxygenation and respiratory function and can facilitate prompt reversal of tissue hypoxia.

REFERENCES

Annat G et al: Mixed venous oxygen saturation in the immediate postoperative period: an index of the increase in oxygen uptake, *Anesthesiology* 77:A495, 1992.

Astiz ME, Rackow EC: Assessing perfusion failure during circulatory shock, *Crit Care Clin* 9:299-309, 1993.

Bartlett RH, Dechert RE: Oxygen kinetics: pitfalls in clinical research, *J Crit Care* 5:77-80, 1990.

Bongard FS, Leighton TA: Continuous dual oximetry in surgical critical care, *Ann Surg* 216:60-68, 1992.

Bowton DL et al: Pulse oximetry monitoring outside the intensive care unit: progress or problem? *Ann Intern Med* 115:450-454, 1991.

Cain SM: Oxygen delivery and uptake in dogs during anemic and hypoxic hypoxia, *J Appl Physiol* 42:228-234, 1977.

Cilley RE et al: Independent measurement of oxygen consumption and oxygen delivery, *J Surg Res* 47:242, 1989.

Cilley RE et al: Low oxygen delivery produced by anemia, hypoxia, and low cardiac output, *J Surg Res* 51:425-433, 1991.

Clarke C et al: Persistence of supply dependency of oxygen uptake at high levels of delivery in adult respiratory distress syndrome, *Crit Care Med* 19:497-502, 1991.

Copel LC, Stolarik A: Continuous Svo_2 monitoring: a research review, *Dim Crit Care Nurs* 10:202-209, 1991.

Danek SJ et al: The dependence of oxygen uptake on oxygen delivery in the adult respiratory distress syndrome, *Am Rev Respir Dis* 122:387-395, 1980.

Dantzker DR, Foresman B, Gutierrez G: Oxygen supply and utilization relationships, *Am Rev Respir Dis* 143:675-679, 1991.

Dantzker DR, Gutierrez G: The assessment of tissue oxygenation, *Respir Care* 30:456-461, 1985.

Dhainaut JF et al: Practical aspects of oxygen transport: conclusions and recommendations of the round table conference, *Intensive Care Med* 16(suppl 2):S179-S180, 1990.

Edwards JD: Practical application of oxygen transport principles, *Crit Care Med* 18:S45-S48, 1990.

Enger EL, Holm K: Perspectives on the interpretation of continuous mixed venous oxygen saturation, *Heart Lung* 195:578-580, 1990.

Epstein CD, Henning RJ: Oxygen transport variables in the identification and treatment of tissue hypoxia, *Heart Lung* 22:328-348, 1993.

Fahey JT, Lister G: Oxygen transport in low cardiac output states, *J Crit Care* 2:288-305, 1987.

Grum CM: Tissue oxygenation in low flow states and during hypoxemia, *Crit Care Med* 21:S44-S49, 1993.

Gutierez G: Summary of the round table conference on tissue oxygen utilization, *Intensive Care Med* 17:67-68, 1991.

Gutierrez G, Pohil RJ: Oxygen consumption is linearly related to O_2 supply in critically ill patients, *J Crit Care* 1:45-53, 1986.

Haglund U: Assessing tissue perfusion, *Intensive Care Med* 17:71-72, 1991.

Hankeln KB et al: Use of continuous noninvasive measurement of oxygen consumption in patients with ARDS following shock of various etiologies, *Crit Care Med* 19:642-649, 1991.

Hayes MA et al: Response of critically ill patients to treatment aimed at achieving supranormal oxygen delivery and consumption: relationship to outcome, *Chest* 103:886-895, 1993.

Kuckelt W, Bohmert F: Disturbed oxygen transport in multiple organ failure—pathophysiology and therapy in clinical practice, *Intensive Care Med* 16:S89, 1990.

Kupeli IA, Satwicz PR: Mixed venous oximetry, *Int Anesthesiol Clin* 27:176-183, 1989.

Leach RM, Treacher DF: Oxygen transport: the relation between oxygen delivery and consumption, *Thorax* 47:971-978, 1992.

Marini CE, Lodato RF, Gutierrez G: Cardiopulmonary interactions in the cardiac patient in the intensive care unit, *Crit Care Clin* 5:533-549, 1989.

Moreno L et al: Mathematical coupling of data: correction of a common error for linear calculations, *J Appl Physiol* 60:335-343, 1986.

Myburgh JA: Derived oxygen saturations are not clinically useful for the calculation of oxygen consumption, *Anesth Intensive Care* 20:460-463, 1992.

Pallares LCM, Evans TW: Oxygen transport in the critically ill, *Respir Med* 86:289-295, 1992.

Ramsing T, Rosenberg J: Pulse oximetry in severe anemia, *Intensive Care Med* 18:125-126, 1992.

Reinhart K et al: Accuracy of two mixed venous saturation catheters during long-term use in critically ill patients, *Anesthesiology* 69:769-773, 1988.

Reynolds LM et al: Changes in oxygen saturation in children are detected earlier by centrally placed pulse oximeter sensors, *Anesthesiology* 77:A1178, 1992.

Samsel RW, Schumacker PT: Determination of the critical O_2 delivery from experimental data: sensitivity to error, *J Appl Physiol* 64:2074-2082, 1988.

Schlichtig R, Pinsky MR: Defining the hypoxic threshold, *Crit Care Med* 19:147-149, 1991.

Severinghaus JW, Kelleher JF: Recent developments in pulse oximetry, *Anesthesiology* 76:1018-1038, 1992.

Shibutani K et al: Critical level of oxygen delivery in anesthetized man, *Crit Care Med* 11:640-643, 1983.

Shoemaker WC: Monitoring and management of acute circulatory problems: the expanded role of the physiologically oriented critical care nurse, *Am J Crit Care* 1:38-53, 1992.

Shoemaker WC, Appel PL, Kram HB: Tissue oxygen debt as a determinant of lethal and nonlethal postoperative organ failure, *Crit Care Med* 16:1123, 1988.

Shoemaker WC et al: Prospective trial of supranormal values of survivors as therapeutic goals in high-risk surgical patients, *Chest* 94:1176-1186, 1988.

Siegel JH: Through a glass darkly: the lung as a window to monitor oxygen consumption, energy metabolism, and severity of critical illness, *Clin Chem* 36:1585-1593, 1990.

Silverman HJ: Lack of a relationship between induced changes in oxygen consumption and changes in lactate levels, *Chest* 100:1012-1015, 1991.

Smithies MN et al: Comparison of oxygen consumption measurements: indirect calorimetry versus the reversed Fick method, *Crit Care Med* 19:1401-1406, 1991.

Swinamer DL et al: Twenty-four hour energy expenditure in critically ill patients, *Crit Care Med* 15:637-643, 1987.

Vincent JL: The relationship between oxygen demand, oxygen uptake, and oxygen supply, *Intensive Care Med* 16(suppl 2):430-435, 1990.

Weg JG: Oxygen transport in adult respiratory distress syndrome and other acute respiratory problems: relationship of oxygen delivery and oxygen consumption, *Crit Care Med* 19:650-657, 1991.

Weissman C, Kemper M: The oxygen uptake-oxygen delivery relationship during ICU interventions, *Chest* 99:430-435, 1991.

Whitney JD: The measurement of oxygen tension in tissue, *Nurs Res* 39:203-206, 1990.

Young D et al: Response time of pulse oximeters assessed using acute decompression, *Anesth Analg* 74:189-195, 1992.

Chapter 11

Circulatory Assist

Numerous methods of assisting the patient's circulation during periods of transient myocardial depression have been attempted. Of these methods, counterpulsation has been the most successful in improving circulation while causing the lowest incidence of complications. The principles and use of counterpulsation devices are discussed in this chapter.

PHYSIOLOGIC BASIS FOR COUNTERPULSATION DEVICES

The two primary goals for the clinical use of circulatory assist devices are to provide temporary assistance to the patient's circulation until the underlying pathophysiologic condition is corrected and to afford optimal conditions for repair of the heart until it can provide adequate circulation unaided. The intraaortic balloon pump employs the principles of counterpulsation as a means of achieving these goals.

The intraaortic balloon consists of a polyurethane balloon (usually 40-cc capacity for adults) mounted on a vascular catheter that contains multiple holes. It usually is inserted into the femoral artery and positioned in the descending aorta just distal (within 1 to 2 cm) to the left subclavian artery (Fig. 11-1). The balloon catheter is connected to a pump console that shuttles helium or carbon dioxide through the catheter into the balloon to inflate it. Inflation is timed to occur during diastole. During isovolumetric contraction, the gas is rapidly withdrawn to deflate the balloon (counterpulsation). The hemodynamic consequences of this action are augmentation of the intraaortic pressure during diastole (inflation) and reduction of the intraaortic pressure during systole (deflation). In this section the physiologic basis for circulatory assist devices and its application to patient care are discussed.

Diastolic Augmentation

Diastolic augmentation occurs as the direct result of the inflation of the balloon during diastole. The primary effect of this action is to displace blood and force some of it back into the aortic root and the coronary arteries and some of it distally into the peripheral circulation. This increase in ascending aortic blood volume is accompanied by a rise in diastolic pressure (diastolic augmentation). Augmenting the diastolic pressure is particularly beneficial for the patient with coronary occlusive disease, because at least 70% of arterial perfusion to the myocardium occurs during the diastolic phase of the cardiac cycle. By augmenting the intraaortic pressure during diastole, the counterpulsation device mechanically increases coronary perfusion of the

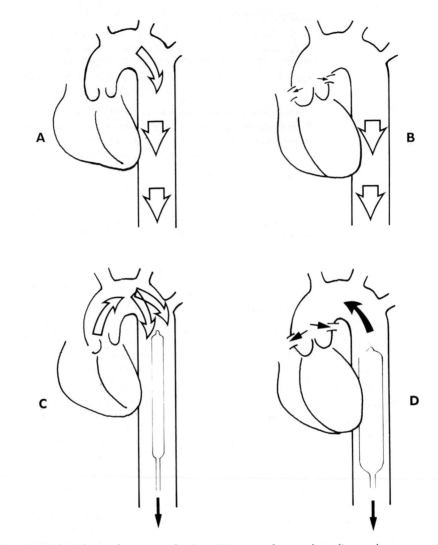

Fig. 11-1. Physiology of counterpulsation. Diagram of normal cardiac cycle pressure flow sequence as compared with the counterpulsed pressure flow sequence. **A,** Normal systole characterized by antegrade volume flow and peak intraaortic pressure. **B,** Normal diastole showing continued antegrade volume flow and adequate intraaortic pressure for coronary perfusion. **C,** Balloon deflation just before systole, allowing antegrade volume flow from the aortic arch (systolic unloading). **D,** Balloon inflation during diastole mechanically boosting volume flow peripherally and retrograde to the aortic arch, heightening diastolic pressure and coronary perfusion.

failing myocardium without increasing myocardial work or oxygen demands. Thus the additional coronary perfusion, at no oxygen expense to the myocardium, may potentially limit the infarction size or reverse the cardiac ischemic dysfunction. In addition, peripheral perfusion is enhanced as aortic blood below the level of the balloon is propelled forward.

Afterload Reduction

The second beneficial effect of counterpulsation is afterload reduction. Afterload, or resistance to left ventricular (LV) ejection, is determined by the residual aortic blood volume and pressure met during LV systole. Afterload reduction is accomplished by the deflation of the balloon just before ventricular ejection. Blood volume leaves the aortic arch to fill the space previously occupied by the inflated balloon or positive pressure. Less effort or work is then required for the left ventricle to empty into the area of lower blood volume. Because blood in the aorta is already moving forward and there is less resistance to flow, afterload reduction can occur with small decreases in systolic pressure.

There are three beneficial effects of afterload reduction by the use of circulatory assist devices. First, myocardial oxygen requirements are reduced as less work is required to eject stroke volume. Second, systolic ejection time is shortened; the duration of diastole is thereby increased, allowing more time for coronary perfusion. Third, the heart can eject more blood per beat because of the decreased resistance (systolic unloading) to forward flow. Thus stroke volume increases while diastolic filling pressure remains the same or decreases.

Although the systolic pressure decreases during balloon pumping, the augmentation in diastolic pressure results in an increase in the mean arterial pressure, which acts as an in-line boost to the general circulation, improving perfusion to other vital organs as well.

Counterpulsation meets the primary goals of circulatory assist by its combined actions of diastolic augmentation and afterload reduction. The overall effect of counterpulsation is to improve both coronary and systemic circulation until the heart can maintain circulation without assistance.

APPLICATION TO PATIENT CARE
Indications

The efficacy of counterpulsation in assisting the circulation provides the basis for an ever-growing variety of indications in a wide range of clinical settings (see box, p. 244). Some of the applications listed are based on theoretic, experimental, or limited data and have not as yet been proved to be clinically effective. This is particularly true of the more recent use of counterpulsation in children.

Contraindications

The two primary contraindications to counterpulsation circulatory assist are aortic valve incompetency and a thoracic or abdominal aortic aneurysm. Diastolic augmentation may aggravate aortic insufficiency and further compromise forward blood flow. Diastolic augmentation is contraindicated in the presence of an aneurysm of the descending thoracic or abdominal aorta, because additional stress would be applied to an already weakened aortic wall.

Severe peripheral vascular disease, although not an absolute contraindication, may present serious technical difficulties in catheter insertion. Counterpulsation also is contraindicated in patients with underlying brain death or advanced or terminal disease states.

Indications for use of counterpulsation devices

- Heart failure or cardiogenic shock resulting from an acute myocardial infarction
- Low cardiac output states
- Cardiac interventional procedures (angioplasty ventriculogram, coronary arteriogram, and cardiac catheterization) in patients at high risk
- Papillary muscle rupture, ventricular aneurysm, and ventricular septal defect (VSD) caused by myocardial infarction
- Removing patients from cardiopulmonary bypass
- Drug-resistant, life-threatening dysrhythmias
- Unstable angina pectoris
- Acute myocardial infarction, (with, without, or with failed thrombolytic therapy)
- High-risk cardiac patients undergoing noncardiac surgery
- Septic shock (hypodynamic stage)
- Cardiac surgery patients who are at high risk preoperatively (severe LV dysfunction, severe coronary artery disease, left main disease)
- Bridge to cardiac transplantation

INTRAAORTIC BALLOON PUMP

The intraaortic balloon pump has been one of the most effective methods of counterpulsation used in the clinical setting. Moulopoulos, Topaz, and Kolff first introduced the basic principles of the intraaortic balloon pump in 1962, and Kantrowitz et al. had further developed these principles by 1967. The device itself consists of a balloon-tipped catheter that is positioned in the descending thoracic aorta via the femoral artery. This catheter is then attached to the gas-driving unit. Counterpulsation is achieved by alternate inflation of the balloon during distole and rapid deflation of the balloon just before systole.

Equipment

Balloon catheters have undergone considerable improvement in design and reduction of size. The single-chambered balloon, by far the most widely used, is assembled on an 8.5-, 9.5-, 10.5- or 12-Fr double-lumen catheter. One lumen has multiple holes that open into the balloon and is used to deliver gas (either carbon dioxide or helium), whereas the other lumen opens at the catheter tip and is used to monitor the aortic pressure. Table 11-1 lists types and sizes of various adult intraaortic balloons (IABs).

Selection of the correct balloon size is an important consideration when therapy is being initiated. Balloon capacities vary from 30 to 50 cc. The more blood volume displaced, the better the intraaortic balloon pump functions. However, total occlusion of the aorta may injure the aortic intima and cause hemolysis of red blood cells. To avoid these complications, the balloon should fill at least 85% to 90% of the diameter of the aorta and yet be nonocclusive. Estimating the aortic diameter is an uncertain process, because the diameter varies with the individual patient and with the mean arterial pressure. Hence the aortic diameter must be estimated from the size of the

Table 11-1. Calculation of intraaortic balloon (IAB) size*

Height (in)	Weight (lb)	Body surface area (BSA)	Balloon size (cc)
60	100	1.38	23.5
64	125	1.60	27.2
68	160	1.87	31.8
72	180	2.04	34.7
74	200	2.18	37.1

From Hartnett TM, Gaffney T. In Quaal SJ, editor: *Comprehensive intra-aortic balloon counterpulsation,* ed 2, St Louis, 1993, Mosby–Year Book.
*Heart rate = 100 beats/min; cardiac index (CI) = 1.5 L/min/m^2.

Table 11-2. Balloon volumes, membrane lengths, and inflated diameters by manufacturer

Manufacturer	IAB volume (cc)	Membrane length (cm)	Inflated diameter (mm)
Aries/St. Jude Medical	30	24.1	15.6
	40	27.5	16.2
	50	27.5	18.3
Datascope Corporation	34	21.9	14.7
	40	26.3	15.0
Kontron Instruments, Inc.	30	19.8	15.0
	40	22.7	16.0
	50	22.7	18.0
Mansfield Cardiac Assist	30	20.0	15.0
	40	22.0	17.0
	40	27.0	15.0
	50	23.0	18.5

From Hartnett TM, Gaffney T. In Quaal SJ, editor: *Comprehensive intra-aortic balloon counterpulsation,* ed 2, St Louis, 1993, Mosby–Year Book.
IAB, Intraaortic balloon.

femoral artery and the patient's body surface area. One formula derived by clinicians at Massachusetts General Hospital calculates the product of the patient's weight (pounds) and age (years). If this product exceeds 6000, a 50-cc balloon is used; if less than 6000, a 40-cc balloon is used. Another method uses a formula based on the patient's body surface area (BSA), an assumed heart rate of 100 beats/min, and a cardiac index (CI) of 1.5 L/min/m^2. Balloon sizes estimated in terms of these variables are listed in Table 11-1. The largest size that can be accommodated by the patient's aorta yet can be inserted easily should be selected.

Another consideration regarding catheter selection relates to the balloon length. Although there are limited choices and most adults can accommodate the longer balloons, in patients of short stature (< 64 inches), the standard balloon length may occlude the mesenteric or renal arteries. Table 11-2 lists currently available adult intraaortic balloons, along with their corresponding balloon volumes, length, and inflated diameter.

Additional equipment needed to insert an intraaortic balloon includes the following:
1. Supplies for skin preparation
2. Catheter insertion kit
3. Resuscitation equipment, including crash cart and defibrillator
4. ECG and arterial pressure monitoring equipment
5. Gas-driving pump with emergency power source

Patient Preparation

The following steps should be taken to prepare the patient for IAB insertion.
1. Explain the procedure to the patient and/or to the family, if appropriate.
2. Obtain informed consent.
3. Obtain and review current laboratory values, including hemogram, platelets, prothrombin time (PT), partial thromboplastin time (PTT), and bleeding time.
4. Secure and maintain an IV line if a pulmonary artery (PA) catheter is not in place.
5. Check and record the presence and quality of the dorsalis pedis pulse.
6. Shave the ilioinguinal area of the side selected for catheter insertion. Cleanse the area with povidone-iodine, and allow to dry. Apply sterile drapes.

Insertion

The introduction of the percutaneous IAB catheter in 1979 greatly increased the overall use of counterpulsation. Because percutaneous insertion is faster than the surgical approach and is not dependent on the availability of a cardiac or vascular surgeon, therapy can be initiated sooner, providing better long-term results.

The percutaneous balloon catheter with a central lumen permits insertion of a guidewire through the lumen and facilitates passage of the balloon through atherosclerotic and tortuous vessels. In addition, contrast medium can be injected through the lumen and intraaortic pressure monitoring can be performed.

Percutaneous balloon insertion

Before insertion, the percutaneous intraaortic balloon should be prepared under sterile conditions and the manufacturer's specific recommendations should be followed. The balloon is prepared by testing the balloon integrity with the injection of air from a 50-ml syringe and wetting the balloon in sterile saline to lubricate it and to check for any leaks. The air is then redrawn into the syringe and discarded. After the syringe is reattached to the balloon port, the plunger is withdrawn to apply negative pressure to the balloon and the balloon is wrapped snugly around the catheter. If the balloon is wrapped while negative pressure is applied to the chamber with the use of a syringe, all the air will be removed and the balloon will wrap more compactly for easier insertion. To facilitate unwrapping when the balloon is positioned in the aorta, it is important that the balloon catheter be moistened with saline before wrapping. The pressure lumen of the balloon catheter should be flushed with sterile, heparinized IV fluid. The length of catheter required for optimal placement in the descending aorta can be estimated by placing the tip of the catheter approximately 1 cm below the sternal angle of Louis and the other end of the catheter at the proposed insertion point.

After appropriate skin preparation and the administration of a local anesthetic, either the right or left common femoral artery is punctured approximately one fingerbreadth below the inguinal crease with an 18-gauge arterial needle. A 0.030- or 0.035-inch J-tip guidewire is advanced through the needle into the abdominal aorta. The needle is removed and dilators of sequentially increasing size (beginning with an 8-Fr Teflon dilator) are inserted over the guidewire to enlarge the puncture site. The final dilator is removed and a 12-Fr Teflon dilator and sheath are inserted over the guidewire into the femoral artery. After removal of the dilator and guidewire, the prepared balloon-catheter is inserted through the sheath and positioned with the tip just distal to the takeoff of the left subclavian artery (Fig. 11-2). Alternatively, the dilator is removed and the inner lumen of the catheter is passed over the guidewire through the sheath and advanced to the aorta.

Correct positioning is confirmed by fluoroscopy or chest radiograph. The guidewire is removed and the central lumen is aspirated, flushed, and connected to a prepared transducer for intraarterial pressure monitoring. The balloon is unwrapped according to directions, and the connector of the balloon lumen is attached to a gas-pumping console for inflation and deflation of the balloon. The balloon-sheath system is sutured to the skin with several sutures to ensure stability.

The development of balloon catheters with smaller diameters (8.5-, 10-, and 11-Fr) has resulted in the ability to insert these catheters percutaneously without the use of an arterial sheath. This reduces the effective occluding diameter and associated complications. The catheter is inserted directly over the guidewire into the artery after substantial dilation of the cutaneous and subcutaneous tissue has been performed.

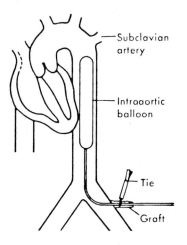

Fig. 11-2. Placement of the intraaortic balloon. Insertion is made through a sidearm graft via a cutdown on the common femoral artery. The balloon position is just distal to the left subclavian artery. Ties around the graft secure the catheter in place without jeopardizing perfusion to the leg distal to the insertion site.

Arteriotomy

The balloon can be inserted into either common femoral artery. The artery with the strongest pulse is chosen to permit easier insertion of the balloon and better perfusion to the limb once the balloon catheter is in position.

After local anesthesia is administered, an arterial cutdown is performed. A beveled Teflon graft is sewn to the side of the artery (see Fig. 11-2). The balloon is inserted through this side graft and advanced to its position in the descending thoracic aorta. Heparin is administered intravenously (maintenance doses are then given every 4 to 6 hours for the duration of counterpulsation). A tie is placed around the side graft (as opposed to the artery itself) to secure the catheter. This method secures the catheter and affords the best opportunity for adequate distal perfusion to the leg.

The percutaneous IAB catheter also can be inserted directly into an exposed femoral artery. This may be performed after cardiopulmonary bypass or if difficulty is encountered with percutaneous insertion. The balloon catheter is prepared in the routine fashion and inserted through the arteriotomy or with the optional use of a Teflon graft. Use of a guidewire through the central lumen of the IAB can aid in passage through tortuous vessels.

The optimal position for the balloon is just distal to the left subclavian artery. This position should be confirmed by fluoroscopic examination after insertion. In this position the balloon is close enough to the aortic valve to optimize diastolic augmentation, yet far enough away to reduce the risk of cerebral embolism. This position also decreases the potential for balloon-tip perforation of the aortic arch during catheter insertion or patient movement.

Operation

Once the balloon is positioned properly, the catheter is attached to the gas-pumping apparatus and therapy is initiated. Several different types of IAB pumps are available for use in counterpulsation. It is recommended that all personnel involved in the care of a patient undergoing counterpulsation receive detailed instruction and carefully follow the specific manufacturer's recommendations and procedures for proper usage. Basic pump setup consists of establishing power, establishing gas pressure, setting controls, and establishing ECG and arterial pressure signals. The two types of gases used to drive the balloon pump are helium and carbon dioxide. Because helium is more lightweight and has a more rapid delivery time, balloon function at faster heart rates and during dysrhythmias is facilitated. Carbon dioxide, on the other hand, is more soluble in blood; therefore the seriousness of gas embolization if the balloon ruptures is reduced.

To safely initiate balloon pumping, it is necessary to display the patient's arterial pressure, observe the appearance of the waveform with a distinct dicrotic notch, and obtain a reliable, artifact-free ECG with a tall (≥ 0.2 mV) positive R wave. Obtaining such a signal depends on properly preparing the skin (shaving the electrode site if necessary and rubbing the site briskly with a dry gauze pad); avoiding electrode placement on bony prominences, joints, or skin folds; and securely attaching pregelled electrodes to the skin. If 60-cycle electric interference is present in the ECG, the interference should be isolated and removed. Anti-dysrhythmic therapy may be necessary to reduce or eliminate premature beats (atrial or ventricular) that would prevent proper timing of counterpulsation.

Timing

Proper timing of balloon inflation, which is based on the electrical and mechanical events of the heart, is essential to obtain optimal circulatory support. The R wave of the patient's ECG is used most commonly as the reference point or "trigger" for balloon inflation and deflation. Other potential "trigger" references to use when the patient's ECG signal is inadequate include the upstroke of the arterial waveform and an electronic internal signal or "trigger" generated by the balloon pump console.

Proper timing can best be achieved when counterpulsation occurs with every other beat (1:2 frequency) so as to compare the assisted with the nonassisted arterial waveform. Inflation should be set and adjusted first; then deflation should be optimized.

Inflation. Fine adjustments should be made to time inflation with the dicrotic notch of the arterial waveform. However, because of the time for arterial wave propagation, the dicrotic notch, which represents aortic valve closure, is somewhat delayed from the causative event by about 20 to 25 msec. In addition, the transmission of the balloon pressure from the catheter to the aortic root is also about 20 to 25 msec. This represents a total delay of 40 to 50 msec with regard to balloon inflation timing. To compensate for these delays, balloon inflation ideally should be timed to occur about 40 msec (one small box on the ECG paper) *before* the dicrotic notch (Fig. 11-3). This results in a change in the contour of the dicrotic notch from a typical U shape to a sharp V shape (Fig. 11-4). This also causes an increase in the pressure that exceeds the patient's unassisted arterial systolic pressure. In consideration of the delays in arterial pulse wave transmission, combined with the importance of precise timing, the use of more central arterial pressures (such as that obtained from the central lumen of the balloon catheter) is preferred over peripheral artery pressures.

Deflation. Balloon deflation should occur during isovolumetric contraction, just before the aortic valve opens. On the arterial waveform this point occurs immediately before the upstroke. Optimal deflation produces (1) a diastolic arterial pressure that is 5 to 15 mm Hg lower than the patient's unassisted end-diastolic arterial pressure, and (2) a balloon-assisted systolic pressure that is lower than the patient's unassisted systolic pressure.

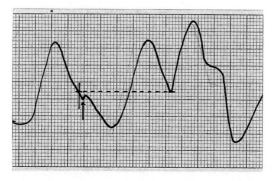

Fig. 11-3. To set proper timing of balloon inflation and deflation, locate the midpoint of the dicrotic notch *(arrow)*, move one box (0.04 sec) to the left, and draw a vertical line. The point at which the vertical line bisects the arterial waveform is the point at which balloon inflation should occur *(dotted line)*.

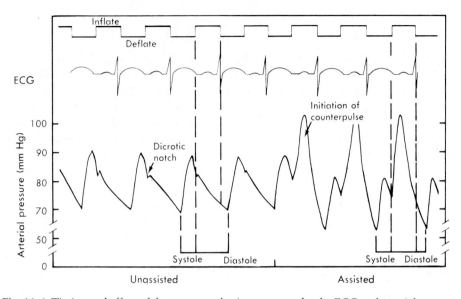

Fig. 11-4. Timing and effect of the counterpulsation sequence by the ECG and arterial pressure waveform. With initiation of counterpulsation, diastolic pressure is heightened and systolic and end-diastolic pressures are lowered.

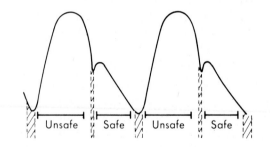

Fig. 11-5. Functional range of safe timing for counterpulsation.

From Quaal SJ: *Comprehensive intraaortic balloon pumping,* ed 2, St Louis, 1993, Mosby–Year Book.

Adjusting and optimizing the timing of balloon inflation and deflation must be based on a clear understanding of when such events are "safe" and when they are "unsafe" (Fig. 11-5). Obviously, during the diastolic phase (from the dicrotic notch, or aortic valve closure, until the next systolic upstroke) balloon inflation or deflation will not interfere with systolic ejection and thus is a safe period. However, even though it may be safe during this time, less than optimal results may be achieved.

Late inflation of the balloon, although safe, is suboptimal and can be identified on the arterial waveform by a widening of the dicrotic notch (Fig. 11-6). Correcting the timing of inflation to occur earlier produces the typical *V*-shaped dicrotic notch (see Fig. 11-4) and improves augmentation.

Early inflation would occur during the unsafe period during systolic ejection. Although most IABP consoles have a safety mechanism that prevents balloon inflation at the peak of systole, it is possible for early inflation to occur during the latter part

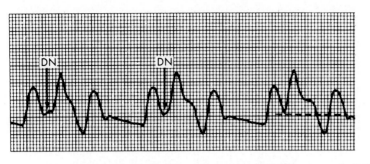

Fig. 11-6. 1:2 assist with late balloon inflation resulting in a wide dicrotic notch *(DN)* on the first arterial waveform. Balloon timing is gradually adjusted until optimal inflation occurs 40 msec before the dicrotic notch producing the desired V-shape dicrotic notch on the last assisted arterial waveform.

From Quaal SJ: *Comprehensive intraaortic balloon counterpulsation,* ed 2, 1993, St Louis, Mosby–Year Book.

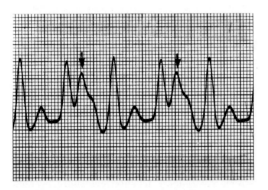

Fig. 11-7. 1:2 assist with early balloon inflation producing shortened systolic ejection time and reduced stroke volume.

of systole, when the aortic valve is still open. This causes the aortic valve to close early and thus prevents adequate ventricular emptying. The net result is a decrease in the stroke volume and an increase in the end-diastolic volume. Early inflation can be identified on the arterial waveform as an increase in arterial pressure occurring shortly after the peak systolic pressure and before the dicrotic notch (Fig. 11-7).

Late timing of balloon deflation is unsafe as the balloon is still inflated when the aortic valve opens and systolic ejection occurs. Not only does this substantially increase ventricular work and myocardial oxygen consumption but stroke volume decreases. Late deflation can be identified on the arterial waveform by a high end-diastolic pressure of the assisted beat and by a prolonged slope of the following unassisted systolic upstroke (Fig. 11-8).

Balloon deflation that occurs too early is not unsafe, but it does not accomplish the goal of unloading the ventricle during systole. Early deflation is characterized by the lack of a plateau on the downslope of the augmented wave and an end-diastolic pressure that equals the patient's unassisted end-diastolic pressure. In addition, the assisted systolic pressure is as high as or higher than the unassisted systolic pressure (Fig. 11-9).

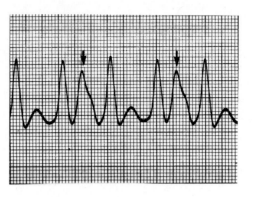

Fig. 11-8. 1:2 assist with late balloon deflation evidenced by a high end-diastolic pressure that equals the unassisted end-diastolic pressure.

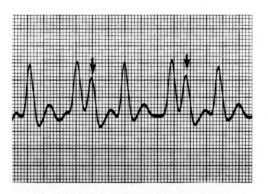

Fig. 11-9. 1:2 assist with early balloon deflation evidenced by rapid equilibration of the augmented end-diastolic pressure to the nonaugmented end-diastolic pressure.

Effects of Dysrhythmias

Manual adjustments in timing may be necessary if the heart rate changes more than 10 or 12 beats/min. Most computerized IAB pumps automatically and instantaneously adjust timing for changes in heart rate and rhythm when operating in the automatic mode. Balloon pumping is most effective if the heart rate is greater than 80 beats/min and less than 110 beats/min in normal sinus rhythm.

Tachycardia. Heart rates above 120 beats/min compromise the duration of diastole and therefore diastolic augmentation. Tachycardia also may pose mechanical problems in the pump's ability to track higher heart rates, resulting in reduced carbon dioxide gas flow and volume. Use of helium, rather than carbon dioxide, as a driving gas is suggested for patients with higher heart rates. For heart rates greater than 120 beats/min, the pumping frequency rate is decreased to 1:2 and appropriate therapy is instituted to lower the heart rate.

Atrial fibrillation. Irregularity of the RR interval poses a severe timing problem, particularly if the R wave appears early. Overall effects of augmentation are best achieved by adjusting the augmentation sequence to the shortest RR interval. It is also prudent to adjust the deflation control, causing the balloon to deflate on the peak of the R wave. This prevents inflation during any systolic event, regardless of timing. Digoxin may be used to slow the heart rate; verapamil also may be used unless there is severe left ventricular dysfunction. Antidysrhythmic therapy or cardioversion may be used to achieve a sinus rhythm and improve augmentation.

Ventricular tachycardia. Ventricular tachycardia usually can trigger the balloon pump if the timing frequency is decreased to 1 : 3. Balloon fill time can be reduced so that balloon inflation and deflation require less time. Antidysrhythmic therapy or cardioversion is used to correct the dysrhythmia.

Ventricular fibrillation. Defibrillation can be carried out in the usual manner, with discontinuation of counterpulsation for a few seconds during delivery of the current. Because the system is not completely isolated from the patient, there is the danger of damaging the unit during defibrillation.

Cardiac arrest. The IAB does not interfere with cardiopulmonary resuscitation (CPR); in fact, balloon inflation during the diastolic phase of CPR would be beneficial. If chest compressions are regular, the balloon pump will be triggered with each compression (or systole). If compressions are not regular, the balloon will automatically deflate. Balloon fill time should be reduced. The IAB catheter can be inserted percutaneously during resuscitation to provide immediate circulatory assistance.

Balloon Pressure Waveforms

In addition to careful evaluation of the arterial waveform, the balloon waveform, which reflects the pressure inside the balloon, must be assessed and compared with the augmented waveform. Fig. 11-10 depicts the components of a normal balloon waveform and its relationship to the augmented arterial waveform. Note that the width of the balloon square wave correlates with the length of the diastolic phase — the period of augmentation. As the duration of diastole varies according to the heart rate, it follows that the width of the balloon square wave will vary according the heart rate (Fig. 11-11). The slower the heart rate, the longer the period of diastole and the wider the balloon square wave. The reverse is true with fast heart rates.

The height of the plateau portion of the balloon pressure waveform indicates the pressure required to overcome the existing intraaortic pressure so that the balloon can

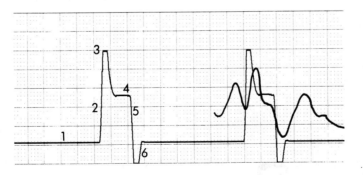

Fig. 11-10. Normal components of the balloon pressure waveform *(left): 1,* fill pressure; *2,* rapid inflation; *3,* peak inflation artifact; *4,* inflation plateau pressure; *5,* rapid deflation; *6,* peak deflation pressure and return to baseline. Right side of figure depicts relationship between the balloon pressure waveform and the augmented arterial pressure waveform.

inflate. In general, the balloon pressure plateau approximates the augmented pressure value. The higher the intraaortic pressure, the higher the balloon pressure, and vice versa (Fig. 11-12).

Whereas changes in the pressure value of the balloon waveform may reflect physiologic changes, accompanying changes in the configuration of the pressure waveform indicate problems within the system that require troubleshooting interventions. A balloon pressure that exceeds the augmented arterial pressure by >25 mm Hg indicates an obstruction or kink in the system. Often the high balloon pressure also appears squared off, or rounded off, with absence of both the inflation overshoot artifact and the deflation undershoot artifact (Fig. 11-13). If the balloon is obstructed, diastolic augmentation will be minimal as evidenced on the arterial waveform. If kinks, occlusions, or inappropriate balloon size are eliminated as causative factors, decreasing the gas fill volume may improve the waveform and still achieve augmentation.

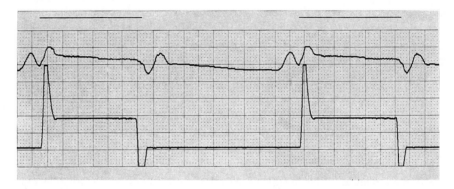

Fig. 11-11. Widened balloon pressure wave as a result of increased diastole in a patient with bradycardia.

Courtesy Kontron Cardiovascular, Everett, Mass.

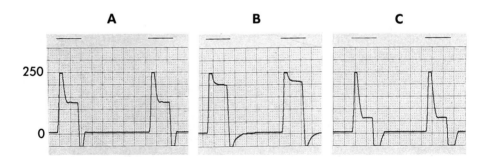

Fig. 11-12. Balloon pressure waveforms. **A,** Normal balloon pressure waveform with plateau pressure approximately 125 mm Hg. **B,** Balloon pressure waveform with a high plateau pressure of approximately 200 mm Hg in a patient with a high arterial pressure. **C,** Balloon pressure waveform with a low plateau of approximately 65 mm Hg in a hypotensive patient.

Courtesy Kontron Cardiovascular, Everett, Mass.

Aortic Pressure Monitoring with the IAB Catheter

Monitoring of the aortic pressure rather than peripheral arterial pressure is essential for accurate timing of counterpulsation. Direct aortic pressure monitoring can be performed through the central lumen of the IAB catheter in the following way:

1. After insertion of the percutaneous IAB catheter, and following removal of the guidewire from the central lumen, aspirate blood from the central lumen and flush with sterile heparinized saline.
2. Attach a three-way stopcock with a continuous flush device, transducer, tubing, and heparinized IV solution to the hub of the inner lumen of the IAB catheter (Fig. 11-14). Carefully ensure that all air bubbles are removed from any of the attached equipment.
3. Maintain a continuous infusion of heparinized solution through the catheter lumen, and activate the "fast flush" on an hourly basis to maintain catheter patency. Discontinue balloon pulsation before fast flushing or blood sampling to reduce the risk of retrograde embolus.

Associated Therapy

When balloon pumping is initiated, other supportive therapies are begun to enhance the effect of counterpulsation. These therapies include the following:

1. Discontinuation of inotropic and vasopressor agents as soon as possible, inasmuch as their therapeutic action may oppose the effect of the balloon pump
2. Fluid administration to maintain adequate filling pressures in the face of reduced vasoconstriction, which lessens diastolic filling pressures
3. Administration of small doses of peripheral vasodilators (sodium nitroprusside) to further decrease the afterload and increase peripheral perfusion, particularly to the kidneys
4. Intravenous administration of heparin for the duration of balloon placement to prevent thrombus formation on the balloon catheter
5. Administration of prophylactic, broad-spectrum antibiotics

Patients require close monitoring if optimal counterpulsation is to be realized.

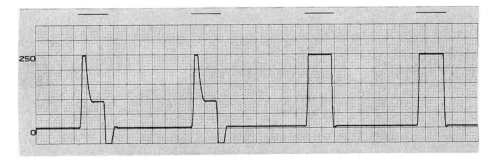

Fig. 11-13. Normal balloon pressure waveform evident in the first two waveforms that suddenly changes to a high, squared-off waveform with absent inflation overshoot and deflation undershoot. This abnormality is caused by a kink in the catheter or tubing.

Courtesy Kontron Cardiovascular, Everett, Mass.

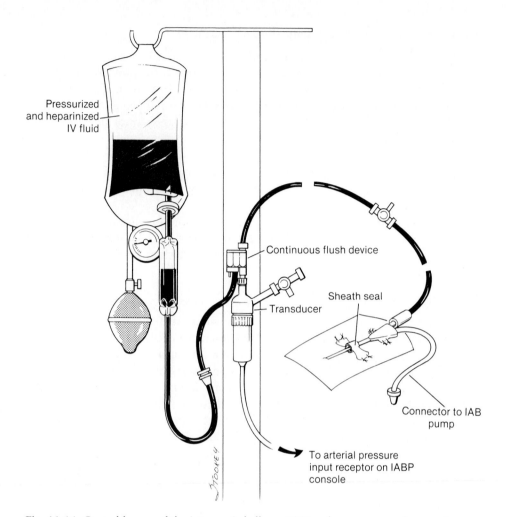

Fig. 11-14. Central lumen of the intraaortic balloon (IAB) catheter connected to continuous-flush device with heparinized solution and a transducer for monitoring of the intraaortic pressure.

Parameters to be monitored include the following:
1. Vital signs (blood pressure, heart rate, respiratory rate, temperature)
2. Hemodynamic pressures, including central venous pressure (CVP) or, preferably, PA pressure (systolic, diastolic, mean), pulmonary artery wedge (PAW) mean pressure, and intraarterial pressure
3. Oxygenation (arterial oxygen saturation [Sao_2] and venous oxygen saturation [Svo_2])
4. Renal function (monitored by urinary flow, specific gravity, and blood chemistries; frequent monitoring is facilitated by the insertion of a urinary catheter)
5. Blood flow to the catheterized limb (monitored for signs of circulatory insufficiency such as cyanosis or decreased pulses and temperature)
6. Anticoagulation (monitored by activated clotting time or partial thromboplastin test)

Table 11-3 lists suggested monitoring parameters during counterpulsation.

Table 11-3. Suggested monitoring schedule of hemodynamic, laboratory, and clinical parameters in patients undergoing IABP

Parameters	Monitoring frequency
HEMODYNAMICS	
RA, PA, PAW or LA pressures Intraarterial pressure (systolic, diastolic, and augmented diastolic)	Every 30 min until stable (and during weaning); every 2 hr thereafter
CI, SVR, SWI	Every 1 hr until stable; every 4 hr thereafter
PERIPHERAL CIRCULATION	
Quality of dorsalis pedis, posterior tibial pulses Color, temperature, movement, and sensation of legs Doppler flowmeter	Every 15 min the first hr; every 30 min the next 2 hr; every 2 hr and as needed thereafter
RENAL CIRCULATION	
Urine output	Every 1 hr
CEREBRAL CIRCULATION	
Mental status	Every 1 hr and as needed
HEMATOLOGIC ASSESSMENT	
Hemogram	Daily and as needed
Platelet count, PTT	Every 8-12 hr and as needed after therapeutic anticoagulation is obtained
OXYGENATION	
Arterial blood gases	Every 8 hr and as needed
Mixed venous oxygen saturation	Continuously (via fiberoptic catheter) or every 8 hr and as needed
VITAL SIGNS	
Heart rate, respiratory rate, temperature	Every hr until stable; then every 2-4 hr and as needed
AUSCULTATORY EXAMINATION	
Heart sounds Breath sounds	Every 2 hr and as needed

IABP, Intraaortic balloon pump; *RA*, right atrial; *PA*, pulmonary artery; *PAW*, pulmonary artery wedge; *LA*, left atrial; *CI*, cardiac index; *SVR*, systemic vascular resistance; *SWI*, stroke work index; *PTT*, partial thromboplastin time.

Table 11-4. Complications of the intraaortic balloon pump

Complication	Incidence	Prevention
Ischemia of the limb distal to the insertion site	Most frequent	Use the largest femoral artery with the best pulse for balloon insertion.
Loss of peripheral pulses	Frequent	Administer heparin for anticoagulation.
		Frequently check the limb for signs of decreased circulation (temperature, color, pulses, movement, and sensation).
		When the balloon is removed, explore the femoral artery with a Fogarty catheter to remove clots.
Aortic or arterial damage (dissection, intimal laceration, or hematoma)	Occasional	Position the balloon catheter in the descending aorta just distal to the left subclavian artery.
		Select the correct balloon size, so that the inflated balloon does not occlude the aorta.
		Never advance the balloon-catheter if resistance is felt.
		Do not elevate head of bed >30 degrees; limit patient movement (leg flexion can move the balloon tip up in the aorta, resulting in possible puncture of the arch).
Emboli from the balloon, catheter, sheath, or graft	Occasional	Administer heparin or low molecular–weight dextran to maintain PTT 1.5 to 2 times normal.
		Do not leave the balloon in place if it is collapsed and motionless.
		Remove percutaneous sheath and catheter together.
		Allow wound to bleed vigorously 1-2 sec after removal of percutaneous balloon catheter.
Infection	Frequent	Use aseptic technique.
		Care for wound daily.
		Use prophylactic antibiotics.
		Change IV tubing every 24-48 hr.
Hemolysis	Minimal	Select the correct balloon size, so that the inflated balloon does not occlude aorta.
Platelet reduction	Frequent	Decrease duration; heparin may help.

PTT, Partial thromboplastin time.

Table 11-4. Complications of the intraaortic balloon pump—cont'd

Complication	Incidence	Prevention
Balloon leak or rupture with gas embolism	Rare	Use careful insertion technique to prevent damage to the balloon. Use carbon dioxide as the inflation gas because it is more soluble in blood. Choose the largest femoral artery for insertion. Avoid exposing catheter to acetone and/or ether.
Pseudoaneurysm or hematoma	Rare	Direct mechanical pressure at puncture site for 30-60 min after balloon removal.
Bleeding at puncture site	Occasional	Same as above.
Compartment syndrome	Occasional	Careful insertion. Avoid use of vasopressors.

Complications

Complications associated with the IABP occur frequently, and many relate to the problem of passing a large catheter into an atherosclerotic vessel. Patients at increased risk for the development of complications with IABP include women, older patients, patients with peripheral vascular disease or diabetes, and prolonged counterpulsation therapy. Other possible risk factors include smoking, obesity, cardiogenic shock, and hypertension.

Approximately half of the 20% to 25% of complications reported are major and include aortic dissection, perforation of the common iliac artery, and thrombotic complications, particularly of the renal artery. Death related to one of these complications occurs in 1% of patients. The use of heparin minimizes but does not prevent peripheral embolic complications. In addition, the prolonged use of heparin is associated with bleeding from the insertion site and frequently requires surgical exploration. Septic complications, including septicemia or an infected wound site, require early removal of the balloon and appropriate antibiotic therapy.

The single most frequently occurring complication of balloon pumping has been vascular insufficiency of the catheterized limb (5% to 47%). Although this complication is usually transient, Fogarty catheterization to restore circulation may be necessary.

The enhanced ease and speed of insertion of the percutaneous intraaortic balloon has not decreased the incidence of complications that occur with balloon pumping. In addition, failure to insert the percutaneous balloon-catheter is not uncommon in patients with arteriosclerotic disease. Occasionally, the introduction of a longer, 15-inch 12-Fr dilator will facilitate insertion, whereas at other times an arteriotomy is necessary for balloon insertion.

Table 11-4 lists possible complications of the intraaortic balloon pump and suggestions for their prevention.

Table 11-5. Clinical and hemodynamic criteria for discontinuation of IABP

Clinical criteria	Hemodynamic criteria
Evidence of adequate perfusion	Cardiac index > 2.0 L/min/m^2
Urine output > 30 ml/hr	MAP > 70 mm Hg with minimal or no pressors
Improved mental status	
Skin temperature warm	
No evidence of congestive heart failure	PAEDP/PAWP or LAP < 18 mm Hg
Rales absent	
S$_3$ absent	
No life-threatening dysrhythmias	Heart rate < 110 beats/min without complex ventricular dysrhythmias

IABP, Intraaortic balloon pump; *MAP*, mean arterial pressure; *PAEDP*, pulmonary artery end-diastolic pressure; PAWP, pulmonary artery wedge pressure; *LAP*, left atrial pressure.

Improved Hemodynamics and Removal

Hemodynamic improvement with the intraaortic balloon pump is rapidly observed within the first hour or two of the therapy. Mean arterial pressure rises, and both coronary and peripheral perfusion improves. Mental confusion decreases, and urinary flow improves. Because of afterload reduction, cardiac output increases and preload (LV end-diastolic volume) decreases. This is evidenced by a decrease in PAW mean and PA diastolic pressures.

The optimal duration for balloon pumping has not been established. However, once circulation is stable, mechanical support should be withdrawn. Table 11-5 lists hemodynamic and clinical criteria for cessation of counterpulsation.

Once it has been established that a patient is to be removed from circulatory assist, a systematic weaning process is begun. One method of weaning the patient from circulatory assist is to alternate the amount of time on the balloon with an equal time off the balloon. Another method is to gradually decrease the volume of the balloon inflation, allowing it to displace less blood each time. A third method is to pump every other heartbeat, then every third or fourth beat, and so on, until the patient is finally weaned. The weaning process may take hours to days, depending on the hemodynamic status of the patient. Dependence on the intraaortic balloon pump is indicated by a reversion to a previous shock state when balloon assistance is discontinued.

Although IABP devices have substantially improved and become increasingly "user friendly," their use in critically ill patients demands advanced knowledge and skills. Nurses who care for patients receiving circulatory assist play a major role in optimizing the risk/benefit ratio of this therapy.

REFERENCES

Alcan KE et al: Current status of intraaortic balloon counterpulsation in critical care cardiology, *Crit Care Med* 12:489-495, 1984.

Alderman JD et al: Incidence and management of limb ischemia with percutaneous wire-guided intraaortic balloon catheters, *J Am Coll Cardiol* 9:524-530, 1987.

Ardire L, Boswell J: Intraaortic balloon pump timing in the patient with hypotension, *Focus Crit Care* 19:146-149, 1992.

Bicking M: The patient on the intraaortic balloon pump, *Crit Care Nurse* 2:50-52, 1982.

Bolooki H: *Clinical application of intraaortic balloon pump,* New York, 1984, Futura Publishing.

Bolooki H: Current status of circulatory support with an intraaortic balloon pump, *Med Instrum* 20:266-275, 1986.

Bregman D et al: Percutaneous intraaortic balloon insertion, *Am J Cardiol* 46:261-264, 1980.

Bullas JB: Care of the patient on the percutaneous intra-aortic counterpulsation balloon, *Crit Care Nurse* 2:40-49, 1982.

Creswell LL et al: Intraaortic balloon counterpulsation: patterns of usage and outcome in cardiac surgery patients, *Ann Thorac Surg* 54:11, 1992.

Estrada-Quintero T et al: Prolonged intraaortic balloon support for septal rupture after myocardial infarction, *Ann Thorac Surg* 53:335, 1992.

Flaherty JT et al: Results of a randomized prospective trial of intraaortic balloon counterpulsation and intravenous nitroglycerin in patients with acute myocardial infarction, *J Am Coll Cardiol* 6:434-446, 1985.

Georgeson S, Coombs AT, Eckman MH: Prophylactic use of the intra-aortic balloon pump in high-risk cardiac patients undergoing noncardiac surgery: a decision analytic view, *Am J Med* 92:665-677, 1992.

Goldberg MJ et al: Intra-aortic balloon pump insertion: a randomized study comparing percutaneous and surgical techniques, *J Am Coll Cardiol* 9:515-523, 1987.

Goldberger M, Tabak SW, Shah PK: Clinical experience with intra-aortic balloon counterpulsation in 112 consecutive patients, *Am Heart J* 111:497-502, 1986.

Goodwin M et al: Safety of intraaortic balloon counterpulsation in patients with acute myocardial infarction receiving streptokinase intravenously, *Am J Cardiol* 64(14):937-938, 1989.

Gould KA: Perspectives in intra-aortic balloon timing, *Crit Care Nurs Clin North Am* 1:469, 1989.

Hartnett TM, Gaffney T: *Intra-aortic balloon size selection.* In Quaal SJ, editor: *Comprehensive intra-aortic balloon counterpulsation,* ed 2, St Louis, 1993, Mosby—Year Book.

Harvey JC et al: Complications of percutaneous intra-aortic balloon pumping, *Circulation* 64(part 2):114-117, 1981.

Kahn JK et al: Supported "high risk" coronary angioplasty using intraaortic balloon pump counterpulsation, *J Am Coll Cardiol* 15:1151, 1990.

Kantrowitz A: Percutaneous intraaortic balloon counterpulsation, *Crit Care Clin* 8:819, 1992.

Kantrowitz A et al: Initial clinical experience with intra-aortic balloon pumping in cardiogenic shock, *JAMA* 203:135-140, 1968.

Lazar JM et al: Outcome and complications of prolonged intraaortic balloon counterpulsation in cardiac patients, *Am J Cardiol* 69:955-958, 1992.

McEnany MT et al: Clinical experience with intraaortic balloon support in 728 patients, *Cardiovasc Surg* 58(suppl 1):124-132, 1978.

Moulopoulos SD, Topaz S, Kolff WJ: Diastolic balloon pumping (with carbon dioxide) in the aorta: mechanical assistance to the failing circulation, *Am Heart J* 63:669, 1962.

Nash IS et al: A new technique for sheathless percutaneous intraaortic balloon catheter insertion, *Cathet Cardiovasc Diagn* 23:57, 1991.

Quaal SJ: *Comprehensive intraaortic balloon counterpulsation,* ed 2, St Louis, 1993, Mosby—Year Book.

Skillman JJ, Kim DS, Baim DS: Vascular complications for percutaneous femoral cardiac interventions, *Arch Surg* 123:1207, 1988.

Subramanian VA: Preliminary clinical experience with percutaneous intraaortic balloon pumping, *Circulation* 62(part 2):123-129, 1980.

Vignola PA, Swaye PS, Gosselin AJ: Guidelines for effective and safe percutaneous intraaortic balloon pump insertion and removal, *Am J Cardiol* 48:660-664, 1981.

Willerson JT et al: Intraaortic balloon counterpulsation in patients in cardiogenic shock, medically refractory left ventricular failure and/or recurrent ventricular tachycardia, *Am J Med* 58:183-191, 1975.

Chapter 12

Clinical Management Based on Hemodynamic Parameters

The care and management of critically ill patients has been enhanced by the advent of bedside hemodynamic monitoring. Knowledge of the patient's individual cardiopulmonary profile gives the clinician the ability not only to direct appropriate therapy to specific abnormal parameters but also to immediately assess the patient's response to such therapy.

A primary goal in the clinical management of all critically ill patients is the maintenance of adequate tissue oxygenation. Fig. 12-1 depicts the determinants of oxygen delivery or transport to the tissues, namely cardiac output, hemoglobin, and arterial oxygen saturation. Furthermore, cardiac output can be broken down into the determinants of preload, afterload, contractility, and heart rate. Viewed in this way, it becomes clear that with the use of invasive monitoring, all the determinants of oxygen delivery can be either measured directly or calculated from direct measurements. Preload is measured clinically by right atrial (RA), pulmonary artery wedge (PAW), or left atrial (LA) pressures or by ventricular end-diastolic volume. Afterload is measured clinically as pulmonary vascular resistance (PVR) or systemic vascular resistance (SVR). Contractility is calculated as left ventricular stroke work index (LVSWI) or right ventricular stroke work index (RVSWI). Heart rate is measured continuously. Arterial saturation is measured continuously with a pulse oximeter, and hemoglobin concentration can be measured intermittently. Monitoring of all these determinants allows the capability of effective intervention to alter whichever of these determinants is abnormal and to bring them into normal or even supernormal range for effective delivery and maintenance of tissue oxygenation. In addition, continuous hemodynamic monitoring permits the clinician to assess the effectiveness of a chosen intervention and to titrate or perhaps discontinue it, depending on the patient's response. Frequently these decisions are left to critical care nurses, who often practice

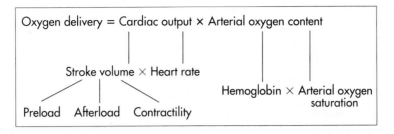

Fig. 12-1. Oxygen delivery ($\dot{D}o_2$) is a product of cardiac output and arterial oxygen content. Cardiac output is a product of stroke volume and heart rate, with preload, afterload, and contractility being the determinants of stroke volume. Arterial oxygen content is the product of the hemoglobin concentration and the oxygen saturation of arterial blood. Monitoring of these parameters, along with the appropriate interventions, comprises the clinical approach to increasing oxygen delivery to the tissues.

with standing orders to maintain certain hemodynamic parameters at specific levels. Thus it is imperative that there be a clear understanding of how certain therapeutic agents are used to alter various hemodynamic parameters, all for the purpose of maintaining a balance between oxygen supply and demand.

PRELOAD

Preload, the diastolic stretch or filling of the ventricles, is an important determinant of stroke volume. Adequate stroke volume requires sufficient myocardial fiber stretch, or preload, according to the Starling law. Inadequate preload of the normal left ventricle, as reflected by left ventricular end-diastolic pressure of < 12 mm Hg, may be associated with reduced stroke volume. Patients with left ventricular dysfunction or decreased compliance of the ventricle usually require a higher filling pressure of 18 to 20 mm Hg for the same volume. However, left ventricular filling pressures higher than 20 or 22 mm Hg often cause pulmonary congestion secondary to transudation of fluid from the vascular network into interstitial, or even intraalveolar spaces. This results in reduced oxygen uptake and overall decreased tissue oxygen delivery.

Low Preload

If signs of hypoperfusion occur in the face of low preload volumes or pressures—RAP or CVP < 6 mm Hg, PAW or LA pressure < 8 mm Hg in patients without cardiac dysfunction, or < 18 mm Hg in patients with cardiac dysfunction—efforts are directed toward increasing preload levels. This can be achieved by the administration of fluid in an attempt to increase circulating volume. In general, patients without cardiac disease do not require a left heart filling pressure > 10 to 16 mm Hg (as measured by the PAWP) to obtain optimal stroke volume. However, patients with cardiac disease and decreased ventricular compliance usually require a higher filling pressure (16 to 22 mm Hg PAWP) and more judicious fluid administration. Yet it must be remembered that relative hypovolemia can exist in the face of elevated filling pressures. Such conditions occur with decreased ventricular compliance, right ventricular (RV) infarction, and cardiac tamponade.

Fluids

IV fluid challenges of 100 to 250 ml crystalloid solution should be administered over 10 minutes until evidence of improved perfusion occurs. Plotting ventricular function curves during this time is helpful to define the optimal filling pressure for the individual patient (i.e., that filling pressure which produces the best stroke volume). In general, left heart filling pressures (PAWP) >22 mm Hg are associated with a flat ventricular response (see Fig. 12-1) and, more important, can cause pulmonary congestion with decreased oxygenation at a time of increased oxygen demands.

High Preload

When left-sided filling pressures become excessively high, pulmonary venous pressure becomes higher than the colloid osmotic pressure surrounding the vasculature. This causes fluid to be driven from the vasculature and into surrounding interstitial or intraalveolar spaces. This backward congestion often manifests clinically by dyspnea and rales, in addition to signs of hypoperfusion, and can occur when the PAW pressure acutely increases to a value >20 to 22 mm Hg. Cardiogenic pulmonary edema usually occurs with a PAW pressure higher than 30 mm Hg. (However, in patients with chronic heart failure, a mean PAW pressure of >30 mm Hg may be seen without evidence of congestion or pulmonary edema.) Fluid in the interstitial or alveolar spaces interferes with oxygen uptake in the lung, and hypoxemia with decreased oxygen delivery results. High ventricular end-diastolic pressure (as measured by the PAWP) also decreases coronary collateral blood flow, an important consideration in the patient with ischemic heart disease. Reductions in preload to the lowest level compatible with adequate stroke volume can be obtained by the following means.

Diuretics

Furosemide, bumetanide, and ethacrynic acid, the three intravenously administered diuretics most commonly used in the critical care setting, are called *loop diuretics* because they inhibit the reabsorption of sodium in Henle's loop. This results in diuresis (usually about 20 to 30 minutes after administration) with resultant decreases in circulating blood volume and decreased preload (RA or CVP and PAWP). In addition, these agents have a pronounced venodilatory effect that occurs within minutes of administration and lasts about 1 hour. This venodilation results in venous pooling, decreased venous return, and therefore decreased preload (CVP or PAW) pressures. The cumulative effective decrease in PAWP reduces pulmonary congestion and pulmonary edema. However, the effect of IV diuretic administration on cardiac output depends on the individual patient's ventricular function. Excessive reductions of preload can result in reduced cardiac output and a clinical picture of cardiogenic shock or low output syndrome. This can be avoided with careful monitoring of the PAWP and cardiac output, as well as construction of ventricular function curves to determine the patient's optimal filling pressure (Fig. 12-2).

Venodilators

Venodilators redistribute blood volume in the capacitance vessels and thus reduce ventricular filling. Nitrate preparations (nitroglycerin) are predominantly venous vasodilators, although they also cause some arteriovasodilation. They reduce venous

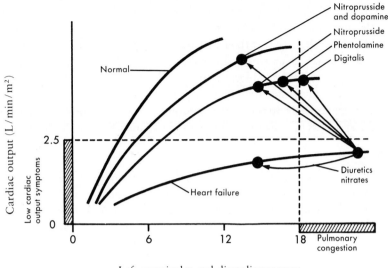

Fig. 12-2. Ventricular function curves depicting effects of various agents used for treating heart failure. Diuretics and nitrates lower filling pressure along the same curve and have little action on forward cardiac output. Positive inotropic agents and arterial vasodilators shift the ventricular function curve upward and to the left, increasing cardiac output for any left ventricular end-diastolic pressure. The combination of an arterial vasodilator and a positive inotropic agent (e.g., nitroprusside and dopamine or amrinone) can augment cardiac output and lower filling pressure to a greater extent.

Modified from Mason DT, editor: *Congestive heart failure,* New York, 1976, Yorke Medical Book.

return and preload (RA/CVP and PAWP) and therefore relieve pulmonary congestion. In addition, nitroglycerin dilates the epicardial coronary arteries and improves collateral coronary blood flow. Because of its rapid action and short half-life, intravenously administered nitroglycerin can be easily and quickly titrated to obtain optimal filling pressure as determined by ventricular function curves. Careful monitoring of arterial blood pressure should be done to avoid significant hypotension, which can occur as preload and, to a certain extent, afterload are reduced.

It is important to remember that the arterial blood pressure measured at a peripheral site is normally higher than the pressure in the central aorta and that this difference becomes exaggerated after nitroglycerin is given. Borderline hypotension as measured peripherally could mean significant central aortic hypotension.

If direct manipulation of preload with the aforementioned measures does not produce an improvement in cardiac output and therefore oxygen delivery to the tissues, therapeutic alterations of the other determinants of cardiac output may be necessary.

AFTERLOAD

True ventricular afterload is a complex measurement of the total force opposing left ventricular ejection. Clinically, afterload refers to the resistance to ventricular ejection that is primarily determined by systemic arterial resistance. A commonly used clinical reflection of the afterload of the left ventricle is the calculated SVR whereas afterload of the right ventricle is the calculated PVR (Table 12-1). Despite changes in resistance, the reserve capacity normally maintains stroke volume fairly constant with either vasoconstriction or vasodilation. In the failing ventricle, however, afterload or impedance is inversely related to cardiac output or stroke volume and directly related to myocardial oxygen consumption ($M\dot{V}o_2$) (Fig. 12-3). The right ventricle, because of its structure, is even more sensitive to increases in afterload than is the left ventricle.

Low Afterload

Arterial vasodilation results in decreased resistance (decreased afterload) and increased blood flow. However, because pressure = flow × resistance, excessive reduction in SVR can result in severe hypotension and consequently inadequate coronary artery perfusion. In this situation, vasopressor agents may be necessary to increase resistance to establish an adequate perfusion pressure. Vasopressors cause

Table 12-1. Derived hemodynamic parameters

Parameter	Abbreviation	Formula	Units	Normal values
Cardiac index	CI	$\dfrac{\text{Cardiac output}}{\text{Body surface area}}$	L/min/m^2	2.5-4.0
Coronary perfusion pressure (left heart)	CPP	Diastolic BP − PAWm	mm Hg	60-80
Left ventricular stroke work index	LVSWI	SVI × (MAP − PAWm) × .0136	g-m/m^2/beat	40-75
Oxygen delivery	$\dot{D}o_2$	Cardiac output × Arterial oxygen content × 10	ml/min	750-1000
Pulmonary vascular resistance	PVR	$\dfrac{\text{PAm − PAWm}}{\text{Cardiac output}} \times 80$	dynes/sec/cm^{-5}	30-100
Pulmonary vascular resistance index	PVRI	$\dfrac{\text{PAm − PAWm}}{\text{Cardiac index}} \times 80$	dynes/sec/cm^{-5}/m^2	70-180
Rate pressure product	RPP	Systolic BP × HR	mm Hg/min	12000
Right ventricular stroke work index	RVSWI	SVI × (PAm − RAm) × .0136	g-m/m^2/beat	4-8
Stroke volume	SV	$\dfrac{\text{Cardiac output}}{\text{Heart rate}} \times 1000$	ml/beat	60-120
Stroke volume index	SVI	$\dfrac{\text{Stroke volume}}{\text{Body surface area}}$	ml/beat/m^2	30-60
Systemic vascular resistance	SVR	$\dfrac{\text{MAP − RAm}}{\text{Cardiac output}} \times 80$	dynes/sec/cm^{-5}	900-1400
Systemic vascular resistance index	SVRI	$\dfrac{\text{MAP − RAm}}{\text{Cardiac index}} \times 80$	dynes/sec/cm^{-5}/m^2	1700-2600

BP, Blood pressure; *PAWm,* pulmonary artery wedge mean; *PAm,* Pulmonary artery mean; *RAm,* right atrial mean; *MAP,* mean arterial pressure; *HR,* heart rate.

vasoconstriction secondary to stimulation of alpha receptors in vascular smooth muscle. This produces an increase in both systolic and diastolic blood pressure. Vasopressor agents include phenylephrine, metaraminol, epinephrine, norepinephrine, ephedrine, and high-dose dopamine (> 10 to 20 μg/kg/min). Of these agents, epinephrine, norepinephrine, ephedrine, and dopamine also possess $beta_1$-stimulating properties that cause an increase in cardiac contractility and ejection. The secondary effects of increased resistance to ejection, or afterload, with the use of vasopressor agents are an accompanying increase in stroke work and $M\dot{V}O_2$. However, when adequate coronary perfusion pressure must be established, vasopressors are used to effectively increase blood pressure by increasing resistance. In general, a *diastolic* blood pressure of 60 mm Hg is necessary to maintain coronary artery perfusion, whereas a *mean* arterial pressure of 65 to 70 mm Hg is required to adequately perfuse the brain, kidney, and splanchnic organs. Although decreased peripheral perfusion may occur with the use of vasopressors, increasing coronary perfusion pressure, and therefore perfusion to the myocardium becomes the primary goal.

High Afterload

When cardiac output and blood pressure fall, reflex sympathetic stimulation causes arterial vasoconstriction to maintain blood pressure. However, such arterial vasoconstriction increases the resistance to ejection and forward blood flow is reduced. In addition, increased afterload increases the work of the heart and therefore $M\dot{V}O_2$. Consequently, oxygen demands are increased at a time when delivery is reduced, an imbalance that may cause ischemia. In such situations pharmacologic afterload reducing agents, or vasodilators, are employed to increase stroke volume and to reduce $M\dot{V}O_2$. This favors a better balance between oxygen supply and demand and thus has become a cornerstone of management of patients with cardiac failure.

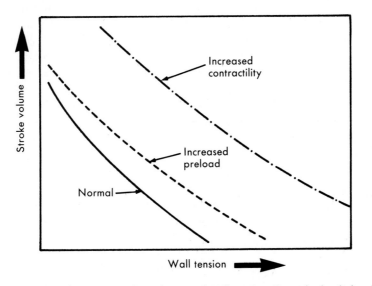

Fig. 12-3. Relationship between stroke volume and wall tension (i.e., afterload) for the intact left ventricle. At constant preload, increases in wall tension result in a decline in stroke volume. Increased preload or increased contractility shifts the curve upward and to the right, resulting in a greater stroke volume for any given afterload.

Vasodilation causes decreases in SVR that usually result in increases in cardiac output with little or no reduction in blood pressure (BP = CO × SVR). Thus, even though the blood pressure may remain the same, the reduction in SVR has unloaded the heart and allowed the LV to increase ejection without an increase in work. However, careful monitoring of both preload (PAW) and blood pressure are necessary to prevent severe hypotension. Maintaining adequate PAW pressures through concomitant volume administration is frequently necessary during afterload reduction. Generally, afterload-reducing agents are not used if the arterial blood pressure is < 90/60 mm Hg.

Arteriovasodilators

Smooth muscle relaxants. Agents that directly activate beta$_2$-adrenergic receptors in the smooth muscle of the arterioles and cause vasodilation include hydralazine, sodium nitroprusside, and nitroglycerin. Hydralazine is solely an arteriovasodilator whereas nitroprusside dilates the smooth muscle in both veins and arteries. Thus nitroprusside reduces both afterload and preload. Because of this, careful attention must be paid to the maintenance of adequate preload levels with sufficient volume administration when nitroprusside is given. The use of nitroprusside in patients with a normal PAWP can result in relative hypovolemia and a consequent fall in cardiac output. Nitroglycerin is, primarily, a peripheral venous dilator that also dilates epicardial coronary arteries and increases collateral coronary blood flow. It does, however, cause some arteriovasodilation, particularly at higher doses, and therefore also reduces afterload. The associated increase in cardiac output is usually small.

Calcium channel blockers

Agents that reduce or block the influx of calcium into arterial smooth muscle result in coronary and peripheral vasodilation and therefore afterload reduction. In addition, extracellular calcium influx into myocardial fibers is inhibited to a certain extent, resulting in a negative inotropic effect with decreased contractility. Certain calcium channel blockers (diltiazem and verapamil) also reduce extracellular calcium influx into atrioventricular (AV) nodal cells, resulting in slower conduction. All of these effects decrease $M\dot{V}O_2$, whereas coronary vasodilation increases myocardial oxygen delivery and thus strikes a more favorable balance between oxygen supply and demand. The use of calcium channel blockers to reduce a high preload or afterload should be undertaken with caution because these agents also possess negative inotropic effects, which could worsen heart failure.

Alpha blockers

Inhibition of stimulation of the alpha-adrenergic receptors in the peripheral vasculature results in vasodilation of both arteries and veins and, therefore, afterload reduction. Prazosin and phentolamine are both alpha blockers that can produce peripheral vasodilation and, thus, afterload reduction.

Angiotensin converting enzyme (ACE) inhibitors

An angiotensin converting enzyme (ACE) converts angiotensin I to angiotensin II, which is a potent vasoconstrictor. Agents that inhibit this enzyme prevent the conversion from angiotensin I to angiotensin II and, thus, produce vasodilation and afterload reduction. In addition, preload is reduced and cardiac output is improved, with variable change in arterial blood pressure. Severe hypotension may occur, particularly in patients who are overdiuresed and hyponatremic. If it occurs, it usually is observed after the first dose. Currently available ACE inhibitors include captopril, enalapril, and lisinopril.

Counterpulsation

Intraaortic balloon pumping with sudden balloon deflation during systole creates a vacuum space in the ascending aorta, which aids in ventricular ejection and therefore reduces ventricular afterload as well as $M\dot{V}o_2$. In addition, balloon inflation during diastole increases coronary blood flow and oxygen delivery to the myocardium (see Chapter 11).

CONTRACTILITY

Contractility refers to the inotropic state of the myocardium or, more specifically, the velocity of fiber shortening during systole. Inasmuch as contractility cannot be directly measured or even approximated in the clinical setting, an index of ventricular work (stroke work index) is used to assess changes in ventricular contractility. Decreased contractility associated with reduced ejection can occur with hypovolemia, myocardial ischemia, or infarction or after the use of certain pharmacologic and anesthetic agents. In such cases, increases in inotropism may be necessary to maintain adequate stroke volume and, more important, oxygen delivery. However, in patients with ischemic heart disease this benefit must be carefully weighed against the associated increase in $M\dot{V}o_2$ that accompanies increased contractility. In fact, decreases in oxygen demands of the myocardium may be the goal in these patients and agents that reduce contractility might be required.

Decreased Contractility

The stroke work indexes of either ventricle can be calculated from traditionally monitored parameters as identified in Table 12-1. Studies by Shoemaker et al. have shown that maintenance of a stroke work index of the left ventricle >55 g-m/beat is associated with improved survival in shock patients. Improvement in myocardial contractility can be obtained with the use of positive inotropic agents, which increase the amount of intracellular calcium available for actin and myosin cross-bridging. The catecholamines (dopamine, dobutamine, isoproterenol, and epinephrine) increase adenosine $3':5'$-cyclic phosphate (cyclic AMP) and thus calcium entry whereas the phosphodiesterase inhibitors (amrinone and milrinone) inhibit the breakdown of cyclic AMP into its inactive form. Increases in contractility are accompanied by increases in ejection fraction, and therefore end-diastolic volume (preload) usually falls. However, increases in contractility usually are associated with an increase in $M\dot{V}o_2$, although other determinants of $M\dot{V}o_2$ (systolic wall stress and heart rate) also affect this response. For example, the use of positive inotropic agents in a patient with a dilated and failing ventricle can produce an increase in stroke volume (secondary change in $M\dot{V}O_2$. On the other hand, the use of positive inotropic agents in patients with a normal-sized ventricle is likely to increase $M\dot{V}O_2$ and negatively affect the myocardium oxygen supply/demand balance.

In addition to the positive inotropic effects of isoproterenol and the phosphodiesterase inhibitors amrinone and milrinone, these agents produce systemic vasodilation through stimulation of beta$_2$-adrenergic receptors in vascular smooth muscle. Hemodynamically, this results in a reduction in SVR (afterload) in addition to the increased contractility. This combined effect may be beneficial.

Certain other positive inotropic drugs possess vasoconstrictor properties (such as epinephrine, norepinephrine, and high-dose dopamine). Thus these agents can increase perfusion pressure as well as augment contractility (Table 12-2).

A special modified PA catheter has been developed that calculates right ventricular volume measurements and cardiac output and, from these measurements, calculates the RV ejection fraction. The ejection fraction can be viewed as an indicator of the overall contractility of the ventricle. Normally, ejection fractions are similar for both ventricles and should be >50%. However, normal RV ejection fraction measured with the modified PA catheter is reportedly about 40%, somewhat lower than with other techniques.

Increased Contractility

Because of the increase in oxygen demands that occur with increased myocardial contractility, patients with myocardial ischemia may benefit from reductions in contractility as well as heart rate and blood pressure. This can be obtained with the use of beta blockers, which inhibit stimulation of beta$_1$-adrenergic receptors in the myocardium (cardioselective) and beta$_2$-adrenergic receptors in the smooth muscle in the arterioles of the lungs (nonselective). Blockage of beta$_1$-adrenergic stimulation results in decreased inotropic and chronotropic response to catecholamine stimulation with consequent reductions in contractility, heart rate, and cardiac output. Blockage of stimulation to beta$_2$-adrenergic receptors results in vasoconstriction. In the acute setting, therapy with beta blockers is begun with an intravenous dose followed by oral maintenance therapy.

HEART RATE

Heart rate (HR) is a major determinant of cardiac output (CO), coronary perfusion, and $M\dot{V}O_2$. Within limits, increases in heart rate can increase cardiac output (CO = stroke volume [SV] × HR). However, heart rates >120 to 125 beats/min may be associated with decreases in stroke volume and cardiac output because of decreased diastolic filling time of the left ventricle. Fast heart rates with shortened diastolic duration also decrease left ventricular coronary perfusion time and increase $M\dot{V}O_2$, causing an imbalance between myocardial oxygen supply and demand. High heart rates markedly increase $M\dot{V}O_2$ in two ways: (1) by increasing the frequency of work per minute and (2) by an accompanying increase in contractility (the Bowditch effect). Pharmacologic agents that are used to decrease heart rate include beta blockers to reduce chronotropism and calcium channel blockers to decrease conduction. In general, heart rates >100 to 110 beats/min are not hemodynamically advantageous.

Bradycardia with heart rates of <50 beats/min results in reductions in cardiac output and overall tissue perfusion. Agents used to increase the heart rate depend on

Table 12-2. Hemodynamic effects of commonly used cardiovascular drugs

Drug	Heart rate	Afterload	Contractility	Preload	Comments
INOTROPIC AGENTS					
Digoxin	− or ↓	±	↑	−	↓ Ventricular rate in AF
Dopamine	± or ↑	− or ↑	↑ ↑	↑ or ↓	Effect on SVR is dose-dependent; ↑ renal blood flow
Dobutamine	− or ↑	±	↑ ↑	↓	
Isoproterenol	↑ ↑	↓ ↓	↑ ↑	↓	Can cause dysrhythmias
Norepinephrine	↑ or ↓	↑ ↑	↑	↑	Can cause dysrhythmias
Epinephrine	↑ ↑	↑ or ↓	↑ ↑	↑	Can cause dysrhythmias
Methoxamine	−	↑ ↑	−	↑	
Amrinone/milrinone	− or ↑	↓	↑	↓	
ANALGESIC AGENTS					
Morphine	−	↓	−	↓	
DIURETICS					
(furosemide, ethacrynic acid, bumetanide)	−	↓	−	↓	May ↓ cardiac output if diuresis excessive
ANTIDYSRHYTHMIC AGENTS					
Lidocaine	−	−	± ↓	−	
Procainamide	−	−	± ↓	−	
Quinidine	−	−	± ↓	−	
Atropine	↑	−	−	− or ↓	
CALCIUM CHANNEL BLOCKERS					
Nifedipine	↑	↓	− or ↓	↓	
Diltiazem	↑	↓	− or ↓	−	
Verapamil	± ↓	± ↓	↓	−	
Amlodipine	↑	↓	−	↓	
Felodipine	↑	↓	−	↓	
BETA BLOCKERS	↓ ↓	− or ↑	↓	↑	
VASODILATORS					
Nitroprusside	− or ↑	↓ ↓	−	↓	↑ Cardiac output by ↓ peripheral resistance
Nitroglycerin	− or ↑	↓	−	↓ ↓	↑ Cardiac output by ↓ peripheral resistance
Hydralazine	−	↓	−	−	↑ Cardiac output by ↓ peripheral resistance
ALPHA BLOCKERS					
Phentolamine	− or ↑	↓	−	− or ↓	↑ Cardiac output by ↓ peripheral resistance
Prazosin	−	↓	−	↓	↑ Cardiac output by ↓ peripheral resistance
ACE INHIBITORS					
Captopril, enalapril, lisinopril	− or ↓	↓	−	↓	May cause hypotension, particularly if urine Na ↓

AF, Atrial fibrillation; *SVR*, systemic vascular resistance; *ACE*, angiotensin converting enzymes; *Na*, sodium; −; no effect; ↑, increase; ↓, decrease.

the underlying cause of the bradycardia. Vasovagal responses usually are managed with atropine and volume administration. A pacemaker (temporary or permanent) may be necessary if heart block is present.

Hemoglobin

Abnormal reductions of hemoglobin can impose a significant threat to tissue oxygenation inasmuch as approximately 98% of the oxygen is carried by the hemoglobin molecules. Maintenance of hemoglobin at normal levels can be obtained with administration of whole blood products, although the risks associated with this

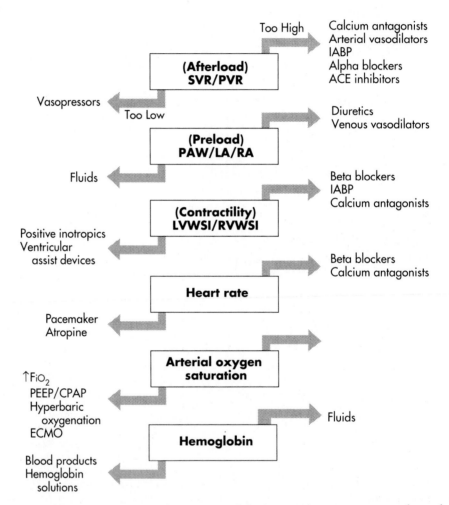

Fig. 12-4. Schematic diagram outlining some of the interventions more commonly used to appropriately affect the hemodynamic parameters that reflect the determinants of oxygen delivery. (See text for complete discussion.) (*IABP,* Intraaortic balloon pump; *ACE,* angiotensin converting enzymes; *SVR,* systemic vascular resistance; *PVR,* pulmonary vascular resistance; *PAW,* pulmonary artery wedge; *LA,* left atrium; *RA,* right atrium; *LVWSI,* left ventricular stroke work index; *RVWSI,* right ventricular stroke work index; *Fio₂,* fractional inspired oxygen concentration; *PEEP,* positive end-expiratory pressure; *CPAP,* continuous positive airway pressure; *ECMO,* extracorporeal membrane oxygenation.)

therapy have resulted in the acceptance of quite low hemoglobin levels (approximately 10 g/L) with manipulation of other oxygen delivery determinants.

Abnormally high hemoglobin concentrations can decrease cardiac output secondary to increased viscosity, again compromising overall oxygen delivery. Hemodilution may be necessary in such situations.

Arterial Oxygen Saturation

Oxygen saturation of arterial blood (Sao_2) can be maintained at normal levels (>97%) with increases in fractional inspired oxygen concentration (Fio_2), with positive end-expiratory pressure (PEEP), with continuous positive airway pressure (CPAP), with hyperbaric treatment, or, when all of the preceding fail, extracorporeal membrane oxygenation (ECMO). Although a Pao_2 of 60 mm Hg can be considered within normal limits, it is associated with an arterial saturation of only 92% to 93% if the oxyhemoglobin dissociation curve is normal. Increasing the Sao_2 to nearly 100% can effectively enhance oxygen delivery. However, consideration must be given to those interventions that also can decrease cardiac output (such as PEEP). If cardiac output is compromised, oxygen delivery can be reduced despite increases in Sao_2 or Pao_2. Maintenance of Pao_2 levels at above 100 mm Hg usually ensures adequate oxygen uptake with complete saturation of the hemoglobin with oxygen.

SUMMARY

Fig. 12-4 is a schematic illustration that depicts the interventions used to manipulate the major determinants of oxygen delivery. In general, critically ill patients suffer from multiple hemodynamic abnormalities, and a variety of agents are used simultaneously to alter them. In addition, a number of therapies can affect more than one hemodynamic parameter. Thus the critical care nurse must possess a sound knowledge of the pharmacologic and hemodynamic effects of agents that are commonly used in critical care. For example, the use of nitroprusside to reduce afterload in a patient with a normal preload may have a deleterious effect on cardiac output secondary to its venodilatory effect. Therefore this agent must be used cautiously with adequate volume administration to maintain preload and thus cardiac output and oxygen delivery. This is only one example of the myriad interactions that necessitate a clear understanding of the goal of all therapies, which is the delivery of adequate oxygen to all tissues.

REFERENCES

Alpert MA: Pharmacotherapy of congestive heart failure, *Postgrad Med* 81:257-267, 1987.

Braunwald E: *The myocardium: failure and infarction,* New York, 1974, HP Publishing.

Braunwald E: *Heart disease,* Philadelphia, 1980, WB Saunders.

Cohn JN: Vasodilator therapy: implications of acute myocardial infarction and congestive heart failure, *Am Heart J* 49:45-59, 1982.

Cohn JN: Treatment by modification of circulatory dynamics, *Hosp Prac* 19:37-52, 1984.

Dalen JE et al: Therapeutic interventions in acute myocardial infarction: survey of the ACCP section on clinical cardiology, *Chest* 86:257-262, 1984.

Davis D, Zelia R: Calcium channel antagonists: what role in the ICU? *J Crit Illness* 4:32-52, 1989.

Deepak V et al: A simplified concept of complete physiological monitoring of the critically ill patient, *Heart Lung* 10:75-82, 1981.

Dracup K et al: The physiologic basis for combined nitroprusside-dopamine therapy in postmyocardial infarction heart failure, *Heart Lung* 10:114-117, 1981.

Hannemann L et al: Dopamine versus dobutamine alone or in combination with norepinephrine in critically ill patients, *Crit Care Med* 18:S211, 1990.

Harvey WP et al: *The year book of cardiology,* Chicago, 1993, Mosby–Year Book.

Karliner J, Gregoratos G: *Coronary care,* New York, 1981, Churchill-Livingstone.

LeJemtel TH, Katz SD, Sonnenblick EH: Newer inotropic agents for managing patients with congestive heart failure, *J Appl Cardiol* 2:361-377, 1987.

Low R et al: The effects of calcium channel blocking agents on cardiovascular function, *Am J Cardiol* 49:547-552, 1982.

Mason DT: *Congestive heart failure,* New York, 1976, Yorke Medical Books.

Murray A: Haemodynamic measurements: a comment on units used, *Eur Heart J* 6:812-814, 1985.

Parmley WW: New calcium antagonists: relevance of vasoselectivity, *Am Heart J* 120:1408-1413, 1990.

Parmley W, Rouleau J: Vasodilators in heart failure secondary to coronary artery disease, *Am Heart J* 103:625-631, 1982.

Rosenthal MH: The appropriate use of inotropes in shock, *Can J Anaesth* 37(4 Pt 2):S1xiv-S1xx, 1990.

Shoemaker WC et al: Clinical trial of survivors' cardiorespiratory patterns as therapeutic goals in critically ill postoperative patients, *Crit Care Med* 10:398, 1982.

Siegl PKS: Overview of cardiac inotropic mechanisms, *J Appl Pharmacol* 8:S1-S10, 1986.

Weber K, Andrews V: Cardiotonic agents in the management of chronic failure, *Am Heart J* 103:639, 1982.

Weber KT, Sundram P, Reddy HK: Managing heart failure with positive inotropic drugs, *J Crit Illness* June 2:14-23, 1987.

Chapter 13

Hemodynamic Monitoring of Children

Mary Fran Hazinski

The critically ill child is both physically and physiologically immature and differs from the critically ill adult in several important ways. As a result, hemodynamic monitoring in children requires both specialized equipment and skills. The equipment used must be available in several small sizes and often requires more careful calibration and maintenance than similar equipment used with adult patients. In addition, the pediatric patient may be unable to understand or cooperate with invasive monitoring procedures, so that it can be difficult to insert and to secure monitoring lines in the child. Careful explanations and use of restraints often will be required. Finally, with any monitoring technique, the data obtained are only as reliable as the professional at the bedside; pediatric monitoring equipment must be carefully calibrated and operated, and the clinician must be able to validate and evaluate the data in light of patient appearance and progress.

PHYSIOLOGIC DIFFERENCES BETWEEN CHILDREN AND ADULTS
Cardiovascular Function

The child's cardiovascular system continues to mature after birth. Changes in the child's cardiac output and myocardial function accompany the child's growth. At birth, cardiac output is higher *per kilogram body weight* than during any other time in life, averaging approximately 400 ml/kg/min; cardiac output per kilogram decreases to 200 ml/kg/min in the infant and ultimately to 100 ml/kg/min in the adolescent. Because the child's body weight is small, the child's *absolute cardiac output* at birth is only approximately 0.6 L/min, but it increases to approximately 6 L/min in the large adolescent male. *Cardiac index* throughout childhood is slightly higher than the cardiac index of the adult and is normally 3.0 to 4.5 L/min/m^2 body surface area.

Table 13-1. Normal pediatric vital signs

NORMAL HEART RATES AND RESPIRATORY RATES

AGE	HEART RATE	RESPIRATORY RATE
Infants	120-160/min	30-60/min
Toddlers	90-140/min	24-40/min
Preschoolers	80-110/min	22-34/min
School-aged children	75-100/min	18-30/min
Adolescents	60-90/min	12-16/min

NORMAL BLOOD PRESSURE RANGES[*]

AGE	SYSTOLIC PRESSURE	DIASTOLIC PRESSURE
Neonate (1 month)	85-100	51-65
Infant (6 months)	87-105	53-66
Toddler (2 years)	95-105	53-66
School age (7 years)	97-112	57-71
Adolescent (15 years)	112-128	66-80

Heart rate and respiratory rate tables reproduced with permission from Hazinski MF, editor: *Nursing care of the critically ill child*, St Louis, 1984, Mosby–Year Book.
*Blood pressure tables taken from the 50th to 90th percentile ranges, extrapolated from graphs published by Horan MJ, chairman, Task Force on Blood Pressure Control in Children: *Pediatrics* 79:1, 1987. These blood pressure ranges were derived by the task force from a sampling of more than 70,000 children.

Cardiac output is a product of heart rate and stroke volume. Heart rate is normally more rapid in childhood than during adult years, and stroke volume averages 1.5 ml/kg. During childhood, cardiac output is very heart rate–dependent (see Table 13-1 for normal pediatric vital signs). The neonatal myocardium contains less contractile elements and has a higher water content than adult myocardium. As a result, the neonatal myocardium is less compliant than adult myocardium and the resting left and right ventricular end-diastolic pressures are higher in the neonate than in the adult. Although early studies of neonatal myocardial function suggested that these differences rendered the neonatal ventricles incapable of increasing stroke volume in response to volume administration, more recent research (Clyman et al.) suggests that neonates are capable of increasing stroke volume in response to volume administration. This increase can occur provided the aortic pressure does not rise precipitously, ventricular function is adequate, and systemic vascular resistance is not elevated. Hypoxemia, acidosis, shock, heart failure, or a rise in pulmonary or systemic vascular resistance may limit the ability of the ventricles to increase stroke volume.

At birth, pulmonary and systemic vascular resistances are approximately equal, and the right and left ventricles have equal thickness. During the first weeks of life pulmonary vascular resistance normally falls from 8 to 10 index units (units/m^2) to 1 to 3 index units as a result of pulmonary vasodilation and regression of the medial muscle layer in the pulmonary arteries. When pulmonary vascular resistance falls, right ventricular muscle mass decreases, and its compliance increases. Systemic vascular resistance gradually rises during childhood and normally ranges between 15 and 30 index units; left ventricular muscle mass increases in a corresponding fashion, and the left ventricle becomes less compliant than the right ventricle (see the box on p. 277 for other normal resting values).

Bradycardia is the most common pediatric dysrhythmia, and it most often occurs as the result of vagal stimulation or hypoxia. Profound or persistent bradycardia in

Normal resting values in children

NORMAL CARDIAC INDEX IN CHILDREN

3.0 to 4.5 L/min/m^2

NORMAL CARDIAC OUTPUT IN CHILDREN*

Age	Cardiac output (L/min)	Heart rate	Normal stroke volume
Newborn	0.8-1.0	145	5 ml
6 mo	1.0-1.3	120	10 ml
1 yr	1.3-1.5	115	13 ml
2 yr	1.5-2.0	115	18 ml
4 yr	2.3-2.75	105	27 ml
5 yr	2.5-3.0	95	31 ml
8 yr	3.4-3.6	83	42 ml
10 yr	3.8-4.0	75	50 ml
15 yr	6.0	70	85 ml

CALCULATION OF SYSTEMIC VASCULAR RESISTANCE

$$SVRI = \frac{\text{Mean arterial pressure} - \text{Mean right atrial pressure}}{\text{Cardiac index}}$$

Normal SVRI in neonates: 10-15 index units (35-50 Wood units; 2800-4000 dynes/sec/cm^{-5})

Normal SVRI in children: 15-30 index units (15-25 Wood units; 1200-2000 dynes/sec/cm^{-5})

NOTE: To convert indexed units to dynes/sec/cm^{-5}, change cardiac index to cardiac output in denominator of equation, and multiply equation by 80.

CALCULATION OF PULMONARY VASCULAR RESISTANCE

$$PVRI = \frac{\text{Mean pulmonary artery pressure} - \text{Mean left atrial pressure}}{\text{Cardiac index}}$$

Normal PVRI in neonates: 8-10 index units (25-40 Wood units; 2000-3200 dynes/sec/cm^{-5})

Normal PVRI in children: 1-3 index units (0.5-4 Wood units; 40-320 dynes/sec/cm^{-5})

NOTE: To convert indexed units to dynes/sec/cm^{-5}, change cardiac index to cardiac output in denominator of equation and multiply the entire equation by 80.

NORMAL OXYGEN CONSUMPTION

Infants <2-3 wk of age: 120-130 ml/min/m^2
Children >2-3 wk of age: 150-160 ml/min/m^2

or

5-8 ml/kg/min

NORMAL ARTERIAL OXYGEN CONTENT

18-20 ml oxygen/dl blood

SVRI, Systemic vascular resistance index; PVRI, pulmonary vascular resistance index.

*Table from Hazinski MF, editor: *Nursing care of the critically ill child*, St Louis, 1984, The CV Mosby Co. Modified from Rudolph AM: *Congenital diseases of the heart*, Chicago, 1974, Year Book Medical Publishers, Inc.

the absence of reversible hypoxia is an ominous finding in the pediatric patient and often indicates impending arrest. In fact, bradycardia (progressing to asystole) is the most common terminal cardiac rhythm in children. Whenever bradycardia is observed, the child's oxygenation, airway, and gas exchange must be carefully evaluated.

Supraventricular tachydysrhythmias also may be observed in the critically ill child. Although tachycardia is an expected response to fever, stress, pain, and critical illness and may help to maintain cardiac output, excessively high heart rates may compromise cardiac output. If the ventricular rate exceeds 180 to 230 per minute, ventricular diastolic filling time and coronary artery perfusion time will be reduced and cardiac output may fall dramatically. Brief episodes of supraventricular tachycardia (SVT) may be tolerated without clinical signs in the normal infant, but they can be expected to produce significant compromise of systemic perfusion in the child with underlying heart disease.

Whenever the nurse cares for the child with an alteration in heart rate or rhythm, attempts should be made to correlate clinical appearance and hemodynamic measurements and calculations with varying heart rates. The nurse should attempt to determine the heart rate at which the child's cardiac output and systemic perfusion are best and should endeavor to maintain that heart rate, if possible.

The normal pediatric myocardium is less likely to develop malignant ventricular dysrhythmias, even during stimulation (such as may occur during placement of a pulmonary artery catheter), than is the adult myocardium. Malignant ventricular dysrhythmias are almost exclusively seen in children with complex heart disease, left ventricular outflow tract obstruction, myocarditis, or cardiomyopathy.

Pulmonary edema in any patient can result either from high pulmonary capillary pressures or from increased pulmonary capillary permeability. Even when congestive heart failure results in increased pulmonary capillary pressures, however, rales may not be appreciated during clinical examination if the child's breathing is shallow. There is evidence that the infant is more likely than the older child or adult to develop increased pulmonary capillary permeability and pulmonary edema during episodes of respiratory dysfunction; thus pulmonary artery wedge pressure in young children is often normal despite evidence of pulmonary edema.

It is thought that biventricular failure is more common in children than is univentricular failure. Although this may be true in the presence of some congenital heart defects, it may not be true of the pediatric patient with shock, myocarditis, or pulmonary hypertension. In these patients, significant discrepancies may exist between right and left ventricular end-diastolic pressures. Therefore, central venous pressure measurements should be used only to evaluate *right* ventricular end-diastolic (or right atrial) pressure; pulmonary artery catheterization should be undertaken if measurement of left ventricular end-diastolic (or left atrial) pressure is necessary.

Circulating Blood Volume

The child's circulating blood volume averages approximately 75 to 80 ml/kg and is smaller than the blood volume of the adult. Unreplaced blood loss of 25 ml will result in a 12% hemorrhage in the 3-kg infant. Therefore it is extremely important to consider any blood lost during procedures or blood drawn for laboratory analysis as a percentage of the child's circulating blood volume (Table 13-2). If unreplaced

Table 13-2. Circulating blood volume in children

Age	ml/kg body wt
Neonates	85-90
Infants	75-80
Children	70-75
Adults	65-70

From Hazinski MF, editor: *Nursing care of the critically ill child*, St Louis, 1984, Mosby–Year Book.

acute blood loss totals more than 5% to 7% of the child's circulating blood volume, transfusion should be considered. *When intravascular or intracardiac monitoring lines are in place, scrupulous attention should be paid to securing all tubing connections.* Loose connections or stopcocks inadvertently turned to allow blood loss may result in significant hemorrhage within a few moments. *All monitoring lines should be connected to monitors with adjustable low pressure alarms, so that line separation or pressure loss will be detected immediately.*

Oxygen Transport and Consumption During Childhood

Oxygen delivery is the product of arterial oxygen content (hemoglobin concentration, which is calculated as g/dl $\times$ 1.34 ml O_2/g saturated hemoglobin $\times$ percent hemoglobin saturation) and cardiac output. Normal arterial oxygen content is 18 to 20 ml O_2/dl blood. The normal cardiac output in the child varies with age, averaging 400 ml/kg/min during the first weeks of life, 200 ml/kg/min during infancy, and 100 ml/kg/min in the adolescent. Cardiac index averages 4.5 L/min/m^2 body surface area (BSA) in the neonate and 3.0 to 4.5 L/min/m^2 in the infant and child. Normal oxygen delivery averages 665 to 1000 ml/min/m^2 during the first weeks of life and 425 to 750 ml/min/m^2 during infancy and childhood. Oxygen consumption averages 180 to 270 ml/min/m^2 during the first weeks of life and 120 to 230 ml/min/m^2 during infancy and childhood.

If either arterial oxygen content or cardiac output falls without a compensatory increase in the other factor, oxygen delivery will fall. When cardiovascular function is good, cardiac output may increase in response to anemia or hypoxemia to maintain oxygen delivery; however, if cardiovascular function is limited, anemia or hypoxemia will result in a fall in oxygen delivery. When cardiac output falls, oxygen delivery usually falls in a commensurate fashion.

In the adult, oxygen delivery is typically about four times the oxygen consumption, and the difference between oxygen delivery and supply provides an oxygen reserve. For this reason a slight increase in oxygen demand or a minimal reduction in oxygen delivery may be well tolerated, unless or until oxygen delivery falls below a critical point. At that point, further decreases in oxygen delivery will be associated with reduced tissue oxygen consumption and tissue oxygenation, and ischemia and metabolic acidosis result.

Oxygen consumption is very high during childhood because the metabolic rate is high in children. This is particularly true during the neonatal period. For this reason, the young child requires a higher cardiac output and oxygen delivery per m^2 than does the adult. Oxygen delivery is only two to three times the oxygen consumption in the young infant, particularly during the first weeks of life. As a result the neonate and young infant have a much smaller oxygen reserve than the normal child or adult; anything that compromises oxygen delivery (e.g., cardiorespiratory failure) or increases oxygen demand (e.g., cold, stress, pain, sepsis) may rapidly result in the development of tissue hypoxia and ischemia. Normal oxygen delivery and consumption during the neonatal period, infancy, and childhood are listed in Table 13-3.

Under some conditions, including sepsis and malignant hyperthermia, oxygen consumption may become supply-dependent. As a result, any fall in oxygen delivery will result in a reduction in tissue oxygenation and oxygen consumption and may contribute to the development of tissue ischemia and metabolic acidosis. In patients with supply-dependent oxygen consumption, oxygen delivery should be supported at levels greater than normal, because normal oxygen delivery may still be inadequate to ensure effective tissue oxygenation. Efforts also should be made to minimize oxygen demands.

Fluid Requirements

The child's metabolic rate is higher than that of the adult, so that the child's maintenance fluid requirements are higher per kilogram than those of the adult. However, the child's body weight is small; thus the child's total fluid needs are less than those of an adult (see Table 13-4 for maintenance fluid requirements in children). For this reason, it is imperative that *all* sources of the critically ill child's fluid intake and fluid loss be recorded on an hourly basis. Fluids used to flush monitoring lines and catheters or dilute medications may be sources of unrecognized fluid overload in the small child.

The infant or young child has high glucose and caloric needs and low glycogen stores. As a result, the critically ill infant requires a virtually constant source of glucose intake, and attempts should be made to ensure that most fluid administered to the child contains glucose or other sources of nutrition. Because most monitoring lines are flushed with glucose-free solution to reduce risk of bacterial growth, the "flush"

Table 13-3. Cardiac output, oxygen delivery, and oxygen consumption in children

Age (wt/BSA)	Cardiac output (CO)* (ml/min)	Oxygen delivery† ($\dot{D}_{O_2}$)		Oxygen consumption ($\dot{V}_{O_2}$)	
		(ml/min)	(ml/min/m²)	ml (min)	(ml/min/m²)
Newborn (3.2 kg/0.2 m²)	700-800	133-200	665-1000	36-54	180-270
6 mo (8 kg/0.42 m²)	1000-1600	200-280	476-667	70-100	167-238
1 yr (10 kg/0.5 m²)	1300-1500	260-300	520-600	85-110	170-220
2 yr (13 kg/0.59 m²)	1500-2000	300-400	508-678	91-123	154-208
4 yr (17 kg/0.71 m²)	2300-2375	460-475	648-669	110-150	155-211
5 yr (19 kg/0.77 m²)	2500-3000	500-600	649-779	115-170	149-221
8 yr (28 kg/0.96 m²)	3400-3600	680-720	708-750	150-208	156-200
10 yr (35 kg/1.1 m²)	3800-4000	760-800	690-727	190-250	122-227
15 yr (50 kg/1.4 m²)	5000-6000	1200	857	300-400	120-200

*Cardiac index (CI) for children: 3.0-4.5 L/min/m²
†Assuming a hemoglobin concentration of 15 g/dl and normal arterial oxygen content.

Table 13-4. Maintenance fluid requirements in children

Body weight increments	Fluid requirements (ml/hr)
First 10 kg	4 ml/kg/hr
Second 10 kg	2 ml/kg/hr (plus 40 ml/hr for kg 1-10)
Third 10 kg	1 ml/kg/hr (plus 60 ml/hr for kg 1-20)
If m² body surface area (BSA) used:	60 ml/m²/hr

fluid will be a source of increased fluid intake of no nutritional value to the child. Therefore the rate of fluid administered to flush the monitoring lines should be no greater than the minimal amount necessary to maintain catheter patency (usually 2 to 5 ml/hr). The use of heparinized flush solutions (in concentration of 1 to 5 units/ml) may contribute to the longevity of monitoring lines.

Inasmuch as small catheters must be inserted into the small vessels of the child, these catheters can quickly become obstructed if they are not flushed appropriately. To guarantee uninterrupted delivery of fluids through the catheter lumen, it is imperative that careful attention be given to the tubing and flush system. If intermittent (rather than continuous) hemodynamic measurements are required, heparin (in concentrations of 20 to 100 units/ml) may be instilled in some catheters to maintain catheter patency between measurements without the need for constant fluid infusion.

If the child has unrepaired cyanotic congenital heart disease, systemic venous blood is allowed to enter the systemic arterial circulation without passing through the lungs. Thus *when the child has unrepaired cyanotic heart disease, absolutely no air can be allowed to enter any intravenous or central venous line*, because it may be shunted into the left heart and ultimately produce a cerebral air embolus. All venous lines should be inspected frequently and thoroughly, and all air must be eliminated.

Thermoregulatory Differences

Infants and small children have large surface area-to-volume ratios, and they can lose a great deal of heat to the environment through evaporation. In addition, the infant cannot shiver to generate heat and must break down brown fat in an energy-requiring process called "nonshivering thermogenesis." If the infant is exposed to a cold environment, oxygen consumption will increase for the purpose of nonshivering thermogenesis; this is clearly undesirable when cardiorespiratory distress or failure is present. For these reasons it is very important to keep young children warm. Incubators are usually impractical thermoregulatory devices in the critical care unit, because they are large enough only for young infants and the inside temperature will fall if the incubator is entered frequently. In addition, the infant must be removed from the incubator during procedures. Over-bed warmers are ideal thermoregulatory devices in the critical care unit, inasmuch as they maintain a warm ambient temperature by heating the air surrounding the child; these warmers enable constant observation of the child and immediate access to the child while preventing cold stress. Such warmers should be used during procedures that require the child to be uncovered for prolonged periods of time.

NONINVASIVE MONITORING
General Assessment

Anyone caring for the critically ill patient of any age should develop the ability to determine at a glance whether that patient "looks good" or "looks bad." *The ability to recognize when the patient "looks bad" is one of the most important observation skills required in the intensive care unit.* When hemodynamic monitoring is performed, it is essential to correlate values obtained with the appearance of the child, so that the monitoring provides quantitative data to support qualitative observations.

To determine the degree of distress the child is demonstrating, the child's color, level of activity, responsiveness, position of comfort, and feeding behavior should be assessed. The healthy child will have pink mucous membranes and nail beds, with consistent skin tones. The skin of the child with cardiorespiratory distress will develop a mottled appearance, and the nail beds and lips may be pale. If the child's condition deteriorates further, a gray pallor, consistent with hypoxemia and poor systemic perfusion, often is observed.

The well-oxygenated, well-perfused child should have warm extremities, with strong peripheral pulses and brisk (instantaneous) capillary refill. It is important to note that *"normal" vital signs are not always "appropriate" vital signs for the critically ill child* (see Table 13-1 for normal vital signs). An early sign of cardiorespiratory distress, pain, or fear is tachycardia, and tachycardia is nearly always more appropriate than "normocardia" when the child is seriously ill or injured. *Bradycardia is usually an ominous clinical sign in the critically ill child.*

The healthy infant or child will be alert and active and will move all four extremities. The normal infant or child will demonstrate good eye contact with parents and health care professionals. The healthy toddler should protest vigorously when separated from parents or touched by strangers and will resist being placed in the supine position. The typical preschooler should be able to converse and may ask questions about treatment or caregivers. The normal school-aged child and adolescent may tolerate examinations if prior explanation is provided and should be able to voice complaints and be able to recall where he or she is hospitalized.

The moderately ill infant or child probably will not demonstrate good eye contact, may be irritable when aroused, and often is unable to find a comfortable position. The extremely ill child will be unresponsive to most stimulation and usually demonstrates flaccid muscle tone. *If the child is unresponsive to pain (such as a venipuncture), severe cardiorespiratory or neurologic compromise should be suspected.* The child's responsiveness should be evaluated during all aspects of critical care, particularly during invasive and noninvasive procedures.

While approaching the child and before touching him or her, it is important to perform a thorough visual inspection, noting all vascular pressures and counting respiratory rate. Resting values should be compared with those obtained after the child is stimulated from tactile and auscultatory examination.

Clinical Signs of Shock

As mentioned earlier, signs of poor systemic perfusion in children include nonspecific signs of distress, such as tachycardia, irritability, and tachypnea. The child whose condition deteriorates further becomes lethargic, with decreased response to painful stimulus. Early signs of cardiorespiratory failure include mottling of the skin, peripheral vasoconstriction and cooling of extremities, prolonged capillary refill, diminished intensity of peripheral pulses, and decreased urine volume (< 1 to 2 ml/kg/hr). If an arterial line is in place, narrowing of the pulse pressure and dampening of the waveform may be noted before hypotension is observed. The child may maintain a "normal" blood pressure despite the presence of shock or significant (up to 20% to 25%) hemorrhage. *Hypotension is only a very late sign of cardiorespiratory distress in children* and indicates the presence of cardiovascular collapse; at this point, cardiorespiratory arrest is imminent.

Clinical Signs of Congestive Heart Failure

Signs of congestive heart failure in the child are similar to those observed in the adult, including signs of adrenergic stimulation and systemic and/or pulmonary venous congestion. In children, however, jugular venous distention cannot be appreciated, so that the most reliable sign of elevated right ventricular end-diastolic pressure and central venous pressure (CVP) is hepatomegaly. When CVP is monitored, attempts should be made to correlate the degree of hepatomegaly with the child's CVP, so that the CVP can be estimated even after the central venous catheter has been removed.

In adult patients, changes in cardiac output, right atrial pressure, and systemic vascular resistance may be accurately estimated approximately 50% of the time on the basis of clinical examination. Prediction of pulmonary artery wedge (PAW) pressure on the basis of clinical examination is even less precise, particularly in the presence of shock. Although the relationship between clinical examination and documented PAW pressure has not been studied in the pediatric population, it generally is thought that clinical appearance does not provide reliable indication of PAW pressure. Pulmonary edema may be caused by high pulmonary capillary pressure (and high PAW pressure), or it may be caused by increased capillary permeability regardless of the PAW pressure. Hence, if determination of the PAW pressure is needed to guide therapy, insertion of a balloon-tipped, flow-directed pulmonary artery catheter will be necessary.

Arterial pressure monitoring can be performed through use of cuff pressure (automatic or manual) or an indwelling arterial catheter, monitoring system, and transducer. If intermittent cuff pressures are obtained, the nurse must frequently evaluate the child's clinical appearance, tissue perfusion, and quality of peripheral pulses to promptly recognize changes in the child's condition that indicate a change in arterial pressure. It is imperative that the blood pressure cuff used be of appropriate size — the width should cover two thirds the length of the upper arm, and the bladder of the cuff should not wrap more than once around the upper arm. (Appropriate blood pressure cuff sizes are listed in Table 13-5.)

Noninvasive blood pressure measurements may be inaccurate when the child's hemodynamic status is unstable; for this reason, intraarterial pressure measurement should be considered to provide the most reliable data in the child with shock or cardiovascular dysfunction. Cuff blood pressure measurements have been shown to provide falsely low pressure measurements when adult patients are hypertensive and falsely high pressure measurements when adult patients are hypotensive; such inaccu-

Table 13-5. Commonly available blood pressure cuffs

Cuff name*	Bladder width (cm)	Bladder length (cm)
Newborn	2.5-4.0	5.0-9.0
Infant	4.0-6.0	11.5-18.0
Child	7.5-9.0	17.0-19.0
Adult	11.5-13.0	22.0-26.0
Large arm	14.0-15.0	30.5-33.0
Thigh	18.0-19.0	36.0-38.0

From Horan MJ, chairman, Task Force on Blood Pressure Control in Children: *Pediatrics* 79:1, 1979.
*Cuff name does not guarantee that the cuff will be appropriate size for a child within that age range.

rate results probably are also present with pediatric cuff blood pressure measurements.

Although noninvasive oscillometric blood pressure monitoring devices have been shown to be accurate when used to evaluate *normotensive* children, these devices may fail to rapidly reflect the development or worsening of hypotension and may be inaccurate in the presence of shock. If there is any doubt as to the accuracy of the oscillometric blood pressure measurement, the blood pressure should be verified with use of a cuff and manometer. Ideally, an intraarterial line should be inserted.

Pulse Oximetry
Hemoglobin saturation

The saturation of hemoglobin in arterial blood may be continuously monitored by means of a pulse oximeter placed on the child's finger, toe, hand, foot, or ear lobe. Pulse oximeters correlate well with measured and calculated arterial oxygen saturations in children over a wide range of clinical conditions. In addition, continuous monitoring of arterial oxygenation may allow recognition and treatment of acute episodes of hypoxemia that may not be detected with intermittent blood sampling alone. Such continuous monitoring can enable modification of nursing care based on the child's response and may allow more prompt confirmation of deterioration (which may result from pneumothorax, endotracheal tube displacement, or airway obstruction) than is possible with intermittent blood sampling.

Unfortunately, the ability of pulse oximeters to reflect hypoxic events varies widely. For this reason the critical care nurse should always rely on clinical assessment of the patient's condition and use the pulse oximeter only as one source of quantitative data. The use of the oximeter probably is most beneficial to evaluate trends in the child's clinical condition.

The pulse oximeter indicates *hemoglobin saturation,* rather than partial pressure of oxygen. To determine the child's approximate arterial oxygen pressure (Pao_2) from the hemoglobin saturation, the nurse must be familiar with (or consult) the oxyhemoglobin dissociation curve (see Fig. 10-2). Under normal conditions, the child's Pao_2 will be adequate once the hemoglobin saturation exceeds 93% to 95%, and hypoxemia is present if the hemoglobin saturation is less than 93%.

Principles of oximetry

Pulse oximeters use two light-emitting diodes that direct a red and an infrared light through the tissue to a photodetector. The diodes and photodetector must be carefully placed so the light is transmitted through tissue perfused by a pulsatile artery to the photodetector. The amount of red light absorbed by the tissue will be inversely related to the saturation of the hemoglobin passing through the pulsatile arterial circulation; hemoglobin that is well-saturated with oxygen will absorb little of the red light, and poorly saturated hemoglobin will absorb a great deal of the red light before it reaches the photodetector (see Chapter 10 for further information).

Pulse oximeters may be inaccurate in the presence of carbon monoxide poisoning, methemoglobinemia, profound anemia (hematocrit <20%), or hypotension. Several pulse oximeters are commercially available, including portable and bedside monitors and those with hard-copy printout of heart rate and hemoglobin saturations. It is important that the nurse be aware of individual differences among brands of pulse oximeters; some oximeters demonstrate more delay in signals with lower heart rates, whereas others demonstrate more delay with higher heart rates. Variability in response to hypoxia also has been documented (Severinghaus and Naifeh; Verhoeff and Sykes). In addition, the cost, accuracy, and reliability of disposable and reusable probes should be considered in the selection of a pulse oximeter.

Differences in the reliability of pulse oximetry may be seen when different types of oximeter *probes* are used. The oximeter probes are most commonly mounted on a disposable adhesive strip or a spring-loaded plastic clip. With either device, it is important to secure the device so that the light transmitters are directly aligned with the photosensors, separated only by well-perfused tissue. Accurate pulse oximetry can be achieved only if the probes are placed and maintained properly.

Clinical use

Disposable probes are most popular for use with infants; these probes consist of the light diodes and photosensors mounted a few centimeters apart on an adhesive strip. The strip is placed on the infant's hand, foot, thumb, or great toe. A well-perfused, warm extremity should always be used. Once the site is selected, positioning of the probe and sensor should be attempted while the oximeter unit is turned on, so that the strength of the pulse signal is displayed. Once a strong, reliable pulse signal is obtained, the adhesive strip is wrapped around the infant's palm, foot, thumb, or toe in such a way that the red light is directly aligned with the photosensor, "sandwiching" the tissue (Fig. 13-1, A). When the probe is correctly positioned, the light will be able to pass directly through the tissue to the photosensor.

A reusable probe may be contained in a hard plastic, spring-loaded clip that can be clamped on the thumb or great toe of a small child or on the middle finger of a large child or adolescent. It is important that the child's digit be large enough so that the clip remains in place, clamped firmly on the digit, or excessive artifact will result. In addition, when any reusable probe is used, the photosensor should be regularly but gently cleansed with an alcohol wipe before use, to remove any oils that may have accumulated during previous use.

Excessive amounts of ambient light can interfere with the accurate detection of light absorption by the photosensor. Therefore, if the infant or child is placed under

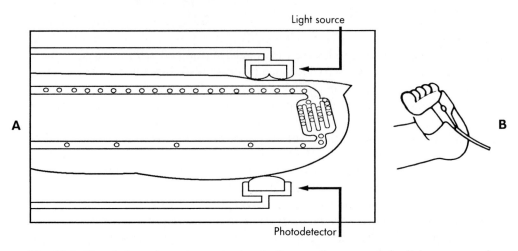

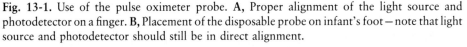

Fig. 13-1. Use of the pulse oximeter probe. **A,** Proper alignment of the light source and photodetector on a finger. **B,** Placement of the disposable probe on infant's foot—note that light source and photodetector should still be in direct alignment.

Courtesy Nellcor, Inc., Hayward, Calif.

warming or phototherapy lights, it is often helpful to loosely wrap gauze around the child's monitored extremity and the pulse oximeter probe to block ambient light from the photosensor.

If the pulse oximeter probe is placed over a finger or thumb tip, all nail polish must be removed from the digit because certain nail polishes can interfere with light transmission and detection. In addition, the digit should be wiped with alcohol to remove excess dirt or oil.

The probe and the oximetry unit should always come from the same manufacturer. The probe of one manufacturer should never be used with the unit from another manufacturer even if the plugs appear to be compatible. Such mixing of equipment may result in inaccurate hemoglobin saturations or in patient burns (Sobel).

Movement artifact is one of the most common causes of inaccurate pulse oximetry results in children. It is often very difficult to secure the pulse oximeter probe properly and to eliminate movement artifact when an active infant is monitored. Such artifact will be reduced if a proximal portion of the infant's extremity is used (e.g., placing the disposable probe around a wrist, hand, ankle, or foot rather than the thumb or toe, as in Fig. 13-1, *B*). If one extremity is restrained with an intravenous line in place, that extremity also should be used for pulse oximetry probe placement. This will eliminate the need for restraint of more than one extremity and will reduce movement artifact. The pulse oximetry probe should not be placed distal to an arterial line if that arterial line has produced any compromise in distal extremity perfusion.

Cautions

Once the hemoglobin is fully saturated, the child's partial pressure of oxygen can be any number *above* 70 to 100 mm Hg. When the neonate's hemoglobin is fully saturated, the Pao_2 may exceed 100 mm Hg, introducing a risk of retrolental fibroplasia. Therefore, if a hemoglobin oxygen saturation of $\geq 96\%$ is observed during supplemental oxygen therapy, the Pao_2 should be checked and the neonate's inspired oxygen concentration adjusted to prevent the Pao_2 from exceeding 80 to 100 mm Hg (Poets et al.).

When pulse oximetry is used to monitor a neonate with a right-to-left (pulmonary artery-to-aorta) *ductal* shunt, the pulse oximeter probe should be placed on an upper extremity if knowledge of the ascending aortic oxygen saturation is desired. If the probe is placed on a lower extremity, the hemoglobin oxygen saturation monitored will reflect that in the right ventricle, pulmonary artery, and descending aorta. Excellent correlation between arterial oxygen saturation and pulse oximetry results in children with cyanotic congenital heart disease has been documented (Boxer et al.).

Pulse oximeters should be used with caution in patients with acute or significant changes in arterial pH, $Paco_2$, or temperature, because these variables will affect the relationship between hemoglobin saturation and Pao_2. In patients with such changing variables, caution should be used when attempting to derive Pao_2 from hemoglobin saturation. Frequently, critically ill children with head injury or pulmonary hypertension are hyperventilated, which produces hypocapnia and alkalosis. *In alkalotic patients, the oxyhemoglobin dissociation curve shifts to the left,* so that the hemoglobin is better saturated with oxygen at even low Pao_2 values. Thus, whereas a hemoglobin oxygen saturation of 93% may be associated with a Pao_2 of 70 mm Hg in the patient with normal pH, it probably will be associated with a Pao_2 of 50 mm Hg or less in the alkalotic patient. Unless the nurse is responsive to even mild reductions in hemoglobin saturation in the alkalotic patient, the detection of severe hypoxemia (and institution of therapy to improve ventilation and alveolar oxygenation) may be delayed.

(Skin Surface) Transcutaneous Blood Gas Monitoring
Principle

Under normal conditions, the oxygen tension measured across the skin is much lower than the arterial oxygen tension (Pao_2). In 1969, Huch, Huch, and Lubbers demonstrated that an approximation of the partial Pao_2 could be measured on the surface of the skin if hyperemia was produced in the skin beneath the electrode. This discovery led to the development of the modified heated Clark electrode that may be mounted to the skin. When the electrode heats the skin to 43° to 45° C, oxygen diffuses rapidly through the skin and blood flow through the dermal capillary bed is stabilized; as a result, as long as cardiac output and skin blood perfusion are adequate, there is good correlation between skin surface, or transcutaneous, oxygen tension ($Ptco_2$) and Pao_2. If blood flow to the tissues is significantly compromised, however, $Ptco_2$ will be much lower than Pao_2; such a discrepancy is commonly seen during periods of low cardiac output.

When a Stowe-Sevringhaus electrode is added to the Clark electrode, monitoring of the child's skin surface (transcutaneous) carbon dioxide may be performed. In neonates, there is good correlation between transcutaneous carbon dioxide pressure ($Ptcco_2$) and arterial carbon dioxide pressure ($Paco_2$), although the skin surface Pco_2 tends to be approximately 2 to 11 torr higher than the $Paco_2$. If skin blood flow is compromised (such as in low cardiac output), the $Ptcco_2$ may become significantly higher than the Pao_2. Because the Stowe-Sevringhaus electrode is pH-sensitive, the $Ptcco_2$ may correlate poorly with the $Paco_2$ when the child is acidotic (pH < 7.3) or profoundly hypoxemic (Pao_2 < 40 mm Hg).

Clinical use

Transcutaneous blood gas monitoring may be used in a variety of clinical settings; however, it has been used to any great extent only in the newborn intensive care unit, and its use has decreased considerably since pulse oximeters have become readily available. When any transcutaneous monitor is used, adequate electrode warm-up time must be allowed, and the unit must be appropriately calibrated, according to the manufacturer's specifications. *Careless or irregular calibration of the transcutaneous blood gas machine and electrode will result in inaccurate monitoring results.*

The electrode should be placed over a well-perfused area of the skin; placement over the trunk or proximal portion of an extremity is preferred, because these areas should remain well perfused even if mild reductions in cardiac output develop. Placement over bony prominences or over large blood vessels should be avoided, inasmuch as these areas do not have consistent capillary density. The electrode should never be placed on the child's face because a burn may develop.

Once the monitor has been warmed up and appropriate calibration performed, the skin at the selected monitoring site is wiped with alcohol to remove oil and dead cells. The electrode is secured on the skin by use of the adhesive mounting ring. After the electrode is in place, adequate skin warming time (up to 25 minutes) should be allowed before $Ptco_2$ or $Ptcco_2$ values are recorded. Unit policy should indicate the frequency of correlation of arterial blood gas values with transcutaneous blood gas values.

Warming of the skin by the electrode results in the development of a circular erythematous area, similar to a sunburn. For this reason, heated electrodes should be moved to new skin sites every 2 to 4 hours (see manufacturer's recommendations). The erythema usually becomes most noticeable several hours after electrode removal and usually fades within 12 to 24 hours.

Correlation between the arterial and transcutaneous oxygen tensions is reduced when cardiac output and systemic and skin perfusion are compromised. As a result, transcutaneous blood gas monitoring may provide an indication of poor systemic perfusion (e.g., during trauma resuscitation) if $Ptco_2$ is less than 90% of the Pao_2. Correlation between transcutaneous and arterial oxygen tension should improve when perfusion improves.

Cautions

The popularity of transcutaneous monitoring devices has decreased dramatically in recent years as the result of consumer frustration with the meticulous and frequent calibration required, as well as the tendency of some monitors to drift. In most institutions, the pulse oximeter has replaced the $Ptco_2$ monitor for noninvasive monitoring of patient systemic arterial oxygenation. Transcutaneous monitors may still provide useful monitoring of trends in infant carbon dioxide levels, particularly in the monitoring of infants with respiratory failure.

There is no question that these devices require proper care to ensure maximal performance and reliability. In addition, the correlation of arterial blood gases to transcutaneous gases varies with the specific brand and model of monitor used. Therefore it is imperative that personnel be familiar with proper operation of the monitor and electrode and interpretation of the transcutaneous blood gas results obtained with each model used.

Correlation of $Ptco_2$ with Pao_2 is definitely best when used in neonates. Older patients or patients with thick skin often demonstrate poor correlation between $Ptco_2$ and Pao_2 values, and machine drift in these patients is significant. Pao_2 also is affected by capillary density in the skin below the transducer.

If the infant's cardiac output is significantly reduced, or if vasoactive drugs result in increased or diminished skin blood flow, transcutaneous blood gas values may vary significantly from arterial blood gases, despite careful monitor calibration and electrode placement. Halothane anesthesia and hypothermia also interfere with accurate transcutaneous blood gas monitoring.

The heated electrode may produce blisters and second-degree burns in infants with extremely sensitive skin. The purposes of the transcutaneous monitoring should be explained to the parents, and the possible development of a reddened area (not unlike a sunburn) should be discussed. The heated electrode should not be applied over the skin of the hypothermic infant, because burns may result and reliable monitoring will not be possible.

If the neonate has a right-to-left shunt at the level of the ductus arteriosus (such as may occur in the presence of some congenital heart defects or persistent pulmonary hypertension of the newborn), it is advisable to place the electrode over the upper portion of the child's trunk (above the nipple line) or on the proximal portion of either arm. With this electrode placement, the $Ptco_2$ should reflect ascending aortic Pao_2.

Some electrodes must be wrapped if they are used under phototherapy lights. Whenever the transcutaneous monitor is used, regular correlation between arterial blood gases and monitored blood gases should be documented.

Automatic Oscillometric Monitoring of Blood Pressure

Oscillometric blood pressure monitoring devices use standard sizes of blood pressure cuffs joined by cables to a monitor unit. The unit inflates and deflates the cuff, and it documents cuff inflation pressures and oscillations in cuff pressure, which are related to systolic, diastolic, and mean arterial pressures.

Principle

The cuff is inflated to a systolic pressure of approximately 200 mm Hg, although this maximal inflation pressure is modified on the basis of the patient's previous systolic pressure readings. As the cuff is deflated, oscillations in cuff pressure are detected as the patient's arterial pressure exceeds cuff pressure and pulsatile flow occurs in the artery under the cuff. Small but recognizable oscillations correspond to the systolic blood pressure, maximal oscillations correspond approximately to the mean arterial pressure, and the recurrence of small oscillations is recognized as corresponding to the patient's diastolic blood pressure.

The accuracy of the blood pressures obtained depends on the programmed characteristics of the monitor—each monitor must recognize oscillations that are caused by arterial pulsations rather than movement or muscle artifact. Yet if small oscillations are discarded, the monitor may be unreliable in the hypotensive or very young patient. Furthermore, the magnitude of the oscillations relate to the patient's systolic, diastolic, and mean arterial blood pressure. If the patient has a narrow pulse pressure, very low cardiac output, or arterial pulsations that are not classic in configuration, inaccurate blood pressure readings may result.

Clinical use

To begin monitoring the patient's blood pressure by oscillometry, one must select a cuff of the proper size (see Table 13-5). The cuff should be wrapped securely around the extremity selected and the monitor turned on. The monitor can obtain the blood pressure immediately or can be programmed to automatically and regularly document the blood pressure at specified intervals (e.g., every 3 minutes or at selected intervals between 1 and 90 minutes). Average elapsed time to display systolic, diastolic, and mean blood pressures and heart rate is approximately 20 to 30 seconds, although a longer time may be required if the patient is hypotensive. If characteristic oscillations are not recognized, an audible alarm may sound and flashing numbers appear on the screen to indicate that the cuff must be repositioned or that the blood pressure is undetectable.

Alarm limits may be set to activate audible and visual alarms for low and high blood pressures (for systolic, diastolic, and mean pressures) and for low or high heart rate. Flashing numbers in any of the display panels usually indicate an alarm condition.

The clinical use of the Dinamap monitor (manufactured by the Critikon Company of Johnson and Johnson) in the pediatric setting has been most extensively documented in the literature. Excellent correlation between auscultatory blood pressures (r = 0.97 for systolic pressure, and r = 0.90 for diastolic pressure) and oscillometrically derived blood pressures have been established in *normotensive* pediatric patients and in normotensive neonates (Park and Menard). However, oscillometric determination of blood pressure may correlate poorly with direct blood pressure measurement or with auscultatory measurement when the patient is hypotensive or when the blood pressure is falling. Such discrepancies have been documented in hypotensive neonates and currently are being studied in hypotensive children (Diprose et al.).

Cautions

When oscillometric pressure measurements are used as the primary source of blood pressure measurements in critically ill children, the recorded pressures should be verified by auscultatory technique at least once every shift and during any change in patient condition. On the basis of the correlation studies published to date, *oscillometric pressure measurements can be used with confidence only in the stable, normotensive neonatal or pediatric patient.*

Movement artifact or seizure activity may produce inaccurate oscillometric pressure measurements in the child with an otherwise stable blood pressure. If movement artifact is suspected, the nurse should wrap the cuff around the child's extremity and hold the extremity in position while the cuff inflates and deflates. Oscillometric blood pressure measurements should not be attempted during seizure activity.

If the patient's condition is extremely unstable, direct arterial monitoring provides a continuous display of the patient's blood pressure and arterial waveform, as well as providing intraarterial access for blood sampling. When intraarterial pressures are obtained with a properly flushed system and a transducer that is properly zeroed, leveled, and calibrated, direct pressure measurements are preferred to indirect oscillometric pressures.

INVASIVE MONITORING

Basic Monitoring Technique

Invasive hemodynamic monitoring in the pediatric patient must be undertaken only by practitioners skilled in establishing and maintaining intravascular access and in interpreting the measurements obtained. It is important to remember that invasive measurements are usually more useful in *trending* changes in patient conditions and responses to therapy than in determining a single measurement in time. Therefore it is imperative that each measurement by every member of the health care team be made under the same conditions; if error cannot be eliminated, it must at least be standardized.

Because arterial blood pressure measurements and cardiac output calculations are smaller in children than in adults, a small error in measurement technique can result in a proportionally large error in data. Monitoring system tubing length should be kept to a minimum so that excellent transmission of pressure waves will occur. All air bubbles, tubing kinks, and loose connections must be eliminated from the system. The number of stopcocks in a monitoring line should be kept to a minimum (preferably less than three stopcocks), and the stopcock must be turned to perfectly align stopcock ports with catheter lumens; this will minimize changes in the radius of the tubing system.

Finally, the transducer must be properly zeroed and mechanically calibrated, and the monitor also must be zeroed and electronically calibrated. Although the transducer may be placed at any level and zeroed, it is essential to consistently place the air-reference port at the level of the right atrium (also called the *phlebostatic axis*). This level is commonly considered to be at the junction of the nipple line and the anterior axillary line. Once the transducer is zeroed, the relationship between the patient's right atrium, the transducer, and the "zeroing" stopcock (which was opened to air) must remain constant; if the relationship changes, the system must be rezeroed. Effects of transducer movement on invasive monitoring measurements are summarized in the box on p. 292.

Proper intravascular monitoring must take into account anatomic and physiologic differences between children and adults. Specific differences that affect invasive monitoring are noted next.

Basic Pediatric Considerations

1. The vessels of the child are small. These vessels may be difficult to cannulate, and small catheters (and introducers and guidewires) are needed. The lumen of a small catheter can become occluded by small kinks or with very small accumulation of fibrin or blood products. It is imperative that the catheter be continuously flushed with 1 to 5 ml/hr of the flush solution and that regular assessments be made of the patency of the catheter. Use of heparinized continuous flush solution (1 to 5 units heparin/ml) has been shown to increase the patency of these small catheters. If the catheter is used for intermittent pressure measurements only, concentrated heparinized flush solution (containing 20 to 100 units of heparin/ml) may be instilled into the catheter to ensure patency. This heparin should be withdrawn, however, before fluid is instilled into the catheter.

2. Even small amounts of blood loss during catheter insertion may represent significant blood loss for the infant or child. As a result, the child's circulating blood

---

Common causes of error in vascular monitoring systems

TRANSDUCER LEVELED INCORRECTLY

Transducer air-reference port placed above right atrium will result in falsely low
vascular pressure readings
Transducer air-reference port placed below right atrium will result in falsely high
vascular pressure readings

DAMPING OF SIGNAL (USUALLY WILL PRODUCE FALSELY LOW RESULTS)

Kink in monitoring tubing or catheter
Air in monitoring line or transducer
Clot in tip of catheter
Clamp or stopcock obstructing waveform transmission
Catheter wedged against vessel wall
Leak or loose connection in monitoring tubing/system
Blood backup in tubing or transducer
Faulty transducer (check mechanical calibration)

SIGNAL ARTIFACT

Catheter fling may result in erroneously high digital pressure readings
60-cycle interference may introduce error in readings
High fluid infusion rate may dampen waveform signal or result in increased pressure
within monitoring system (reduce flow rate in monitoring line and ensure that
flow-limiting valve is in place)
Excessive tubing length, stopcocks

---

volume should be calculated and blood replacement given if acute blood loss totals
more than 5.0 to 6.0 ml/kg body weight (5% to 7% of the child's total circulating
blood volume). After catheter insertion, the nurse should monitor the child closely for
evidence of bleeding or hypovolemia (including tachycardia with compromise of
systemic perfusion). All blood withdrawn for laboratory analysis should be totaled,
and blood replacement should be considered if the hematocrit level falls or if blood
drawn totals 5% to 7% of the circulating blood volume.

3. Fluid overload can result from excessive fluid administration through
monitoring lines. It is imperative that this source of fluid intake be meticulously
totaled each hour and added to the child's total fluid intake for that hour. Fluids used
to flush monitoring lines should be infused only through a volume infusion pump, so
that the exact volume of fluids administered may be calculated. Intermittent flushing
of the catheter and tubing should be performed with a syringe, rather than through
a fast-flush device, so that the exact volume of such "flushes" can be added to the
child's recorded fluid intake (refer to discussion of central venous pressure
monitoring). The health care team should be aware of the heparin and electrolyte
content of all fluids infused through monitoring lines.

4. Most children move all extremities vigorously. Therefore all tubing connections should have Luer-Loks in place to reduce the possibility of inadvertent
disconnections. In addition, all tubing connections should be taped securely, and

---

Procedure for mechanical calibration of transducer

NOTE: This procedure uses the principle that a column of water 27.2 cm high exerts a pressure equal to 27.2 cm H_2O pressure (27.2 cm H_2O = 20 mm Hg).

1. Assemble flushed transducer, tubing (with appropriate stopcocks and syringes), monitor cable, and tape measure. Be sure that a 12-inch piece of flushed, noncompliant tubing is attached to transducer. Prepare monitor printer.
2. Join transducer to bedside monitor via the monitoring cable.
3. Turn bedside monitor on, and select appropriate pressure monitoring scale.
4. Place air-reference stopcock at level of phlebostatic axis.
5. Open stopcock port to *air,* and depress *zero* button on bedside monitor (this will zero the transducer and monitor to atmospheric pressure).
6. If an electronic calibration button is present on the bedside monitor, depress it after transducer is zeroed—this will electronically calibrate the bedside monitor.
7. Begin printing pressure display.
8. Turn stopcock off to air port, and close this port with sterile dead-end plug. Turn transducer stopcock open to the fluid-filled 12-inch noncompliant tubing.
9. With the free end of the 12-inch tubing open to air, and its tip at the level of the phlebostatic axis, the digital display should read "O" ($\pm$1 mm Hg).
10. Raise the free end of the noncompliant tubing 27.2 cm above the transducer (and phlebostatic axis); this applies a pressure equal to 20 mm Hg on the transducer; the monitor digital display should read "20 [$\pm$1] mm Hg," and the graphic reading should display a signal equal to 20 mm Hg.
11. Return tubing free end to level of phlebostatic axis, and ensure that digital and graphic displays return to "O" level.
12. Adjust monitor or printer as needed to ensure appropriate calibration. If transducer is faulty, change it.

For further information refer to Civetta JM: Pulmonary artery catheter insertion. In Sprung CL, editor: *The pulmonary artery catheter: methodology and clinical applications,* Baltimore, 1983, University Park Press.

catheters should be taped or sutured into place. Whenever possible, the nurse should tape an additional loop of tubing to the patient so that vigorous movement will be more likely to place tension on the loop of tubing rather than on the catheter itself. The transducer, catheter insertion site, and all tubing and connections should be visible at all times. "High" and "low" pressure monitoring alarms should be set so that sudden changes in patient condition or tubing separation will immediately trigger an audible alarm. The bedside nurse should carefully check the entire monitoring system and all connections at least every hour to ensure that loose connections will be detected.

5. The child's arterial blood pressure is usually much lower than the blood pressure of the adult. Therefore small errors in blood pressure measurement may be relatively more significant in the child. For this reason, it is imperative that transducers used in children be carefully zeroed, leveled, and mechanically calibrated before use, so that the data obtained with the transducer will be reliable (see box above).

6. There is a general conception that the child is immunologically immature and

is at greater risk for infection than the adult. Certainly the critically ill child is susceptible to infection. However, extensive studies of invasive hemodynamic monitoring in children have failed to document a higher incidence of catheter-related septicemia in children than that reported for adults (Smith-Wright et al.). There is no question that the combination of a prolonged ICU stay and multiple invasive monitoring lines will make any patient's risk of nosocomial infection extremely high. It is therefore imperative that these lines be established under strict sterile conditions and maintained under strict aseptic conditions.

7. Children often are frightened and unable to cooperate with invasive procedures. Careful explanations should be provided (at an age-appropriate level) before initiation of any procedure. Because children often interpret intentional pain as punishment, the child should be assured that he or she is "good." In addition, adequate analgesia must be provided during any painful procedure.

The child should be securely restrained to prevent the dislodging or separating of essential therapeutic or monitoring equipment. The parents should be allowed to remain with the child and provide comfort once the sterile insertion procedure has been completed.

Central Venous Pressure Monitoring

Insertion of a central venous catheter may be performed to enable fluid or drug infusion or to allow measurement of central venous pressures. Central venous pressure (CVP) monitoring will reflect right atrial pressure unless superior or inferior vena caval obstruction is present. Right atrial pressure will, in turn, reflect right ventricular end-diastolic pressure (RVEDP) unless tricuspid valve stenosis is present.

Very often, if myocardial function and vascular resistances are normal, the child's right and left ventricular end-diastolic pressures will be equal. Then the CVP will be approximately equal to the pulmonary artery wedge (PAW) and left atrial (and LVED) pressures. This equality, however, cannot be assumed when the child is critically ill. Sepsis, septic shock, respiratory disease, cardiomyopathy, myocarditis, and congenital heart disease can all depress right *or* left ventricular contractility and function and may result in a discrepancy between right and left ventricular end-diastolic pressures. For this reason, the CVP should be interpreted only as reflecting RVEDP. Indirect assessment of left ventricular end-diastolic pressure (LVEDP) may be made through echocardiography, and further assessment of LVEDP may be obtained through use of a flow-directed balloon-tipped pulmonary artery catheter (see Chapters 5 and 6 for further information about central venous and pulmonary artery pressure monitoring).

The CVP will be low if the child has inadequate intravascular volume relative to the vascular space. Such low pressures may be observed following absolute volume loss as a result of hemorrhage, dehydration, capillary leak, or other causes of hypovolemia. In addition, a low CVP may result from expansion of the vascular space, with development of a relative hypovolemia. This may occur with early septic shock or administration of vasodilatory agents.

An elevated CVP reflects an increase in RVEDP. This may be caused by hypervolemia, such as occurs with excessive intravenous fluid administration in the presence of renal failure. However, an elevation in CVP more commonly occurs when there is right ventricular failure, with a decrease in right ventricular compliance, contractility, and ejection fraction. Such right ventricular failure may result from congenital heart disease, myocarditis, cardiomyopathy, sepsis, or increased pulmonary vascular resistance (e.g., pulmonary hypertension).

The CVP measurement aids in titration of fluid administration for the pediatric or adult patient in shock (see Chapter 12 for further information). During fluid administration, the nurse should attempt to identify the CVP associated with optimal systemic perfusion (including blood pressure, capillary refill, and urine output). This optimal CVP may then be maintained through careful fluid administration.

As noted, the critically ill child's PAW pressure and LVEDP may be normal, low, or elevated in the presence of a high, normal, or decreased CVP. Therefore, when the nurse monitors the CVP during shock resuscitation, attempts should be made to evaluate left ventricular function and systemic perfusion. Two-dimensional echocardiogram may reveal dilation of the left ventricle if significant left ventricular failure is present. The development of pulmonary edema also can indicate the presence of elevated (>20 to 25 mm Hg) LVEDP, but this clinical sign also may be caused by increased capillary permeability in the presence of a normal or low LVEDP or PAW pressure. If assessment of LVEDP is necessary, a flow-directed, balloon-tipped pulmonary artery catheter should be inserted.

The appearance of the CVP pressure tracing is identical in the child and the adult. The normal mean CVP in the infant is 0 to 4 mm Hg, and the normal mean CVP in the child is 2 to 6 mm Hg.

CVP measurements may be affected by positive pressure ventilation and high levels of positive end-expiratory pressure. The effects observed depend on the compliance of the child's lungs and the amount of positive pressure provided. If the child's lungs are extremely compliant, intrapleural pressure created by the ventilator is likely to be transmitted to the pleural space and vessels, including any vessels in the chest. Thus the CVP may rise during the inspiratory phase of positive pressure ventilation. If the child's lungs are noncompliant (i.e., they are very stiff), the effects of changes in the intrapleural pressure created by the ventilator may be minimal. Higher peak inspiratory pressures and end-expiratory pressures are more likely to affect the CVP than are lower pressures. (Effects of respiratory disease on hemodynamic monitoring also are discussed in Chapter 15.)

Indications

Indications for use of CVP catheters in children include the following:
1. Measurement of CVP for the purposes of determining
   a. Intravascular volume status (and venous return)
   b. RVEDP
   c. Ideal RVEDP (and CVP) necessary to optimize systemic perfusion
2. Rapid delivery of resuscitative and vasoactive drugs to the right atrium
3. Administration of hypertonic fluids (such as parenteral alimentation)
4. Rapid infusion of intravenous fluids
5. Venous access for blood sampling

CVP catheters may be inserted percutaneously or by cutdown through several sites (Fig 13-2): umbilical vein, external or internal jugular vein, femoral vein, basilic vein, or subclavian vein. The site is determined by the experience of the clinician, the age of the child, and the acuity of the child's condition. Umbilical venous, subclavian vein,

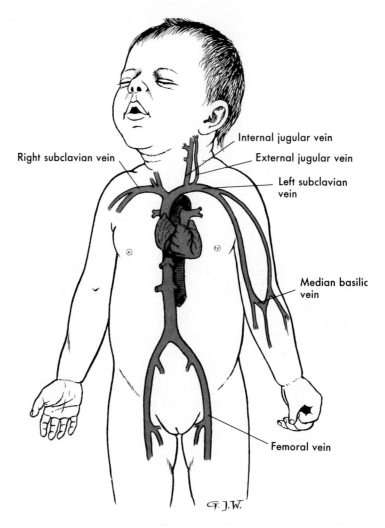

Fig. 13-2. Location of veins used for placement of CVP catheters.

external and internal jugular venous, and femoral venous catheterization are discussed in detail in subsequent sections.

Umbilical venous catheterization is possible during the first weeks of life. External jugular venous cannulation is relatively easy, but this site is often impractical to use during resuscitative efforts. Internal jugular or subclavian vein catheterization should be attempted only by a clinician experienced in the technique, because these procedures may result in bleeding or pneumothorax, respectively.

Femoral vein catheterization may be most appropriate during resuscitative efforts, because this site is distant from the child's airway and chest. Although resuscitative drugs administered into the inferior vena cava may theoretically pool below the diaphragm during cardiac compression unless the catheter is sufficiently long to allow the tip to pass above the diaphragm, the medications can be delivered into the central circulation (and to the right atrium) if they are followed by a bolus (2 to 3 ml) of flush solution. Because femoral venous lines may easily become contaminated by urine or stool, they usually are removed as quickly as possible.

Equipment needed for umbilical venous or artery catheterization

---

Appropriate catheter and blunt needle
Povidone-iodine solution
Sterile hat, mask, gown, and gloves for clinician
Sterile towels
Gauze sponges
Sterile container (for povidone-iodine)
A #11 surgical blade
Scalpel handle
4-0 or 5-0 silk suture on cutting needle
Needle holder
Two small (5-inch), curved mosquito hemostats
Small toothed forceps
4-inch curved forceps
4-inch straight forceps
Small scissors
Sterile umbilical tape (several 6-inch lengths)
Sterile measuring tape
Several syringes
Flush solution for catheter
Monitoring system (with calibrated transducer)

Before insertion of any central venous catheter, the nurse should explain the procedure to the child (if the child is conscious) and the parents, and informed consent should be obtained from the parents or legal guardian (unless the procedure is performed under emergent conditions). Adequate analgesia should be provided, and the child should be restrained before the procedure.

Many clinicians use the Seldinger technique to insert a catheter percutaneously into the child's vein. This technique involves insertion of a large-bore hollow needle into the desired vein. A small-gauge guidewire is then threaded through the needle until several centimeters of the wire are within the large vein. Once the guidewire has been inserted, the needle is withdrawn over the guidewire. Finally, the central venous catheter is threaded over the guidewire, into the vein, until it lies in proper position. The guidewire is then withdrawn, the intravenous fluid infusion system is joined to the catheter, and the catheter is sutured into place. The Seldinger technique is especially effective for percutaneous insertion of catheters of relatively large size into infants and young children.

Umbilical venous catheterization

The umbilical venous catheter (UVC) may provide immediate intravascular access during neonatal resuscitation and allows central venous access for blood sampling and pressure monitoring. The equipment needed for umbilical venous or arterial catheterization is listed in the box above.

Before catheter insertion, the neonate is securely restrained. Electrocardiographic monitoring is provided throughout the procedure. The proper depth of catheter insertion is estimated by adding 4 cm to the distance (in centimeters) between the distal ends of the infant's clavicles and the umbilicus. A sterile piece of cord tape should be tied around the catheter at the calculated insertion depth. The sterile catheter is then irrigated with the flush solution and attached to a fluid-filled transducer and monitoring system to enable monitoring of the umbilical venous waveform during catheter insertion. The umbilical area is draped with sterile towels and scrubbed with a povidone-iodine solution.

Using sterile technique, the clinician examines the umbilical stump and identifies the umbilical vein as the largest vessel in the umbilical cord (the two smaller umbilical arteries have thicker walls). The vein usually is located on the superior portion of the umbilicus.

Sterile umbilical cord tape is placed around the umbilicus and tied loosely; this tie should prevent bleeding during the procedure, although it may be necessary to loosen it as the catheter is inserted. The cord should be pulled upright, with slight tension, and a scalpel should be used to cut the cord horizontally. This cut enables catheterization of nondistorted, uncontaminated umbilical vessels.

Sterile forceps should be used to remove any fibrin or clots from the lumen of the vein; then the forceps should guide the catheter into the umbilical vein. As the catheter is advanced into the vein, the pressure waveform should be displayed on the monitor oscilloscope.

As the umbilical catheter is passed into the subdiaphragmatic portion of the umbilical vein and portal vein, only respiratory pressure variations will be visible on the oscilloscope. However, as the catheter enters the inferior vena cava, a characteristic CVP waveform will be visible on the oscilloscope. The appearance of a CVP waveform should coincide with insertion of the catheter to the measured (and marked) maximal insertion point. The catheter should be marked with indelible ink at this insertion point, and the catheter should be carefully taped in position.

Proper location of the distal tip of the umbilical venous catheter in the inferior vena cava should be verified by chest radiograph. It is essential that proper placement of the catheter be confirmed before any drugs or fluids are infused through the catheter. Once proper placement is ensured, the catheter is sutured and firmly taped in place.

The tape used to secure an umbilical artery or venous catheter should hold the catheter in a straight line from the umbilicus, perpendicular to the anterior plane of the infant's body. This requires creation of a tape "bridge." Two pieces of tape (one on either side of the umbilicus) are placed vertically, anchored at each end to the infant's abdomen. These two pieces of tape are used to brace a third, horizontal piece of tape that suspends the catheter upright between the vertical tapes (the horizontal piece of tape creates the appearance of the crossbar of football goal posts, or the letter H).

The neonate may be placed in the prone position while umbilical artery or venous catheters are in place as long as the nurse is able to observe the umbilicus for evidence of bleeding at all times. Care must be taken to avoid tension on the catheter or the insertion site.

When the umbilical venous catheter is removed, pressure is applied over the umbilicus for at least 5 minutes or until bleeding stops. A sterile gauze pad is then taped over the umbilical site. The nurse should monitor for bleeding from the vein for several hours after catheter removal.

Subclavian vein catheterization

The subclavian vein is gaining in popularity as a site for pediatric vascular access because the catheter may be taped securely in place on the child's chest and it will not interfere with positioning of the child or movement of the child's extremities. Placement of this catheter should be attempted only by clinicians skilled in the technique. Potential complications include tension pneumothorax or hemothorax.

When subclavian vein catheterization is performed, the child should be placed in the Trendelenburg position, with the head 20 to 30 degrees lower than the heart and turned away from the site. This position will distend the subclavian vein and minimize the possibility of an air embolus during catheterization. The site should be draped with sterile towels and scrubbed with povidone-iodine solution. Local anesthetic (1% lidocaine) should be instilled subcutaneously.

The subclavian vein is cannulated at the point where it crosses over the first rib, just before it passes under the clavicle. The clinician's index fingertip is placed in the suprasternal notch to provide a reference point. A needle attached to a syringe will be inserted just under the clavicle at the distal margin of the medial third of the clavicle (a distance equal to one third the length of the clavicle, measured from the junction of the clavicle and the sternum). The syringe and needle should be held parallel to the frontal plane of the body, and the needle is inserted in a medial, cephalad direction, pointing toward the suprasternal notch and the reference fingertip (Fig. 13-3). The syringe plunger should be aspirated as the needle is advanced, and insertion should stop when blood is aspirated freely into the syringe inasmuch as this indicates entrance into the subclavian vein.

Once the needle is in the subclavian vein, it should be rotated so that the bevel of the needle faces downward. The syringe is detached from the needle, and to prevent entry of air into the central venous system, the needle hub is covered with the clinician's (gloved) thumb. During patient spontaneous exhalation or positive pressure ventilation, a guidewire is passed through the needle and advanced to the approximate length required to enter the superior vena cava. Once the guidewire is successfully passed, the needle is withdrawn over the guidewire. Finally, the catheter is passed over the guidewire and into the subclavian vein and, ultimately, into the superior vena cava (and right atrium, if desired). The guidewire is then withdrawn and the catheter is sutured into place. A sterile dressing is applied to the site. The catheter should be intermittently flushed to maintain patency, but it should not be attached to infusion fluids until appropriate placement is verified by chest radiograph.

External jugular venous catheterization

External jugular venous catheterization is generally popular for use in children older than 5 years of age. Because the vein is superficial and visible, this vessel may be used when emergency venous access must be achieved rapidly.

When external jugular venous catheterization is performed, the child is positioned as described for subclavian vein catheterization (30-degree head-down position, with the head turned away from the catheterization site, as already noted). The child must be properly restrained, and 1% lidocaine should be injected to anesthetize the

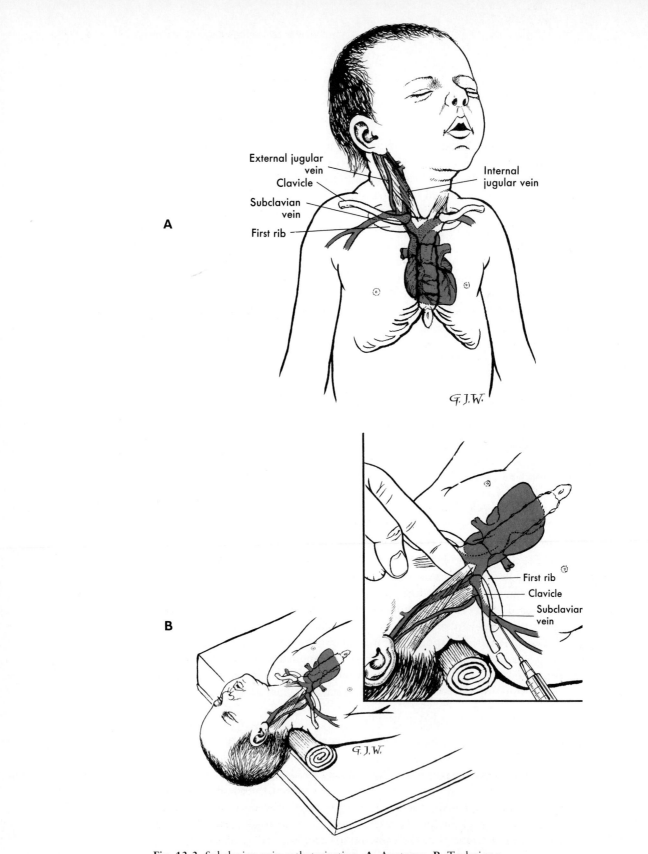

Fig. 13-3. Subclavian vein catheterization. **A,** Anatomy. **B,** Technique.

Modified from Chameides L: *Textbook of pediatric advanced life support*, ed 2, Dallas, American Heart Association (*in press*).

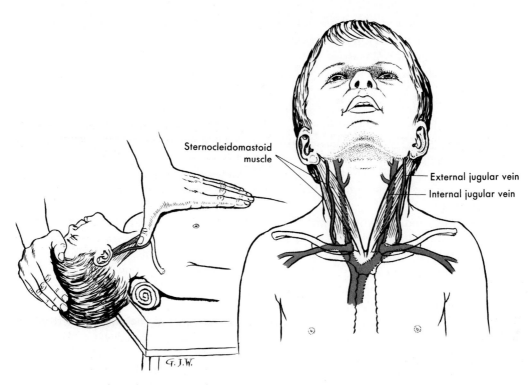

Fig. 13-4. External jugular venous catheterization.

Modified from Chameides L: *Textbook of pediatric advanced life support*, ed 2, Dallas, American Heart Association (*in press*).

insertion site. The right external jugular vein is preferred over the left for the initial approach.

After the insertion site is draped with sterile towels and scrubbed with a povidone-iodine solution, the external jugular vein is visualized; visualization may be enhanced by occluding the vein proximally, just above the clavicle (Fig. 13-4). The skin over the insertion site should be broken by a large (16- to 18-gauge) needle. Then a catheter with stylet, or a large hollow catheter attached to a syringe, is inserted directly into the external jugular vein, several centimeters above the clavicle. As soon as free flow of blood appears in the syringe, insertion of the needle should stop. If a catheter with stylet is used, the stylet is withdrawn and the catheter is advanced and sutured into place; hand irrigation of the catheter is performed. If a hollow needle has been inserted into the vein, the needle is held carefully in place (with the clinician's thumb covering the needle hub), and a guidewire is threaded through the needle and inserted several centimeters into the vein. There may be some difficulty threading the guidewire below the clavicle. If resistance is encountered, it may be helpful to keep the needle in place, remove the initial guidewire, and substitute a small J-wire.

Once the guidewire has been successfully passed well into the jugular vein, the needle is withdrawn over the guidewire, and a catheter is then threaded over the guidewire, into the vein. Once the catheter is in place, the guidewire is withdrawn and the catheter is sewn into place. The catheter should be only gently flushed by hand, and no medications should be infused through the catheter until proper position is verified by radiograph. Reported success rate of external jugular venous catheterization in children is approximately 60% to 75%, and the success rate is highest in children beyond 5 years of age. Failure of proper external jugular venous catheter placement most often results in advancement of the catheter up into the neck.

Internal jugular venous catheterization

Catheterization of the internal jugular vein should not be attempted by unskilled clinicians, because faulty technique may result in puncture of the right carotid artery, with subsequent hemorrhage. The incidence of this complication in children is approximately 8%. The risk is apparently higher than during catheterization of adults because the internal jugular vein and the carotid artery are virtually side by side in the neck of the child.

The child is positioned with the head 15 to 45 degrees below the trunk, with the head turned to the left to facilitate right jugular venous catheterization. The right internal jugular vein is preferred because it joins the right subclavian vein and enters the right atrium in a straight path. In addition, the apex of the right lung is lower beneath the clavicle than the apex of the left lung, and the right approach prevents injury to the thoracic duct.

The internal jugular vein courses between the sternal and clavicular heads of the sternocleidomastoid muscle, above the medial end of the clavicle. The major landmarks to identify before the procedure include the sternal and clavicular heads of the sternocleidomastoid muscle, the external jugular vein, the right nipple, and the suprasternal notch. Once the landmarks have been identified, the area is scrubbed with povidone-iodine solution (leaving the landmarks visible) and draped. The skin entrance site is anesthetized with a 1% lidocaine solution.

If a *posterior* approach is used, the internal jugular vein will be cannulated from a needle directed under and behind the external jugular vein. A hollow needle attached to a syringe is inserted at a 30- to 45-degree angle from the skin, just above the point where the external jugular vein crosses the sternocleidomastoid muscle (Fig. 13-5, *A*). The needle should be pointed toward the suprasternal notch during insertion. Once the vein is entered, the Seldinger technique is used to insert the catheter.

If the *anterior* route of insertion is used, the needle enters between the sternocleidomastoid muscle and the right common carotid artery. It is necessary to retract the artery medially so that it is not punctured. The needle is introduced just lateral to the right common carotid artery, but medial to the sternocleidomastoid muscle. It is inserted at a 30- to 45-degree angle from the skin, directed toward the right nipple (Fig. 13-5, *B*). Once free flow of blood is observed in the syringe, the needle is held carefully in place and the syringe is removed. If the patient is breathing spontaneously, the needle hub should be immediately covered with a thumb to prevent air intake. The Seldinger technique is then used to insert a guidewire and the catheter into the internal jugular vein.

If the catheter threads freely, it almost certainly will pass into the superior vena cava (and, if desired, into the right atrium). Proper placement is verified by chest radiograph and by the observation of a CVP tracing when the catheter is connected to a monitor.

A *central* route of internal jugular venous catheterization requires insertion of the

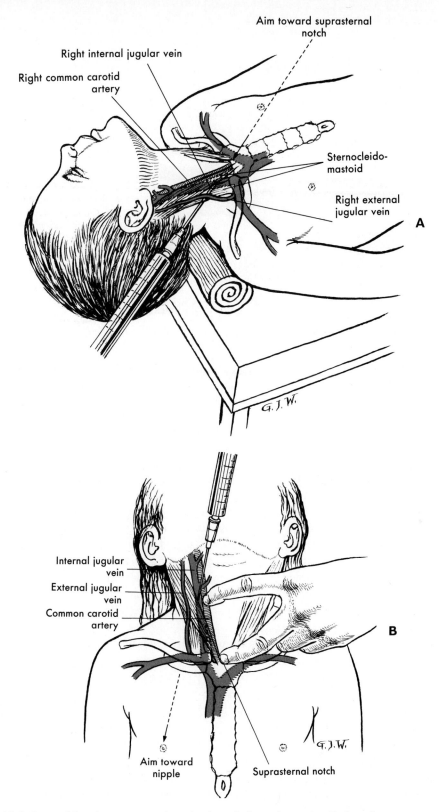

Fig. 13-5. Internal jugular venous catheterization. **A,** Posterior route. **B,** Anterior route.

Modified from Chameides L: *Textbook of pediatric advanced life support,* ed 2, Dallas, American Heart Association (*in press*).

Continued.

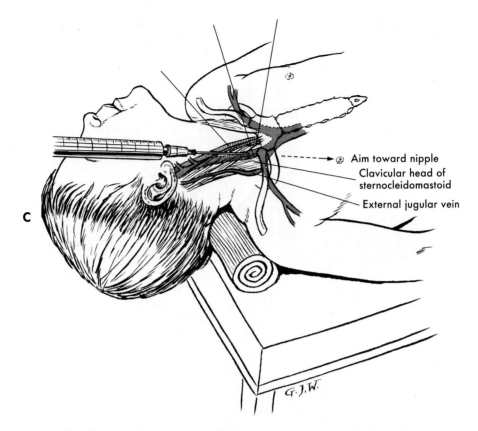

> → (3) Aim toward nipple
> Clavicular head of sternocleidomastoid
> External jugular vein

C

Fig. 13-5, cont'd. Internal jugular venous catheterization. C, Central route.

needle at the apex of the triangle formed by the sternal and clavicular heads of the sternocleidomastoid muscle and the clavicle. The needle is inserted just medial to the clavicular head of the sternocleidomastoid, angled 15 to 30 degrees above the skin, and aimed at the right nipple (Fig. 13-5, C). If immediate blood return does not occur, the needle should be aimed more laterally, toward the right shoulder. The needle should not be directed medially from this approach, because the right common carotid artery may easily be punctured inasmuch as it courses just medial to the internal jugular vein.

Once free blood return into the syringe is observed, the needle is held in place and the syringe is removed. The needle hub is covered until the patient exhales spontaneously or until delivery of a positive pressure inspiration; then the Seldinger technique is used to thread the guidewire and next the catheter into the vein. The catheter should thread easily, directly into the internal jugular vein, the superior vena cava, and toward the right atrium.

If the catheter advances easily, and free blood return occurs whenever the catheter is aspirated, the catheter is almost certainly in place. In addition, a typical CVP waveform should be observed when the catheter is joined to a monitoring system. However, radiographic confirmation will be necessary before infusion of large volumes of fluids or medications.

During internal jugular venous cannulation, everyone at the bedside should observe the patient closely for signs of carotid artery puncture. This complication should be immediately recognized by the appearance of bright red blood into the syringe when the needle is initially inserted. However, if unrecognized carotid arterial catheterization is performed, the arterial waveform should be identified when the vascular waveform is displayed on the monitor. Occasionally, the carotid artery is inadvertently nicked as the internal jugular vein is catheterized, which results in immediate hematoma formation. Whenever the carotid artery is punctured, the needle should be withdrawn immediately, and pressure should be applied over the artery for 10 minutes or until bleeding has stopped.

Femoral venous cannulation

The child's leg should be rotated externally and restrained. The upper portion of the leg is scrubbed with an iodine solution and draped with sterile towels. Using sterile technique, the clinician locates the inguinal ligament and then palpates femoral arterial pulsations approximately midway between the anterior superior iliac spine and the symphysis pubis. A large needle attached to a syringe is inserted one fingerbreadth below the inguinal ligament, just medial to the femoral arterial pulsations. The needle is directed cephalad and in a 45-degree angle downward (Fig. 13-6). As the needle is inserted, the plunger is withdrawn until blood flows freely into the syringe; at this point, insertion should stop. The syringe is detached from the needle while the needle is held carefully in place. The Seldinger technique is then used to insert a guidewire and then the catheter into the femoral vein and the inferior vena cava. The catheter is sutured in place, and a sterile dressing is applied. Infusion of fluid and drugs may begin once the proper placement of the catheter is confirmed radiographically.

Maintenance

Any central venous line must be inserted under sterile conditions and covered with a sterile dressing. The simple monitoring catheter should be continuously flushed with heparinized saline. The addition of 0.5 to 2 units of heparin/ml flush solution reduces the incidence of catheter thrombus formation. If the catheter is used only for intermittent access for blood sampling, it may be "heparin-locked" with instillation of 1 to 2 ml of higher concentrations of heparin (20 to 100 units/ml). However, this heparin should always be withdrawn from the catheter and tubing (rather than "flushed" into the patient) whenever the catheter is used for blood sampling or fluid infusion.

Continuous irrigation of central venous and arterial catheters in children should be accomplished only through use of volume-controlled pumps and syringes (Fig. 13-7). The use of pressurized irrigation bags without volume-controlled infusion for pediatric monitoring is discouraged, because it is impossible to verify the exact quantity of fluids delivered to the child on a continuous basis (although approximately 3 ml/hr will be delivered through standard flow-limiting devices, if they are functioning properly). In addition, any rapid "flushing" of lines with the flow-limiting devices will deliver an unknown quantity of fluid under extremely high pressure. This can result in fluid overload, as well as in damage to the catheterized vessel. Monitoring catheters should be flushed only with gentle irrigation via a syringe. This enables documentation of the exact quantity of fluids delivered and reduces trauma to the catheterized vessel.

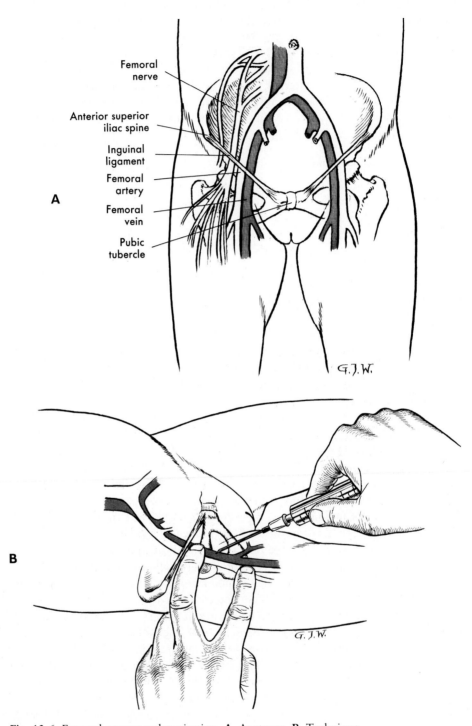

Fig. 13-6. Femoral venous catheterization. **A,** Anatomy. **B,** Technique.

Modified from Chameides L: *Textbook of pediatric advanced life support*, ed 2, Dallas, American Heart Association (*in press*).

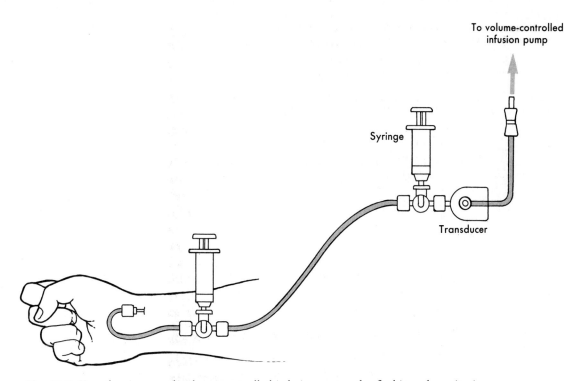

Fig. 13-7. Use of syringes and volume-controlled infusion pumps for flushing of monitoring lines.

If the CVP catheter is used for monitoring and for infusion of intravenous fluids, the fluid, tubing, and transducer are joined to the catheter with a three-way stopcock. With this configuration, pressure measurements may be obtained intermittently when the stopcock is turned off to the fluid infusion and opened to the transducer (Fig. 13-8, *A*).

If large-volume (up to 30 ml/hr) fluid infusion is required while CVP measurements are made, it will be necessary to administer the fluid with a volume-controlled pump through a 30-ml/hr flow-limiting device. Such a device may prevent the fluid infusion from interfering with pressure measurements (Fig. 13-8, *B*). The central venous fluid and monitoring (flush) line fluid and tubing should be changed every 48 to 72 hours. More frequent tubing and fluid changes will be required if parenteral alimentation is administered through the CVP line.

Central venous catheters often are used for administration of drugs and parenteral alimentation. When parenteral alimentation is administered, attempts should be made to avoid entry into the alimentation line. Several small (4-, 5.5-, and 7-Fr) multilumen catheters are now commercially available for central venous insertion in the pediatric patient. These catheters are often preferable to single-lumen catheters in that they allow uninterrupted delivery of parenteral alimentation through one lumen while a second, or even third lumen remains available for blood sampling, monitoring, and drug administration. To ensure placement of the most suitable catheter in the most logical site, it is important to consider the complete monitoring and intravenous access needs of the child before a central venous catheter is inserted.

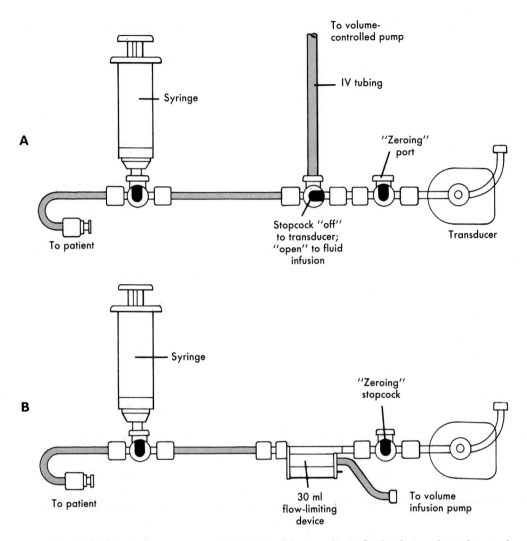

Fig. 13-8. Systems for pressure monitoring and large volume fluid infusion through use of stopcock with intermittent pressure measurements **(A)** and through continuous monitoring and infusion with use of flow-limiting device **(B)**.

Complications

Potential complications after central venous catheterization in children include infection, bleeding, ventricular dysrhythmias (if the catheter enters the right ventricle), and thromboembolus. Additional complications include those related to insertion: pneumothorax and hemothorax are possible complications of subclavian vein catheterization, and bleeding may complicate internal or external jugular venous, umbilical venous, or femoral venous catheterization.

Infection of central venous lines can be prevented by using good hand-washing technique before and after patient contact, by preventing catheter contamination, and by minimizing the duration of catheterization. It is imperative that everyone responsible for catheter insertion adhere to the use of strict sterile technique and that flawless aseptic technique be used when the catheter, tubing, or stopcock is handled.

The risk of catheter-related nosocomial infections increases with the duration of central venous catheterization—most notably with catheter placement beyond 3 to 5 days. Risk of infection also is increased if the catheter is used for blood sampling.

Early signs of sepsis in children include the development of tachycardia and tachypnea associated with a respiratory alkalosis. In addition, thrombocytopenia (or other early signs of disseminated intravascular coagulation), leukocytosis, or leukopenia may develop in the child. Fever also may be present, although temperature instability is a common sign of sepsis in the neonate.

The catheterization site should be observed daily and evidence of inflammation reported to a physician. Use of vapor-permeable, occlusive, transparent dressings may facilitate continuous observation of the entrance site without interruption of the occlusive dressing.

Bleeding is an unusual complication after central venous catheterization in children. It occurs most frequently in critically ill children with preexisting coagulopathies. If the CVP line is used for pressure measurements, it should be joined to a monitor with a high- and low-pressure audible alarm. This alarm should be activated if the patient's CVP falls by 10% or more. This will ensure rapid detection of changes in patient condition or tubing separation.

The entire CVP monitoring system should be joined with only Luer-Lok connections, so that the risk of inadvertent tubing separation is minimized. The catheter entrance site and all tubing connections should be visible at all times; thus tubing separation or blood loss will be immediately detected.

Central venous catheter migration may result in vascular perforation and resultant hydrothorax or hemothorax. This complication should be suspected if the characteristic CVP waveform disappears and is replaced by a signal that varies only with respirations. In addition, evidence of free fluid in the thorax should be apparent on clinical examination. If extravascular catheter migration is suspected, fluid infusion through the catheter should be discontinued and a physician contacted. The extravascular catheter will be removed.

Central venous catheter migration into the right ventricle may produce ventricular dysrhythmias. This migration is apparent when a right ventricular waveform appears on the oscilloscope. If migration into the right ventricle occurs, the catheter should be withdrawn into the right atrium.

Right atrial thrombus formation has been reported in infants and young children with long-dwelling right atrial catheters. Septic or aseptic thrombi should be suspected in any child with an indwelling catheter who develops fever or evidence of vena caval obstruction, and it usually can be confirmed by use of echocardiography. The thrombus often will require surgical evacuation, although occasional success in clot dissolution has been reported with the use of urokinase (Delaplane et al. and Mandoza et al.).

Arterial Pressure Monitoring

Institution of intraarterial pressure monitoring should be considered if shock is present or likely to develop, and whenever continuous evaluation of the arterial pressure is required (e.g., during administration of medications with cardiovascular effects). Intraarterial monitoring also facilitates arterial blood sampling for blood gas and other laboratory analyses. Use of the Seldinger technique allows percutaneous insertion of catheters in even small arteries.

If the monitoring system is appropriately zeroed and calibrated, intraarterial pressure monitoring is more accurate than auscultated or oscillometric blood pressure measurements. The mean arterial pressure calculated by the monitor from the actual area under an arterial waveform is also more accurate than arithmetic estimations of the mean arterial pressure from the systolic and diastolic pressures (see Chapter 7 for further information).

The appearance of the child's arterial waveform is slightly different from that observed in the adult (refer to Chapter 7). As depicted in Fig. 13-9, the contour of the radial artery pressure wave in the first decade of life typically shows two prominent fluctuations following the early systolic peak. The first fluctuation occurs in late systole, and the second fluctuation occurs in diastole immediately after the dicrotic notch. These wave reflections are less apparent in the femoral artery wave and

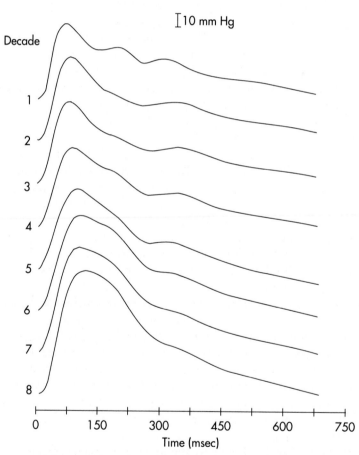

Fig. 13-9. Change in contour and amplitude of the human radial artery pressure wave with age.
From Kelly RP et al: *Circulation* 80:1652–1659, 1989. With permission of the American Heart Association.

normally are not seen in the older adult. (See Chapter 7 for a detailed discussion of arterial pressure waves.) The normal arterial pressure in the child is much lower than that observed in the adult (see Table 13-1 for review of normal blood pressures in children).

Some congenital heart defects produce characteristic changes in the arterial waveform. In a patent ductus arteriosus or aortic insufficiency the arterial waveform may demonstrate rapid aortic run-off with low diastolic and mean pressures, and a widened pulse pressure. Significant aortic valvular stenosis characteristically produces a biphasic pulse (with an anacrotic notch noted during the systolic upstroke of the waveform). Coarctation of the aorta results in hypertensive pulses and associated arterial pressure in the upper extremities (or any arterial circulation arising from the aorta proximal to the narrowed segment), with hypotensive and damped arterial pulses and pressure in the lower extremities. Just as in the adult, the child with tamponade may manifest pulsus paradoxus (if the child's respiratory rate is sufficiently slow), and the child with myocarditis and very low cardiac output may manifest pulsus alternans.

The most common arteries used for intraarterial monitoring in children include radial artery, dorsalis pedis artery, posterior tibial artery, femoral artery, and umbilical artery. Technique for insertion of an umbilical artery catheter is discussed in the next section. The technique for insertion of the catheter into a peripheral artery with the Seldinger technique is identical to that described for adults; for this reason the technique for catheterization of all peripheral arteries is discussed only briefly (see Chapter 7 for further details).

Umbilical artery catheterization

Umbilical artery catheterization may be performed in the critically ill neonate and can be accomplished by an experienced clinician within moments. However, because the procedure can be associated with significant complications, including hemorrhage, thromboembolic phenomena, and infection, it is not recommended for routine intraarterial or vascular access in the neonate.

Long catheters must be used for umbilical artery insertion, because the catheter must pass through the umbilical artery (approximately 7 cm in length in the full-term neonate) into the internal iliac artery, and then retrograde into the common iliac artery and into the aorta. Inasmuch as the catheter lies in the descending aorta, it is useful as a standard arterial line, and it also may enable administration of intravenous fluids and drugs if another intravenous line is not available.

Insertion. An umbilical artery catheterization tray should be obtained (see the box on p. 297). The catheter used should be smooth and radiopaque, with a single hole at the tip. A 5-Fr catheter is used if the infant weighs more than 1200 g, and a 3.5-Fr catheter is used if the infant weighs less than 1200 g.

Before insertion, the proper depth of catheter insertion should be estimated from published charts or by adding 4 cm to the measured distance from the distal end of the clavicle to the umbilicus plus the length of the umbilical stump. The estimated depth (length) of insertion should be marked on the catheter (using sterile umbilical artery tape).

The neonate should be placed in the supine position and restrained, and electrocardiographic monitoring should be performed throughout the procedure. The umbilical cord and surrounding area are cleansed with a povidone-iodine solution, and the umbilical area is draped with sterile towels in such a manner that the infant's face remains visible and chest wall movement can still be observed. The entire procedure is performed with use of strict sterile technique.

A sterile segment of umbilical tape is placed around the umbilicus and knotted loosely—this will reduce bleeding from the cord during cord trimming and catheterization. The tape should not be tied too tightly, or it will be impossible to thread the catheter through the umbilical vessels. The distal end of the cord is held upright, and a scalpel is used to cut the cord horizontally, producing a perfect horizontal view of the vessels. Two curved hemostats are used to grasp the umbilical cord on each side, holding it taut and immobile, while the two umbilical arteries are identified (they are the two smaller, thick-walled vessels). The outer wall of the cord is grasped with forceps, near one of the arteries, and the artery is probed gently with curved forceps. The forceps are inserted two or three more times, to a depth of approximately 1 cm, and the tips of the forceps are spread to dilate the artery. While the curved forceps hold the artery open, the catheter is inserted gently into the arterial lumen. Once the catheter is inserted to a depth of approximately 2 to 3 cm, the forceps may be removed. To enable the catheter to be threaded beyond the depth of the stump, it may be necessary to loosen the umbilical tape that is wrapped around the base of the umbilical cord stump.

The catheter should be advanced gently to the appropriate depth (as indicated by the umbilical tape mark on the catheter). The catheter should not be forced if resistance is felt. If the catheter is in proper position, blood can be readily aspirated from the catheter. When the catheter is connected to the transducer and monitoring system, a characteristic arterial waveform should be displayed.

Some umbilical artery catheters (UACs) are equipped with standard intravenous tubing connections so that they may be directly connected to a fluid-filled monitoring system. However, many umbilical catheters require insertion of a blunt-tipped needle into the distal end of the catheter to provide the proper connection to a tubing system. An 18-gauge blunt-tipped needle is used with a 5-Fr catheter, and a 20-gauge blunt-tipped needle is used with a 3.5-Fr catheter.

After successful catheter insertion, the umbilical tape is removed from the base of the umbilicus, and a purse-string suture is placed around the cord to prevent bleeding from the umbilical vein or the noncatheterized umbilical artery. The catheter should be secured in place by means of a bridge taping system (refer to the preceding discussion under Umbilical Venous Catheterization). It is important to keep the umbilicus and catheter entry site free of dressings or ointment. The nurse should be able to inspect the site at all times to detect any bleeding or inflammation.

Radiographic confirmation of proper catheter placement is mandatory. The tip of the catheter should be either near the diaphragm (usually at the level of the sixth thoracic vertebra) or within the lumbar aorta at the third or fourth lumbar vertebra. *The umbilical artery catheter tip should not remain between the tenth thoracic and the second lumbar vertebrae, because a catheter in this position may obstruct renal and mesenteric arterial blood flow.*

Maintenance. The UAC must be flushed continuously or intermittently with a saline or heparinized saline solution. Continuous infusion heparinized with 0.5 to 1 unit of heparin/ml may increase longevity of the catheter and improve catheter patency. Occasionally, hypernatremia develops in the critically ill neonate. If this occurs, the umbilical catheter may be flushed with heparinized 0.45% normal saline instead of heparinized 0.9% normal saline.

If the catheter is flushed continuously, a volume-controlled infusion pump should be used to ensure delivery of a known quantity of fluid at a constant rate. Use of pressure bags and rapid flush flow-limiting devices is *not* recommended because it is impossible to determine the exact amount of fluid delivered. In addition, the use of the rapid-flush device may produce arterial spasm and may result in retrograde flow into the aortic arch vessels (see the following discussion in the Maintenance section of Peripheral Artery Catheterization). If intermittent irrigation of the catheter is necessary, a syringe should be used to gently flush the catheter over several minutes.

Medications may be administered through an umbilical artery line, if no other route of administration is available. However, complications of such medication administration will depend on the pH and osmolality of the medication and on the adequacy of the infant's cardiac output. If cardiac output is critically low, there will be inadequate blood flow in the aorta to effectively dilute the administered medication, and the drug may flow undiluted into the lower extremity arterial circulation. The nurse should refer to unit and hospital policy before administering any medication or blood product through an umbilical artery catheter.

All connections in the umbilical arterial monitoring system should have Luer-Loks to reduce the risk of inadvertent separation. The entire arterial line should be visible at all times, and the infant should not be covered with blankets, which can prevent or delay the detection of bleeding. The arterial pressure monitor with digital display and oscilloscope should be equipped with an audible low-pressure alarm. This alarm should be set to sound whenever the neonate's systolic or diastolic arterial pressure falls by 10%; this will ensure that tubing separation is detected immediately. Any alarm-silence features should be only temporary; it should be impossible to permanently disable such an alarm.

The most common complication of umbilical artery catheterization is obstruction of renal, mesenteric, and femoral artery blood flow, caused by catheter obstruction of these vessels or by thromboembolic events. Whenever a UAC is in place, the neonate's urine output and perfusion of the lower extremities should be evaluated closely. Lower extremity pulses (including femoral, dorsalis pedis, and posterior tibial arteries) should be palpated hourly, and the quality of the pulses, temperature of the feet and legs, color, and briskness of capillary refill should be documented at least hourly.

Blanching, mottling, cyanosis, pallor, decreased pulses, or cooling of the legs should be reported to a physician immediately. Such developments usually indicate arterial obstruction, and removal of the catheter is usually necessary. These clinical signs also may be observed if a thrombus forms in the descending aorta. Surgical removal of the thrombus may be necessary.

Blood should be drawn from the UAC as from any arterial catheter in the infant or child; very little blood should be wasted, and it should not be necessary to flush any additional fluid after blood drawing (see the following section, Blood Sampling from Indwelling Lines). If irrigation of the catheter is necessary because of suspected catheter obstruction, gentle irrigation and aspiration should be performed.

The catheter always should be taped securely in place so that accidental dislodgement is impossible. The nurse should measure the distance from the umbilicus to the first tubing connection and record this distance on the nursing care plan, so that catheter migration can be detected easily.

The neonate should not receive enteral feedings while the UAC is in place. The catheter may result in compromise to mesenteric blood flow, and feeding may then increase the risk of development of necrotizing enterocolitis. Feeding may be resumed several hours after the catheter has been removed if bowel sounds and respiratory status are satisfactory.

Removal. Before the UAC is removed, the purse-string suture is cut at the umbilical cord stump rather than at the catheter. Sterile umbilical tape is wrapped around the umbilicus and tied loosely. As the catheter is slowly withdrawn, the umbilical tape is tightened to reduce bleeding. In many hospitals the UAC is withdrawn in stages over a period of several hours. During the withdrawal period, the nurse observes the patient closely for evidence of bleeding from the umbilicus.

Complications. The most common complications associated with umbilical artery catheterization include hemorrhage, peritoneal perforation, compromise of lower extremity perfusion, thromboembolic complications (including occlusion of renal, mesenteric, or spinal cord arteries), and infection. Paraplegia and leg necrosis have been reported after UAC use, and intimal damage to the aorta also may occur. These complications often can be prevented or detected with careful observation of the catheter entrance site, arterial waveform, and tubing connections combined with frequent assessment of urine output and lower extremity perfusion.

Peripheral artery catheterization

Insertion of a pediatric peripheral artery catheter is accomplished with techniques identical to those used for adult peripheral artery catheterization (see Chapter 6 for details of peripheral artery catheter insertion). In all but the smallest neonates, the radial artery is the preferred site for arterial cannulation, and the dorsalis pedis and posterior tibial arteries also are used frequently. Femoral artery catheterization usually is performed only under emergent conditions, because the entrance site is likely to become contaminated and limb ischemia also may result. Temporal artery catheterization has been largely abandoned inasmuch as cerebral embolization has been reported after use of this site (Prian et al.).

Insertion. Before insertion of a radial artery catheter, the Allen test should be performed to assess adequacy of collateral circulation to the hand. The radial artery is occluded as the patient's hand is curled into a fist. The radial artery should remain occluded as the patient's hand is opened to the relaxed position; if the hand remains blanched for longer than 3 seconds, collateral circulation is inadequate, and that radial artery should not be catheterized. If the hand reperfuses quickly despite occlusion of the radial artery, the collateral circulation is adequate, and the radial artery can be catheterized without risk of hand ischemia.

The entrance site over the artery is scrubbed with a povidone-iodine solution and draped. A small amount of 1% lidocaine should be instilled subcutaneously at the anticipated catheterization site. Using sterile technique, the clinician palpates the artery. A small nick in the skin may be made with use of a 20-gauge needle.

A 22-gauge catheter is suitable for peripheral artery catheterization for all but the smallest neonates. A 24-gauge catheter may be used in the newborn. If a catheter with stylet is used, it may be inserted directly into the artery at a 30-degree angle from the plane of the arm. Once the artery is entered, the catheter is threaded over the stylet into the artery and the stylet is removed.

The Seldinger technique also may be used to achieve percutaneous arterial catheterization. A needle is used to puncture the artery; then a guidewire is threaded through the needle, well into the artery, and the needle is withdrawn. The catheter is then threaded over the guidewire into the artery. The guidewire is removed, and once the catheter is properly positioned, it should be sutured into place.

If percutaneous entry into the artery fails, an arterial cutdown may be performed. The technique for arterial catheterization through direct cutdown is identical to that performed in the adult patient.

Once the catheter is in the artery, it is irrigated gently with a syringe that contains normal saline and the catheter is connected to the monitoring system and transducer. Placement of a short T-connector between the catheter and the monitoring tubing (Fig. 13-10) may reduce movement of the catheter and facilitate blood sampling (see the following section, Blood Sampling from Monitoring Lines). Use of this T-connector usually will not reduce the quality of the arterial waveform signal (Fig. 13-11), but the nurse should ensure that no damping of the displayed arterial waveform occurs.

Maintenance. Catheter patency is improved if peripheral pediatric arterial catheters are flushed continuously rather than intermittently. Use of heparinized flush solution rather than nonheparinized solution also will prolong catheter patency; most commonly, 1 unit of heparin/ml concentration is used, although concentrations ranging from 0.25 to 5 units/ml have been reported.

The arterial line should be flushed at a rate of 1 to 3 ml/hr to prevent clot formation. Pediatric catheters should *not* be flushed by use of pressure bags and continuous flush devices; such devices will deliver an unknown quantity of fluid at a rapid rate when the flush valve is opened. Catheter irrigation should be accomplished with use of a volume-controlled infusion pump with noncompliant tubing. The infusion should be delivered through the valved continuous flush device (see Fig. 13-6); the flush device may prevent damping of the waveform signal by the continuous infusion.

If intermittent flushing of the pediatric arterial catheter and tubing is necessary (as a result of waveform damping or blood back-up into the tubing), only gentle irrigation should be provided through use of a syringe. Rapid, forceful irrigation with a syringe or a flush device may result in retrograde flow of irrigant (and possibly air or thrombus) into the arch of the aorta and cerebral circulation. Such retrograde flow has been documented during irrigation of radial artery catheters in neonates, children, and adults (Butt et al.). All fluids used to flush the arterial line must be totaled and added to the child's hourly fluid intake.

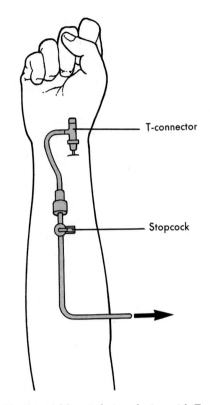

Fig. 13-10. Arterial line infusion device with T-connector.

Throughout the time the arterial catheter is in place, assessment of distal extremity perfusion and appearance of the catheter entry site must be performed and documented. Signs of distal limb ischemia include cooling, mottling, blanching, or cyanosis of the limb, as well as reduced arterial flow assessed by Doppler measurements. Such signs should be reported to a physician immediately, and removal of the catheter is usually necessary. If arterial spasm is suspected to be causing distal limb ischemia, a warm compress may be applied to the *contralateral* extremity to induce reflex vasodilation (heat should *never* be applied to the ischemic extremity because it will increase oxygen demand and worsen the ischemia).

While the catheter is in place, blood loss may occur if tubing connections separate. Luer-Lok connections always should be used in monitoring systems to prevent inadvertent tubing disconnection. Significant blood loss can occur as a result of only brief seconds of tubing separation; a 25-ml blood loss in a 3-kg infant is equivalent to a 12% hemorrhage. The monitor used to display digital arterial pressure and waveform should have a high- and low-pressure alarm. These alarms should be set to alert the clinician if the systolic or diastolic blood pressure falls by 10%. Thus an alarm will sound as soon as pressure loss occurs from a loose connection — before significant blood loss has occurred. The low-pressure alarm on the monitor should be active at

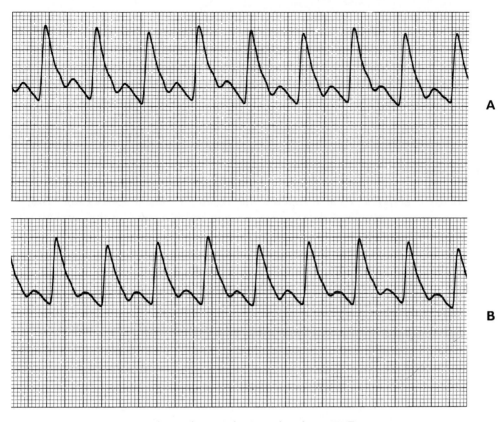

Fig. 13-11. Arterial waveform with **(A)** and without **(B)** T-connector.

all times. If the alarm is silenced during blood sampling or tubing changes, a temporary alarm silence option should be used; such temporary options will automatically reactivate the alarm within 90 seconds, and they are much safer than options that may permanently disable the alarm. The catheterization site and all tubing connections should be visible at all times (never covered by blankets), so that tubing separation and blood loss will be detected immediately.

The catheter insertion site should be dressed with sterile gauze and occlusive tape or with use of transparent, vapor-permeable occlusive film. Routine use of povidone-iodine ointment is not recommended because it has not been shown to alter the incidence of catheter-related infection. Throughout the catheterization period, the entrance site should be observed closely for evidence of inflammation, including local tenderness, drainage, erythema, or warmth. The development of fever, leukocytosis, lymphangitis, and thrombocytopenia would strengthen the suspicion of infection or sepsis. The use of a transparent dressing enables continuous observation of the catheter entrance site without the need for dressing changes.

Arterial line tubing and fluid are routinely changed every 48 hours. Although some studies (Ducharme et al.) have documented that such frequent changing of tubing may not be necessary, current Centers for Disease Control guidelines and published standards recommend the 48-hour tubing and fluid change to reduce the incidence of system contamination and septicemia (Maki et al.). Aseptic technique must be employed whenever the tubing or line is handled. Blood sampling from arterial lines is reviewed in the following section, Blood Sampling from Indwelling Lines.

Complications. Distal extremity ischemia, infection, and bleeding are the most common complications reported after peripheral artery catheterization in infants and children. Hypotension, the administration of vasoactive agents, small patient size (younger than 5 years) and prolonged (more than 4 to 6 days) catheterization time are consistent variables associated with increased risk of distal arterial occlusion and embolic complications. Major ischemic/embolic complications are reported in approximately 1% to 3% of children who require peripheral artery catheterization; these include the loss of distal pulses, cooling and blanching of the extremity, and decreased capillary refill. Such complications should be detected quickly, and the catheter should be removed immediately. Embolic complications may require heparin therapy or surgical treatment. Minor reduction in distal limb blood flow may occur in as many as 57% of children who have undergone catheterization.

Catheter-related infection is most likely to develop in the pediatric patient if breaks in aseptic technique occur during catheter insertion or maintenance, if the catheter remains in place longer than 4 to 6 days, or if the patient has multiple invasive monitoring lines. Infection should be suspected if local tenderness, drainage, or erythema are noted at the insertion site. In addition, infection should be suspected if fever, leukocytosis, thrombocytopenia, or lymphangitis develops. The septic neonate may demonstrate temperature instability.

Bleeding related to arterial catheterization in the child is most commonly caused by loose catheter connections, although excessive bleeding may occur during catheter insertion. The catheterized extremity and the entire length of monitoring tubing should be visible at all times, and all connections should have Luer-Loks in set position. At least hourly, every portion of the monitoring system should be closely inspected and palpated, so that kinks or loose connections will be detected immediately. If blood loss occurs as the result of catheterization or tubing separation, the quantity of blood loss should be estimated and considered as a percentage of the child's circulating blood volume. Significant blood loss (more than 5% of circulating blood volume) must be reported to a physician immediately, and blood component therapy may be required. (See Table 13-3 for calculation of circulating blood volume.)

Blood Sampling from Indwelling Lines

When blood is withdrawn from the pediatric patient for laboratory analysis, attempts must be made to minimize blood loss and fluid administration. Laboratory analysis must be performed by means of "micro" techniques, so that blood sample volume is minimal (e.g., arterial blood gas analysis should require no more than 0.3 to 0.5 ml of blood). Everyone who cares for the child should be aware of the minimal volume of blood required for each laboratory test and for typical combinations of tests (e.g., the volume required for CBC, electrolytes, and arterial blood gas values is probably less than the sum of volumes required for each test). Minimal sample volumes should be posted in a prominent area in the unit; in some hospitals the director of laboratory services is asked to sign a copy of the notice, so that there will be no dispute about the sample volumes required. The entire blood withdrawn for laboratory analysis should be totaled daily for infants less than 6 months of age, and blood replacement should be contemplated if this amount approximates 5% to 7% of the child's circulating blood volume or if the hematocrit is critically low.

Of course, all blood sampling must be performed with use of strict aseptic technique. Good hand washing is performed before and after each patient contact, and gloves must be worn whenever blood or bodily fluids are handled.

During blood sampling, an adequate volume of discarded blood must be used to clear the sample tubing and stopcock of irrigant fluid; yet the child's actual blood loss for each sample should be limited, if possible, to the sample volume itself (not the sample volume plus the discard volume). In many hospitals the discarded blood is withdrawn from the sampling tubing into a syringe and then is reinfused into the patient after the blood sample is withdrawn. This practice is undesirable because the discarded blood may begin to clot in the syringe and may mix with bits of fibrin; reinfusion of this partially clotted blood may result in thromboembolic phenomena.

The child should not receive an undetermined or large volume of irrigant fluid to clear the tubing of blood after the sampling procedure. Any net fluid administered after blood sampling must be added to the child's total hourly fluid intake. Excessive irrigant fluid administration may necessitate reduction of other sources of fluid intake and may result in reduction of the volume of nutritional fluid administered to the child.

Use of the two-stopcock or closed, needle-less system for blood sampling allows blood sampling without significant blood loss and without net fluid administration.

Blood sampling from a proximal and distal stopcock

The tubing and monitoring system should be constructed with two stopcocks; a proximal stopcock is positioned near the entrance of the catheter, and a distal stopcock is positioned adjacent to the transducer. The two stopcocks are separated by at least 6 inches, but preferably no more than 24 inches of noncompliant tubing (Fig. 13-12, A). The greater the space between stopcocks, the larger the effective discard volume displaced during blood sampling.

1. Syringes are attached to both stopcocks, with the stopcocks turned off to the syringes (see Fig. 13-12). The syringe attached to the distal stopcock should contain exactly 2 ml of irrigation (flush) liquid (the fluid should be identical to that in the monitoring tubing).
2. The *distal* stopcock is turned off to the transducer, and irrigant fluid from the monitoring tubing is withdrawn into the distal syringe. This fluid aspiration will result in movement of patient blood into the monitoring tubing; this blood will act as the discard blood volume. It is extremely important that fluid be aspirated to draw blood toward *but not into* the distal stopcock; the distal stopcock and syringe should contain only irrigant fluid (Fig. 13-12, B).
3. The *proximal* stopcock is now turned off to the transducer. This will allow aspiration of blood from the patient into the proximal syringe. However, before sampling is performed, a small amount of blood (0.1 ml) should be withdrawn and

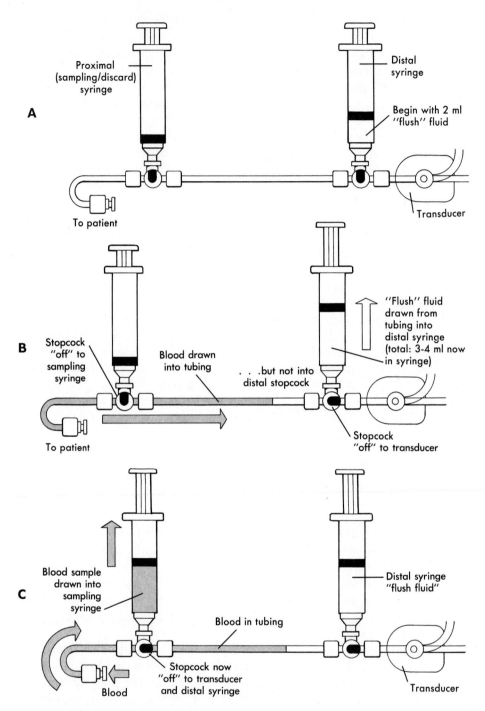

Fig. 13-12. Blood sampling from monitoring line using two-stopcock technique. **A,** Initial setup. Begin with 2 ml of irrigation (flush) fluid in distal syringe. **B,** Turn distal stopcock off to transducer, and aspirate until patient blood is drawn into monitoring tubing into distal syringe. **C,** Turn proximal stopcock off to transducer and distal syringe, and draw blood sample into syringe (after discarding initial 0.1 ml).

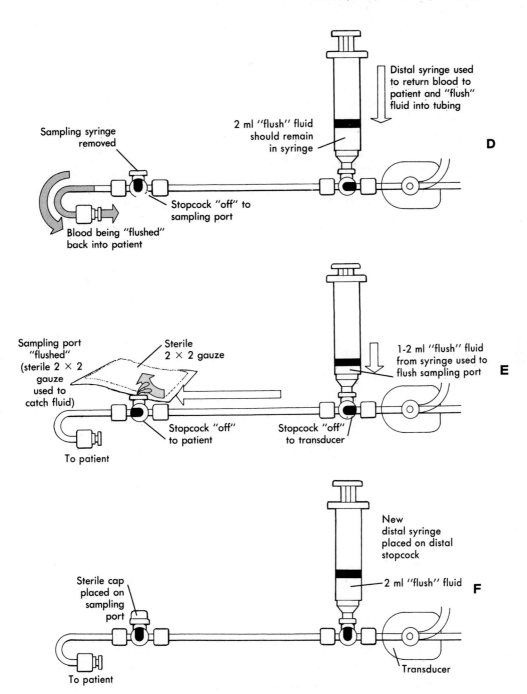

Fig. 13-12, cont'd. D, Turn proximal stopcock off to sampling port. Flush irrigation fluid from distal syringe into tubing and patient, until blood is cleared from monitoring tubing; 2 ml of fluid should remain in distal syringe. **E,** Turn proximal stopcock off to patient, and use remaining fluid from distal syringe to irrigate sampling port. **F,** Turn proximal stopcock off to sampling port. Turn distal stopcock off to syringe. Waveform should be visible on monitor. Place sterile occlusive cap on sampling port of proximal stopcock and syringe containing 2 ml of irrigant on distal stopcock.

discarded (this clears irrigation fluid from the stopcock port), and a second syringe is attached to the proximal stopcock for actual sampling of blood.

4. The blood sample is withdrawn into the proximal syringe (Fig. 13-12, C).
5. The proximal stopcock is turned off to the sampling port, and fluid from the distal syringe is used to flush patient blood back into the patient and irrigation fluid back into the tubing. Gentle irrigation should be provided, and 2 ml of irrigant fluid should remain in the distal syringe at the end of the procedure (Fig. 13-12, D). Thus no net fluid administration has occurred.
6. The proximal stopcock is turned off to the patient, and a small amount of the irrigant fluid in the distal syringe is used to flush out the sampling port of the proximal stopcock (Fig. 13-12, E).
7. When the sampling is complete, a sterile cap is placed on the sampling port of the proximal stopcock. A fresh syringe (containing exactly 2 ml of irrigant fluid) may be placed on the distal stopcock (Fig. 13-12, F).

This sampling procedure results in patient blood loss equal to the sample volume plus 0.1 ml. If care is taken to begin and end the procedure (before flushing of the sampling port) with exactly the same volume of irrigation fluid, no net fluid is administered to flush the monitoring line.

Recently, several blood-drawing tubing systems have become commercially available. The sampling ports replace stopcocks, cumbersome manipulation of the stopcocks is avoided, and exposure to blood is minimized.

Flow-Directed Balloon-Tipped Pulmonary Artery Catheterization

The assessment and manipulation of cardiac output are presented in Chapter 8. This section is designed to summarize essential aspects of the use of flow-directed balloon-tipped pulmonary artery catheters and thermodilution cardiac output measurements in children, with particular reference to techniques and typical errors in measurements and derived calculations unique to the pediatric patient.

Indications

The flow-directed, balloon-tipped pulmonary artery (PA) catheter is used to measure PA and PAW pressures. If the catheter is wedged in an appropriate segment of the lung and if no anatomic or physiologic (e.g., caused by mechanical ventilation) pulmonary venous obstruction is present, PAW pressure will approximate left atrial pressure. In the absence of mitral valve disease, left atrial pressure may equal left ventricular end-diastolic pressure (LVEDP). Measurement of PA pressure is useful in the treatment of the child with pulmonary hypertension, and estimation of LVEDP is helpful in the management of the child with shock or cardiovascular dysfunction. Under these conditions, right ventricular end-diastolic pressure (and right atrial and central venous pressures) cannot be expected to resemble LVEDP.

In general, when use of the PA catheter is indicated, a PA catheter that contains a thermistor is used; thus thermodilution cardiac output determinations may be obtained from the same catheter. Consideration also may be given to use of a fiberoptic PA catheter to allow continuous display of the mixed venous (pulmonary artery) oxygen saturation ($S\bar{v}o_2$). The $S\bar{v}o_2$ may trend directly with the child's cardiac output, but more important, changes in the $S\bar{v}o_2$ may indicate changes in oxygen delivery or consumption.

Indications for the use of the thermodilution balloon-tipped PA catheter in children are as follows:

1. Shock unresponsive to volume therapy and short-term inotropic support
2. Septic shock with low cardiac output (myocardial dysfunction can play an important role in deterioration of condition)
3. Any time precise tracking of hemodynamic parameters is required (e.g., during treatment with a drug that may produce myocardial depression, with use of new antidysrhythmic or vasoactive drugs, or during treatment of a child with severe cardiovascular instability)
4. Postoperative monitoring in the unstable patient
5. Any time precise tracking of oxygen transport parameters (arterial oxygen content × cardiac output) is required; for example, evaluation of oxygen transport is useful during manipulation of positive end-expiratory pressure (PEEP) in the treatment of severe respiratory failure
6. The catheter also may be used in the treatment of the child with severe pulmonary hypertension. However, the risks of using the catheter in these patients may be greater than the potential benefits.

Contraindications

In general, the PA catheter should be inserted only when the information it will yield is expected to influence therapy. Specific contraindications for its use in children include the following:

1. Presence of large intracardiac shunts — the PA catheter may inadvertently pass into the left side of the heart, and the balloon could wedge in the mitral or aortic valve, resulting in severe compromise in cardiac output and cerebral perfusion.
2. Presence of serious dysrhythmias — malignant dysrhythmias may develop during catheter passage through the right ventricle
3. Presence of severe coagulopathies — bleeding at the insertion site may be impossible to control
4. Presence of a very low cardiac output — the balloon may fail to float out of the right ventricle if cardiac output is extremely low
5. Any time the potential risks of the procedure outweigh the potential benefits

Insertion

The PA catheter is inserted into a large vein, most commonly the right internal jugular vein, the left subclavian vein, or the right femoral vein. The right internal jugular venous approach may be favored because it does not introduce the risk of pneumothorax; however, bleeding at this site is very difficult to control. The internal jugular vein should not be used if increased intracranial pressure is present, because the catheter may obstruct cerebral venous return.

The left subclavian venous approach is preferred over the right subclavian venous approach, because the curve of the vein toward the superior vena cava facilitates catheter entry into the right atrium and right ventricle. The right subclavian venous approach may be used, however, if the left subclavian vein has already been used for venous access. The femoral venous approach is most often used in infants inasmuch as the catheter may not be long enough to float into the pulmonary artery if this approach is used in older patients.

If the child weighs less than 15 to 18 kg, a 5-Fr catheter is used, and if the child weighs more than 15 to 18 kg, a 7-Fr catheter is used. A 5- or 5.5-Fr catheter is inserted through a 6.0-Fr introducer, and a 7- or 7.5-Fr catheter is inserted through an 8.5-Fr introducer sheath.

The 5- and 5.5-Fr catheters contain small lumens that may readily become occluded by fibrin material so that these catheters require scrupulous attention to lumen irrigation. In addition, the thermal injection lumen of the 5- or 5.5-Fr catheter is very small and provides a great deal of resistance to rapid injection of the thermal indicator. Finally, insertion and proper placement of small catheters may take a long time (much longer than insertion of 7-Fr catheters in adult patients).

The procedure should be explained simply (as age-appropriate) to the child and informed consent obtained from the parents before catheter insertion. If possible, the child should receive premedication with an analgesic, and appropriate restraints should be applied. Strict sterile technique must be maintained during catheter insertion. Absolute aseptic technique is then maintained during manipulation of the catheter monitoring and irrigation system. The placement technique is summarized in the following steps.

1. Prepare the fluid-filled monitoring system, and flush the transducer and all tubing. Zero and mechanically calibrate the transducer (see box on p. 293), and zero and electronically calibrate the monitor. The display scale should be set at 0 to 30 or 0 to 60 and preparations made to obtain a paper printout of the waveforms from the cardiac chambers and the pulmonary artery wedge. (The printer also should be calibrated.)

2. The vascular insertion site is scrubbed with a povidone-iodine solution and draped. A 1% lidocaine solution is injected into the subcutaneous tissue surrounding the insertion site. If the neck veins are used, the child should be placed in Trendelenburg's position to reduce the possibility of air entry into the right atrium.

3. A needle is used to enter the desired central vein (see previous section, Central Venous Pressure Monitoring, for further information about catheterization of specific veins), and the Seldinger technique is applied to insert a guidewire into the large vein.

4. Once the guidewire is in place, a catheter introducer sheath is threaded over the guidewire and into the large vein, and the sheath is sutured in place. This sheath facilitates entry of the PA catheter into the large vein and also provides an additional fluid administration port. Most introducer kits include a sterile, transparent sleeve that can be attached to the sheath; when the catheter is threaded through the sleeve into the sheath, it permits subsequent advancement and withdrawal of the catheter without compromising its sterility.

5. Once the introducer sheath and sleeve are in place, the PA catheter is prepared for insertion. Each lumen of the PA catheter is flushed with normal saline, and the distal lumen is connected to the transducer and monitoring system, so that a digital display as well as the waveform can be observed on the monitor.

6. The air-reference port of the system is placed at the level of the right atrium, and the tip of the catheter is held within the sterile field at the same height as the air-reference port and the patient's right atrium. The pressure reading from the transducer should be zero at this time. The tip of the catheter is then elevated 27.2

cm above the zero-reference point, and the pressure reading should be 20 mm Hg ($\pm$1 mm Hg). If accurate readings are not obtained, the transducer and monitoring system should be checked.

7. The catheter balloon is inflated in a sterile container of normal saline or water. If bubbles are visible or the balloon fails to inflate or inflates asymmetrically, a new catheter should be obtained (and steps 5 and 6 repeated). Carbon dioxide is the preferred gas for balloon inflation because it is easily dispersed in the blood should balloon rupture occur. However, because this gas is not readily available in the clinical setting, room air generally is used for balloon inflation. The maximum balloon inflation volume is printed on the catheter and should be written on the nursing care plan.

8. If a thermodilution catheter is used, the thermistor connector cable from the cardiac output computer (or from the monitor, if cardiac output calculations are performed by the bedside monitor) should be connected to the thermistor hub of the catheter. The cardiac output computer or monitor should be turned on. If the thermistor is faulty, this will be indicated by the computer or monitor, and a new catheter should be obtained (and steps 5 and 6 repeated).

9. If a fiberoptic PA catheter is used, the fiberoptic port must be joined to the optical module and microprocessor and adequate computer warm-up time allowed. The fiberoptic catheter must be calibrated before insertion in the patient.

10. While the pressure waveform obtained through the distal port is monitored, the catheter is advanced through the introducer sheath. Once a venous waveform appears, the balloon may be inflated to half its normal inflation volume. The catheter is then advanced until it reaches the right atrium. Some clinicians prefer to leave the balloon deflated until the catheter is clearly in the right atrium. Once the catheter is in the right atrium and a typical right atrial waveform is achieved (Fig. 13-13, A), the balloon is completely inflated with the recommended volume.

11. The catheter is then gently advanced as the balloon floats into the right ventricle and pulmonary artery, as illustrated by the appearance of corresponding waveforms (Fig. 13-13, B and C). During passage of the catheter through the right ventricle, everyone at the bedside should monitor the patient's electrocardiogram for evidence of premature ventricular contractions. If these develop, the catheter should be quickly moved out of the right ventricle.

12. Once a characteristic pulmonary artery wedge (PAW) waveform is visualized (Fig. 13-13, D), advancement of the catheter should stop. The balloon is deflated, and a PA waveform should reappear. The balloon is again inflated, and the PAW waveform should again become apparent. If the PAW waveform occurs only intermittently during balloon inflation, it may be necessary to advance the catheter 1 to 2 cm further.

13. Once the catheter is in place, the length of catheter insertion is noted on the nursing care plan and in the patient's chart. It is not possible to suture the catheter to the sleeve; thus care must be taken to avoid any tension on the catheter or tubing.

14. Radiographic confirmation of proper catheter placement is necessary.

15. The proximal right atrial port should be joined to a fluid infusion transducer and monitoring system. It is possible to join the proximal and distal ports to the same

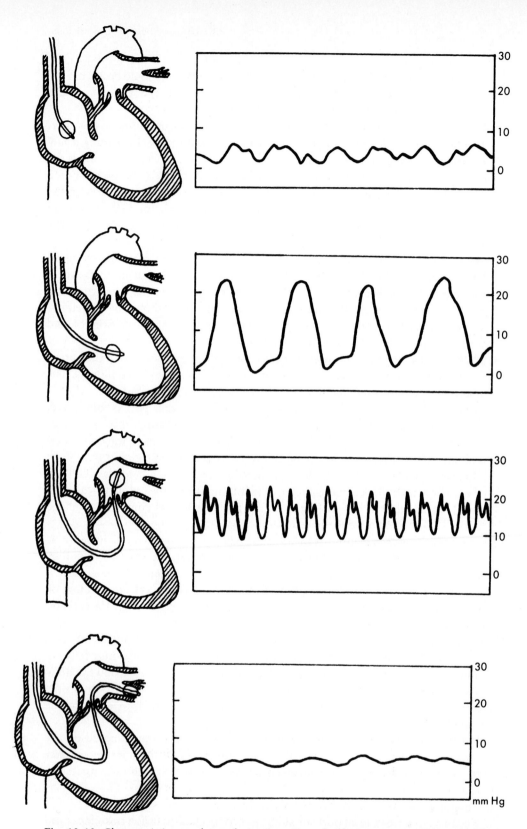

Fig. 13-13. Characteristic waveforms during insertion of pulmonary artery (PA) catheter. **A,** Right atrial position and waveform (normal mean pressure is 0 to 5 mm Hg). **B,** Right ventricular position and waveform (normal pressure is approximately 30/5 mm Hg). **C,** PA position and waveform (normal pressure is approximately 30/15 mm Hg). **D,** Pulmonary artery wedge position and waveform (normal mean pressure 4 to 8 mm Hg).

monitoring line, so that both pressures can be monitored with the use of a single transducer (with the turning of a stopcock).

16. If thermodilution cardiac output calculations will be performed, the proximal right atrial port should be joined to the injection syringe and injection system. If a second right atrial port is present, it should be connected to a fluid infusion system.

17. If a fiberoptic PA catheter has been inserted the mixed venous oxygen saturation ($S\bar{v}o_2$) will be displayed on the microprocessor. If the patient's length and weight are entered into the microprocessor, the patient's expected cardiac output is displayed. The $S\bar{v}o_2$ is normally approximately 75%, and a fall in this saturation usually indicates a fall in oxygen transport (as a result of an uncompensated fall in arterial oxygen content or cardiac output, or both, or an increase in oxygen consumption). If the fiberoptic catheter utilizes two light wavelengths (e.g., the Baxter catheter), it will be necessary to enter the patient's hemoglobin concentration into the microprocessor data base. This information should be reentered whenever the patient's hemoglobin concentration changes. If the fiberoptic catheter utilizes three light wavelengths (e.g., the Abbott catheter), entry of the patient's hemoglobin concentration is not necessary.

18. PA and PAW waveforms should be recorded on graphic paper, and the patient's end-expiration should be marked. Both pressure measurements should be taken at end-expiration.

Maintenance

Care must be taken to ensure that the transducer and monitoring system are appropriately leveled, zeroed, and calibrated and that they are free of air or kinks. Small, disposable transducers may be taped to the chest at the phlebostatic axis. The transducer and monitor should be zeroed to air at least once every shift and whenever there is a change in patient or transducer position. The transducer should be mechanically calibrated (see box on p. 293) once every day. Irrigation fluid and intravenous tubing should be changed, with use of aseptic technique, every 48 to 72 hours.

The PA waveform should be displayed at all times, so that spontaneous wedging of the balloon or catheter movement into the right ventricle will be immediately detected. If such wedging or movement occurs, a physician should be contacted immediately, and the catheter should be repositioned. High- and low-pressure alarms should be set carefully so that spontaneous wedging or tubing disconnection (and resultant fall in PA pressure) or change in patient condition will immediately trigger an audible alarm.

The lumens should be flushed continuously with 1 to 3 ml/hr of heparinized normal saline (1 unit of heparin/ml is standard), and all fluids administered through the catheter should be added to the child's hourly fluid intake totals. Because the lumens are very small, they can easily become occluded by fibrin, clots, or crystals from intravenous solutions. The distal lumen should be used for pressure measurements only and should *not* be used for infusion of antibiotics or drugs. It may be used as a lumen of last resort for vasoactive drug infusion.

Mixed venous blood samples from the pulmonary artery may be drawn from the distal port, but such sampling may lead to the development of clot occlusion of the lumen. If blood sampling is performed, the catheter should be irrigated several times after the sampling is performed.

Pulmonary artery measurements

PA pressure measurements should be obtained only if the system is appropriately zeroed, leveled, and mechanically calibrated. The measurement should *not* be taken from the digital display on the bedside monitor unless the patient's end-expiration can be determined by the monitor. The display, which represents the average pressure over a several-second sampling period, may not reflect the pressure at end-expiration. If the monitor cannot be programmed to determine the pressure at end-expiration, the PA and PAW pressures should be derived from a graphic printout of the waveforms. Inspiration and expiration should be marked on the waveform, and the pressures at end-expiration should be calculated. A graphic printout of the PA waveform should be added to the patient's chart every 8 hours to document appropriate catheter placement and catheter patency.

When PAW pressure measurements are obtained, the balloon should be inflated with the minimal volume necessary to wedge the catheter. The catheter should be in the wedge position only long enough to obtain a graphic printout of the PAW waveform. The balloon should never be inflated with a larger volume than that recommended by the catheter manufacturer.

If pulmonary vascular resistance is normal, PA end-diastolic pressure will approximate the mean PAW pressure. If PA end-diastolic pressure is significantly higher than PAW pressure at end-expiration, pulmonary vascular resistance must be elevated (Fig. 13-14).

If PAW pressure is to accurately reflect left atrial pressure (and LVEDP), there must be patent, fluid-filled, vasculature between the tip of the catheter and the left atrium. Therefore, accurate PAW pressure measurements require that the catheter be wedged in a physiologic zone III pulmonary artery (anatomically identified as relating to the posterior, inferior portion of the lung below the level of the left atrium). In this area of the lung, both PA and venous pressures are greater than alveolar pressure so

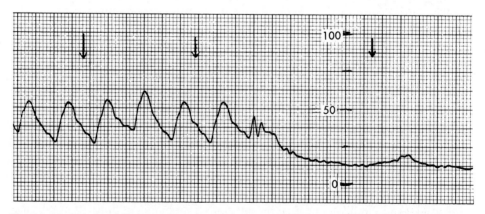

Fig. 13-14. Relationship between pulmonary artery end-diastolic pressure and pulmonary artery wedge pressure when pulmonary vascular resistance is elevated. Pulmonary artery end-diastolic pressure is 27 mm Hg and pulmonary artery wedge pressure is 12.5 mm Hg. All pressures are recorded only at end-expiration *(arrows)*. Patient is on positive pressure ventilation, and all pressures are recorded only at end-expiration *(arrows)*.

Typical errors in pediatric thermodilution cardiac output calculations

---

INACCURATE COMPUTER CALIBRATION CONSTANT

INAPPROPRIATE INJECTATE VOLUME/TEMPERATURE

Falsely high cardiac output calculations will result from:
    Inaccurately smaller injectate volume than programmed
    Dead space between injectate syringe and right atrial injectate port
    Warming of injectate temperature before injection
    Large volume infusions into right atrium or introducer sheath
    Injectate exit port within introducer sheath instead of right atrium

Falsely low cardiac output calculations will result from:
    Inaccurately larger injectate volume than programmed
    Iced injectate with calibration constant set for room temperature injectate

POOR INJECTION TECHNIQUE

COMPUTER OR CATHETER MALFUNCTION

---

calculation. If possible, the fluid infusion should be briefly interrupted during determinations.

Anything that artificially increases the magnitude of the temperature change in the pulmonary artery will result in erroneously low cardiac output calculations. If, for example, the computer programming or calibration constant is set for a 3-ml injection and a 3.5- or 5-ml injection is given, an inaccurate low cardiac output calculation will result. If iced injectate is used, and the computer programming or calibration constant is set for room-temperature injectate, the cardiac output calculation will be falsely low.

The thermodilution curves should have the same height and configuration (see Fig. 13-17, *A*). Changes in curve configuration from injection to injection or from clinician to clinician indicate lack of standardization or error in injection technique (Fig. 13-17, *B*).

Slow or uneven injection technique also produces error in cardiac output determinations. The computer or monitor records the temperature change only after the start button or foot pedal is depressed; therefore, false calculations could result if the injection begins before the computer begins recording (Fig. 13-17, *C*) unless the cardiac output is very low. Slow injection usually results in inaccurate cardiac output determinations; injections should take no longer than 4 seconds.

Continuous monitoring of mixed venous oxygen saturation ($S\bar{v}o_2$)

Mixed venous oxygen saturation ($S\bar{v}o_2$) is the percentage of hemoglobin that is saturated with oxygen in a well-mixed systemic venous blood sample. The most accurate $S\bar{v}o_2$ is obtained in the pulmonary artery, because superior and inferior vena caval blood are well-mixed in the pulmonary artery.

When a fiberoptic catheter is placed in the child's pulmonary artery and the catheter is joined to a microprocessor, a continuous display of the child's $S\bar{v}_{O_2}$ can be obtained in a manner similar to that employed during pulse oximetry. Fiberoptic PA catheters are now available in sizes as small as 5.5-Fr, and fiberoptics as small as 4-Fr may be inserted into vessels.

Normal $S\bar{v}_{O_2}$ is approximately 75%. The $S\bar{v}_{O_2}$ is influenced by arterial oxygen saturation, cardiac output, and tissue oxygen consumption, although there may be a direct relationship between changes in $S\bar{v}_{O_2}$ and cardiac output. $S\bar{v}_{O_2}$ also will fall if significant hypoxemia develops, such as may be observed in the child with severe respiratory disease or cyanotic heart disease that is not compensated by a rise in cardiac output. The $S\bar{v}_{O_2}$ usually rises when cardiac output rises, but it also may increase in the presence of sepsis (and resultant maldistribution of blood flow).

Continuous display of the $S\bar{v}_{O_2}$ may provide an immediate indication of changes in the child's oxygen supply-demand relationship. The $S\bar{v}_{O_2}$ monitor may be useful during titration of PEEP therapy; when arterial oxygen content is improved significantly without a compromise in cardiac output, the $S\bar{v}_{O_2}$ will rise. If, however, PEEP therapy compromises cardiac output proportionately more than it improves arterial oxygen content, oxygen delivery and, consequently, the $S\bar{v}_{O_2}$ will fall.

Transthoracic Right or Left Atrial or Pulmonary Artery Catheterization

During cardiovascular surgery, catheters may be inserted through the chest wall and placed directly into the right atrium, left atrium, or pulmonary artery. Generally, a 2- to 3-Fr catheter is used, and the principles of monitoring the use of these catheters are the same as those discussed for any invasive intravascular catheter.

The right atrial catheter is used as a CVP line and accurately reflects right ventricular end-diastolic pressure. This catheter may be used for right atrial pressure measurements, infusion of fluids, or administration of medications. Care should be taken to prevent air or clot entry into the catheter. *If the child has unrepaired cyanotic congenital heart disease, any air entering the right atrial catheter may be shunted to the left side of the heart and into the systemic circulation, ultimately producing a cerebral air embolus (stroke).*

The left atrial catheter is used to monitor left ventricular end-diastolic pressure when the surgeon wishes to avoid the need to place a PA catheter. When the left atrial catheter is joined to the monitoring and flush system—and throughout the use of this catheter—scrupulous care must be taken to prevent air entry into this line. *Air entry into the left atrial catheter can result in cerebral air embolus.* This catheter should *not* be entered once it is joined to the monitoring system, and only irrigation fluid should be flushed through the catheter. If damping of the left atrial waveform occurs, a physician should be consulted, and the line should be aspirated and then irrigated gently *only* with physician approval, if no particulate matter is observed in the catheter or tubing.

A PA catheter may be placed directly into the pulmonary artery to allow postoperative monitoring of PA pressure. Use of the catheter in this way does not allow PAW pressure measurements. However, if the child's pulmonary vascular resistance is normal, PA end-diastolic pressure will equal mean PAW pressure (note that normal pulmonary vascular resistance will *not* be present in most children with congenital heart disease and pulmonary hypertension).

Small (2.5-Fr) PA catheters are available with thermistor beads. During cardiovascular surgery, while the chest is open, the tip of the catheter is passed through a small incision in the child's chest and placed directly in the pulmonary artery. The catheter is joined to a cardiac output computer and a monitoring/fluid infusion system. Thermodilution cardiac output calculations may be performed with use of this catheter if a right atrial or CVP line is in place to allow right atrial fluid injections. However, it will be necessary to check with the catheter manufacturer to determine the appropriate calibration constant, as well as the precise recommended volume and temperature of right atrial injections. Such information is also available in the literature (Baskoff and Maruschak).

Transthoracic catheters generally are left in place for several days. After this time, a small tract has formed through the chest wall. If bleeding occurs after catheter removal, the blood can be evacuated through the tract instead of accumulating in the mediastinum. The catheters are removed only with a physician's order, and the patient should be monitored closely for evidence of bleeding or tamponade after catheter removal.

SUMMARY

Accurate hemodynamic monitoring of pediatric patients requires careful attention to construction of a reliable monitoring system and standardization of measurement techniques. Measurements and derived calculations of hemodynamic variables should always be evaluated in light of the patient's condition and general appearance. The best monitoring system is the presence of a skilled clinician at the bedside.

REFERENCES

Aherne W, Hull D: Brown adipose tissue and heat production in the newborn infant, *J Pathol Bact* 91:223, 1966.

American Association of Critical-Care Nurses: Evaluation of the effects of heparinized and non-heparinized flush solutions on the patency of arterial pressure monitoring lines: the Thunder Project, *Am J Crit Care* 2:3, 1993.

Baskoff JD, Maruschak R: Correction factor for thermodilution determination of cardiac output in children, *Crit Care Med* 9:870, 1981.

Boxer RA et al: Noninvasive pulse oximetry in children with cyanotic congenital heart disease, *Crit Care Med* 15:1062, 1987.

Buntain WL, Lynch FP, Ramenofsky ML: Management of the acutely injured child, *Adv Trauma* 2:43-86, 1987.

Butt WW et al: Complications resulting from use of arterial catheters: retrograde flow and rapid elevation in blood pressure, *Pediatrics* 76:250, 1985.

Butt WW et al: Effect of heparin concentration and infusion rate on the patency of arterial catheters, *Crit Care Med* 15:230, 1987. NOTE: this article refers to pediatric catheters.

Cannon K, Mitchell KA, Fabian TC: Prospective randomized evaluation of two methods of drawing coagulation studies from heparinized arterial lines, *Heart Lung* 14:392, 1985.

Carroll GC: Blood pressure monitoring, *Crit Care Clin* 4:411, 1988.

Chameides L, Hazinski MF, editors: *Textbook of pediatric advanced life support,* ed 2, Dallas, American Heart Association and the American Academy of Pediatrics (in press).

Clyman R et al: How a patent ductus arteriosus affects the premature lamb's ability to handle additional volume loads, *Pediatr Res* 23:316-320, 1988.

Cohn JN: Blood pressure measurement in shock: mechanisms of inaccuracy in auscultatory and palpatory methods, *JAMA* 199:188, 1967.

Delaplane D et al: Urokinase therapy for a catheter-related right atrial thrombus, *J Pediatr* 100:149, 1985.

Diprose GK: Dinamap fails to detect hypotension in very low birthweight infants, *Arch Dis Child* 61:771, 1986.

Ducharme FM et al: Incidence of infection related to arterial catheterization in children: a prospective study, *Crit Care Med* 16:272, 1988.

Eisenberg PR, Jaffe AS, Schuster DP: Clinical evaluation compared to pulmonary artery catheterization in the hemodynamic assessment of critically ill patients, *Crit Care Med* 12:549, 1984.

Fanconi S et al: Pulse oximetry in pediatric intensive care: comparison with measured saturations and transcutaneous oxygen tension, *J Pediatr* 107:362, 1985.

Friedman WF: *The intrinsic physiologic properties of the developing heart.* In Friedman WF, editor: *Neonatal heart disease,* New York, 1973, Grune & Stratton.

Green GE, Hassell KT, Mahutte CK: Comparison of arterial blood gas with continuous intra-arterial and transcutaneous PO_2 sensors in adult critically ill patients, *Crit Care Med* 15:491, 1987.

Hansen TN, Tooley WM: Skin surface carbon dioxide tension in sick infants, *Pediatrics* 64:942, 1979.

Hazinski MF: Nursing care of the critically ill child: the 7-point check, *Pediatr Nurs* 11:453, 1985.

Hazinski MF: *Children are different.* In Hazinski MF, editor: *Nursing care of the critically ill child,* ed 2, St Louis, 1992, Mosby–Year Book.

Hazinski MF, Barkin RM: *Shock.* In Barkin RM, editor: *Pediatric emergency medicine: concepts and clinical practice,* St Louis, 1992, Mosby–Year Book.

Horgan MJ et al: Effect of heparin infusates in umbilical arterial catheters on frequency of thrombotic complications, *J Pediatr* 111:774, 1987.

Huch R, Huch A, Lubbers DE: Transcutaneous measurement of blood PO_2 ($tcPO_2$): method and application in perinatal medicine, *J Perinat Med* 1:183, 1973.

Katz RW, Pollack MM, Weibley RE: Pulmonary artery catheterization in pediatric intensive care, *Adv Pediatr* 30:169, 1983.

Kelly RP et al: Non-invasive determination of age-related changes in the human arterial pulse, *Circulation* 80:1652-1659, 1989.

Lister G et al: Oxygen delivery in lambs: cardiovascular and hematologic development, *Am J Physiol* 237:H668, 1979.

Lock JE: Hemodynamic evaluation of congenital heart disease. In Lock JE, Kean JF, Fellows KE, editors: *Diagnostic and interventional catheterization in congenital heart disease,* Boston, 1987, Martinus Nijhoff.

Maki DG et al: Prospective study of replacing administration sets for intravenous therapy at 48- vs 72-hour intervals, *JAMA* 258:1777, 1987.

Mandoza GJB et al: Intracardiac thrombi complicating central total parenteral nutrition: resolu-

tion without surgery or thrombolysis, *J Pediatr* 108:610, 1985.

Milliken J et al: Nosocomial infections in a pediatric intensive care unit, *Crit Care Med* 16:233, 1988.

Miyasaka K et al: Complications of radial artery lines in the pediatric patient, *Can Anaesth Soc J* 23:9, 1979.

Morris AH, Chapman RH, Gardner RM: Frequency of wedge pressure errors in the ICU, *Crit Care Med* 13:705, 1985.

Nicolson SC et al: Comparison of internal and external jugular cannulation of the central circulation in the pediatric patient, *Crit Care Med* 13:747, 1985.

Park MK, Menard SM: Accuracy of blood pressure measurement by the Dinamap monitor in infants and children, *Pediatrics* 79:907, 1987.

Poets CF et al: Reliability of a pulse oximeter in the detection of hyperoxemia, *J Pediatr* 122:87-90, 1993.

Prian GW et al: Apparent cerebral embolization after temporal artery catheterization, *J Pediatr* 93:115, 1978.

Ricard P, Martin R, Marcoux A: Protection of indwelling vascular catheters: incidence of bacterial contamination and catheter-related sepsis, *Crit Car Med* 13:541, 1985.

Riggs CD, Lister G: Adverse occurrences in the pediatric intensive care unit, *Pediatr Clin North Am* 34:93, 1987.

Rudolph AM: Cardiac catheterization and angiocardiography. In Rudolph AM, editor: *Congenital diseases of the heart,* Chicago, 1974, Mosby–Year Book.

Selden H et al: Radial arterial catheters in children and neonates: a prospective study, *Crit Care Med* 15:1106, 1987.

Severinghaus JW, Naifeh KH: Accuracy of response of six pulse oximeters in profound hypoxia, *Anesthesiology* 67:551-558, 1981.

Smith-Wright DL et al: Complications of vascular catheterization in critically ill children, *Crit Care Med* 12:1015, 1984.

Snydman DR et al: Intravenous tubing containing burettes can be safely changed at 72-hour intervals, *Infect Control* 8:113, 1987.

Sobel DB: Burning of a neonate due to a pulse oximeter: arterial saturation monitoring, *Pediatrics* 89:154-156, 1992.

Sprung CL, Rackow EC, Civetta JM: Direct measurements and derived calculations using the pulmonary artery catheter. In Sprung CL, editor: *The pulmonary artery catheter: methodology and clinical applications,* Baltimore, 1983, University Park Press.

Verhoeff F, Sykes MK: Delayed detection of hypoxic events by pulse oximeters: computer simulations, *Anaesthesia* 45:103-109, 1990.

Walsh MC et al: Relationship of pulse oximetry to arterial oxygen tension in infants, *Crit Care Med* 15:1102, 1987.

Wareham JA et al: Prediction of arterial blood pressure in the premature neonate using the oscillometric method, *Am J Dis Child* 141:1108, 1987.

West P, George CF, Kryger MH: Dynamic in vivo response characteristics of three oximeters: Hewlett-Packard 47201A, Biox III, and Nellcor N-100, *Sleep* 10:263, 1987.

Chapter 14

Hemodynamic Monitoring of the Patient with Acute Myocardial Infarction

PATHOPHYSIOLOGY

The actual event that precipitates the dramatic, sudden onset of an acute myocardial infarction (AMI) is poorly understood. In more than 95% of patients who die of myocardial infarction (MI), there is associated severe occlusive atherosclerosis in the coronary arteries that supply the area of infarction. Most investigators who have performed coronary arteriography within a few hours of onset of angina in patients suspected of having an MI have found complete occlusion of those coronary arteries supplying the infarcted area. In many instances the clot appeared fresh, as evidenced by staining with the angiographic dye. These findings have set the stage for early intervention with the use of thrombolytic therapy. The evidence of fresh thrombus in most patients with AMI suggests that a platelet thrombus, caused either by disruption of the endothelium over an atherosclerotic plaque or perhaps by focal spasm, is an important etiologic factor in the onset of MI. Clinical investigations indicate that aggressive treatment with thrombolytic agents to dissolve the occluding clot results in improved myocardial function and survival. The role of immediate angioplasty of the underlying stenotic lesion is an alternative method to establish maximal flow to the ischemic myocardium as quickly as possible. In addition, some clinicians have taken a highly aggressive approach and use emergency coronary arteriography and coronary bypass surgery in the treatment of patients with AMI. It has been difficult to document the efficacy and extent of infarct reduction accomplished with these treatment approaches. It is certain that the longer the patient has angina and myocardial ischemia before these interventions can be accomplished, the less myocardium can be salvaged.

A rare event that may precipitate infarction is hemorrhage beneath an atherosclerotic plaque, resulting in sudden occlusion of the coronary artery. Spasm of a severely atherosclerotic vessel also can cause irreversible ischemia. If this event occurs, there is a vicious cycle of ischemia → decreased myocardial function → further ischemia → decreased myocardial function → decreased coronary perfusion and infarction.

Within 30 seconds of the onset of ischemia, metabolic changes occur in the myocardial cells that affect their function. Effective ventricular contraction ceases almost immediately, and there are changes in membrane electropotential. These changes are associated with ECG changes, including marked ST elevation and peaking of the T waves, probably resulting from the loss of sodium pump activity and a change in transmembrane potassium gradient. Cessation of oxidative phosphorylation results in a rapid fall in myocardial temperature. Anaerobic glycolysis is initiated for cellular high-energy phosphate production in lieu of the aerobic Krebs' cycle. This anaerobic process results in lactate production from glucose.

In experimental animals these ischemic changes are reversible up to 15 or 20 minutes after the onset of coronary occlusion. When the occlusion is released, function is restored within a few minutes, and after several hours cellular structure is essentially normal. The time period of reversible ischemia can be markedly prolonged, however, by lowering the temperature of the myocardium during the ischemic result. This procedure is commonly performed during cardiac surgery, particularly for congenital heart disease, in which regional and total body hypothermia is used on infants too young to be placed on cardiopulmonary bypass. In cardiac transplantation the intact denervated heart can be preserved with iced saline for several hours during the interval before coronary blood flow is reinstituted in the recipient's body.

Attempts at reversing myocardial ischemia, decreasing infarct size, or stabilizing the electrophysiologic system require an understanding of the acute metabolic effects of ischemia. The point at which these anaerobic processes become associated with irreversibility is more difficult to analyze. Irreversibility relates to a number of pathologic processes, including rupture of lysozymes, structural defects in sarcolemma, marked rises in intracellular acidity that may result in protein denaturation, and other irreversible changes in the structure of the cell. Although initially these abnormalities may be reversible, after approximately 20 minutes they become irreversible. One can attempt to prevent irreversible damage by delivering oxygen, stabilizing cell membranes, and administering hydrogen receptors to combat lactic acidosis. It is important to note, however, that irreversible infarction occurs in the center of the infarcted zone; there is an increasing number of normal or near-normal cells toward the periphery, and it is this borderline or "twilight" zone that is the most susceptible to pharmacologic and physiologic intervention to maintain myocardial function and prevent necrosis.

The clinical picture of the patient with AMI may not necessarily indicate the status of the patient's myocardial function unless the ischemic area is extensive. Decreased coronary blood flow, resulting in ischemia and segmental akinesia, leads to myocardial dysfunction that manifests as a decreased rate of left ventricular (LV) pressure development (dp/dt, i.e., rate of pressure rise per unit of time), decreased LV ejection rate, and decreased stroke volume. These abnormalities are accompanied by an increase in LV end-diastolic volume and filling pressure. The extent of the infarction can be closely related to the degree of LV dysfunction. This correlation is particularly accurate in the patient with a single infarction and no evidence of previous ventricular damage. The full spectrum of LV dysfunction seen in patients with MI ranges from cardiogenic shock or pump failure (which occurs when over 40% of the left ventricle is infarcted) to essentially normal or near-normal pressures and cardiac output.

Our understanding of LV function and dysfunction after an AMI has been broadened by the development of the pulmonary artery (PA) catheter for indirect monitoring of LV filling pressures—pulmonary artery wedge (PAW) pressure and perfusion (cardiac output). Table 14-1 outlines the variety of hemodynamic abnormalities that can be seen after an AMI. In the patient with a small infarction, whose clinical condition is uncomplicated, hemodynamic measurements, if obtained, are usually normal, although approximately 25% of these patients have a slight increase in their LVEDP or PAW pressure. In the majority (45%) of patients who develop a transient mild LV failure (usually during the first 4 days after the infarction), hemodynamic measurements reveal an elevated PAW pressure, reflecting an abnormal LVEDP. These patients experience further deterioration with any challenge, such as an increase in afterload as a result of a rise in blood pressure. Of the remaining 25% of patients with acute infarction, about 15% develop severe LV failure, of which approximately one half will show marked improvement after a week's convalescence. These patients exhibit serious elevations in LVEDP and PAW pressure, with abnormally low stroke volume and cardiac output.

The hemodynamic pattern of the patient who has developed cardiogenic shock from severe LV failure typically consists of an increase in the central venous pressure (CVP) and PAW pressure, associated with a low arterial blood pressure and cardiac output. However, a small percentage of patients have a low cardiac output with normal, or even decreased, CVP and PAW pressure. These patients require fluid challenge to separate hypovolemic shock from the true low-output cardiogenic shock. (This is discussed in the section on cardiogenic shock.) In most circumstances the range of hemodynamic patterns can be correlated with the extent of the infarction.

The hemodynamic pattern of the patient in cardiogenic shock from right heart failure resulting from right ventricular (RV) infarction shows an elevated CVP or right atrial (RA) pressure, with a normal or low PAW pressure, low arterial blood pressure, and low cardiac output. (See p. 356 for a more detailed discussion.)

Table 14-1. Hemodynamic findings after a myocardial infarction

Clinical status (% of patients)	Blood pressure	Cardiac output	Heart rate	Peripheral vascular resistance	CVP	PAW or PADP (mm Hg)
Uncomplicated (30)	N	N	↑ or ↓	N	N	3-12
Mild LV failure (45)	N	N	↑ or ↓	N	N	12-15
Severe LV failure (15)	N or ↓	↓	↑	↑	N or ↑	15-20
Cardiogenic shock (10)	↓	↓	↑	↑	↑ or ↓	15-30

CVP, Central venous pressure; *PAW*, pulmonary artery wedge; *PADP*, pulmonary artery diastolic pressure; *N*, normal range; ↑, increased; ↓, decreased.

PHYSIOLOGIC CONCEPTS OF TREATMENT
Maintenance of Optimal Cardiac Function
Maintaining electrophysiologic stability

More than 90% of patients who have an AMI develop dysrhythmias some time during the first 72 hours of the infarction. As many as 50% of patients with an infarction develop a lethal ventricular dysrhythmia at the onset of the infarction, and this dysrhythmia precipitates sudden death before hospital admission. Fortunately, malignant dysrhythmias occur in only a small percentage of hospitalized patients with acute infarction. The seriousness of any dysrhythmia depends not only on the type of dysrhythmia but on the degree of myocardial dysfunction.

A number of clinical factors are associated with an increased potential for the development of dysrhythmia:
1. Myocardial ischemia
2. Systemic hypoxemia
3. Cardiomegaly
4. Conduction abnormalities
5. LV failure
6. Acidosis
7. Increased sympathetic tone
8. Hypokalemia
9. Hypomagnesemia

Myocardial ischemia increases vulnerability to ventricular fibrillation by altering conduction velocity, automaticity, and membrane potentials. Systemic hypoxemia associated with LV failure may aggravate myocardial ischemia, further enhancing susceptibility to dysrhythmias. Other factors associated with dysrhythmias (and probably reflecting the severity of the cardiac disease) include an enlarged heart, preexisting impairment in conduction, and pacemaker abnormalities. The degree of either systemic or local acidosis caused by peripheral or cardiac anaerobic metabolism is believed to cause changes in transmembrane potassium potential and cellular function, which may alter the potential for cardiac dysrhythmias. Anxiety, fear, and pain cause increases in catecholamine secretion. Experimental studies have shown that sympathetic activity markedly affects susceptibility to ventricular fibrillation. Metabolic abnormalities, particularly hypokalemia and hypomagnesemia, also can cause dysrhythmias.

Atrial dysrhythmias occur less frequently than ventricular dysrhythmias in the patient with an AMI. Their development is critical, however, inasmuch as the loss of atrial systole can result in a 20% or greater decrease in cardiac output. In the undigitalized patient, atrial fibrillation and the associated rapid ventricular rate, decreased diastolic filling period, and increased myocardial oxygen demand may precipitate a fatal outcome. The occurrence of atrial dysrhythmias reflects a serious prognosis and may be caused by extensive infarction involving the atrium, atrial distention resulting from ventricular failure, or pericarditis.

Ventricular dysrhythmias may be caused by alterations in automaticity, or abnormalities in conduction that allow a reentry mechanism to develop, or a combination of the two. Normal cardiac conduction tissue (not myocardial contractile cells) is characterized by a phase IV depolarization, which at a given threshold triggers depolarization of the cell. Abnormalities may occur either in the

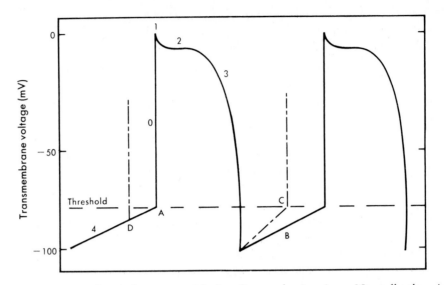

Fig. 14-1. Transmembrane electropotential of cardiac conduction tissue. Normally, there is a gradual rise in voltage from the low point of − 90 mV. At a given threshold the cell depolarizes; then myocardial contractile cells depolarize and contract. During repolarization, a peak negative transmembrane voltage is again attained, and the sequence recurs. *A,* Normal threshold for depolarization; *B,* normal slope of depolarization; *C,* increased slope of depolarization reaching threshold for firing prematurely (as might occur with ischemia); *D,* decreased threshold also causing premature firing.

rate (slope) of phase IV depolarization or in the *threshold* for depolarization (Fig. 14-1). It is thought that ischemia, as well as local metabolic factors, can affect this rate and threshold of depolarization.

Altered conduction of the cardiac impulse, rather than increased automaticity, probably accounts for most occurrences of dysrhythmias related to ischemia. Concepts about the development of these dysrhythmias are based on the premise that there is a unidirectional conduction block in the ischemic tissue surrounding the infarction area. Thus a given propagating cardiac impulse may be blocked or slowed through a zone of ischemic injury, but the impulse spreads normally through the terminal branches of nonischemic tissue. Because of slowed conduction through the ischemic muscle, the normal conduction tissue has had time to repolarize, so that when the propagating impulse finally leaves the ischemia area, it can repolarize the normal conductive tissue, giving rise to a premature ventricular beat. A reentry tachycardia can develop from this mechanism, precipitating ventricular tachycardia or ventricular fibrillation.

The therapeutic goal is to achieve optimal electrophysiologic function, by eliminating or decreasing factors known to be associated with increased susceptibility to ventricular fibrillation. Administering oxygen and treating LV failure may be important in eliminating or decreasing the frequency of premature contractions.

The development of a second- or third-degree block complicates AMI in about 10% of patients. When the heart block is associated with an anterior wall infarction, the prognosis is poor because of the implication of extensive septal damage. In most patients with a heart block caused by an inferior MI, the dysrhythmia resolves within 1 to 2 weeks after the infarction. When the heart block is complete, or 2:1, a temporary pacemaker may be required to maintain an adequate heart rate and cardiac output.

Maintaining adequate coronary perfusion

Sufficient coronary circulation is important not only for electrophysiologic stability but also for maintenance of myocardial contraction. Approximately 70% to 85% of the coronary blood flow occurs during the diastolic phase of the cardiac cycle. Normally, a certain degree of autoregulation of coronary flow occurs, so that an increase in aortic diastolic pressure without an increase in myocardial demand will result in an increase in resistance to the coronary circulation. This autoregulation is operative until a mean arterial diastolic pressure of 80 mm Hg is reached. Below this level there is complete vasodilation of the coronary bed, and flow through the coronary circulation is more linearly related to the perfusion pressure at the coronary ostia (the central aortic pressure). Although coronary blood flow may be normal in patients with occlusive coronary disease, there are inadequacies or inequities in the distribution of the blood flow, determined by the severity and distribution of the occlusive disease. It has been demonstrated that an atherosclerotic plaque has little impact on blood flow through the artery until the vessel becomes approximately 75% occluded. After this point, however, rapidly increasing resistance to flow occurs, and greater pressure falls across the partially occluded area. The length of the occluded area also affects blood flow.

Because most of the coronary flow to the left ventricle occurs during diastole, the heart rate, which determines the length of diastole, is an important factor in myocardial oxygen delivery. With an increasing heart rate, there is less time for diastole and therefore less time for coronary perfusion. This problem is aggravated by the increased myocardial oxygen required for the increased work of a faster heart rate.

Studies in animal coronary circulation indicate that the coronary circulatory bed can regulate itself (autoregulation) and vasodilate in response to decreased flow or increased metabolic demands. In the diseased human coronary arterial system, however, evidence suggests that inappropriate increase in vasomotor tone or even occlusive spasm may occur in the setting of an anginal attack or acute infarction. Therefore the use of vasodilators such as nitroglycerin sublingually or as a paste may improve coronary perfusion when hypovolemia or excessive diastolic hypotension are not present. Nitrates thus may improve myocardial ischemia by decreasing afterload via peripheral arterial vasodilation, by decreasing preload via peripheral venodilation, and by direct coronary artery dilation.

Decreasing myocardial oxygen demands

The four major factors that determine myocardial oxygen demand are (Fig. 14-2): heart rate; afterload—arterial systolic pressure or systemic vascular resistance (SVR) for the left heart, PA systolic pressure or pulmonary vascular resistance (PVR) for the right heart; preload—PAW pressure or PAEDP for the left heart, CVP or RA for the right heart; and ejection time or contractility.

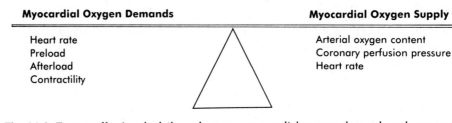

Fig. 14-2. Factors affecting the balance between myocardial oxygen demands and myocardial oxygen supply. Efforts are directed at decreasing those determinants that affect myocardial oxygen consumption (left side of balance) and increasing the arterial oxygen content and coronary perfusion pressure (CPP) to increase myocardial oxygen supply. Increasing heart rate, however, not only increases myocardial oxygen demands but also decreases the period for coronary perfusion.

Bedside monitoring of these factors provides a basis for maintaining optimal myocardial oxygen delivery and cardiac function while attempting to decrease myocardial oxygen demands in the critically ill patient.

The patient with minimal LV dysfunction can tolerate a wide range of *heart rates* without a serious effect on the cardiac output. Many patients with inferior infarction have a heart rate as low as 55 beats/min in the early phase of acute infarction. Normally this low rate achieves adequate compensation by an increase in stroke volume as a result of a prolonged diastolic filling period. In the patient with a compromised left ventricle, however, the heart rate is an important determinant of cardiac output. An increase in heart rate to maintain output and coronary perfusion must be balanced against its adverse effect on increasing myocardial oxygen demands and decreasing diastolic filling time.

Afterload is particularly relevant in assessing myocardial oxygen demands. Even in the patient with long-standing systemic hypertension, both diastolic and systolic pressure usually can be lowered to reduce $M\dot{V}o_2$ without seriously impeding adequate renal or coronary blood flow. A systolic pressure decrease of 30 to 40 mm Hg may have a dramatic effect on cardiac function directly (by allowing an increase in stroke volume) and indirectly (by decreasing myocardial oxygen demands) and, therefore, on cardiac ischemia. Increased right heart afterload (elevated PVR or pulmonary hypertension) is particularly relevant in patients with RV dysfunction, inasmuch as the thin-walled RV is much more sensitive to afterload elevations than is the thicker-walled LV. In addition, elevated RV (and PA) systolic pressures may compromise myocardial blood flow, which occurs during both systole and diastole through the right coronary artery.

Preload, or end-diastolic volume, is the third determinant that affects myocardial oxygen demands. Preload can be monitored with a PA catheter by use of either the PA diastolic pressure or the PAW pressure as a reflection of the LV diastolic filling pressure, and the CVP or RA pressure as the RV filling pressure. Again, changes in filling pressures must be related to their effect on cardiac output. If the LV is compromised, a left-side filling pressure between 16 and 22 mm Hg is thought to be optimal for maintaining stroke volume. An LV diastolic filling pressure above 22 mm Hg probably has deleterious effects because of increased pulmonary congestion and myocardial oxygen demands occurring with minimal further increase in stroke volume.

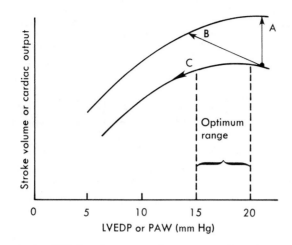

Fig. 14-3. Left ventricular (LV) function curves showing an index of LV performance such as stroke volume or cardiac output on the vertical axis and pulmonary artery wedge (PAW) pressure as a reflection of LV filling pressure on the horizontal axis. As the PAW (or LVEDP) pressure rises, myocardial fiber shortening increases (Frank-Starling law), resulting in increased cardiac output (CO). Increases in PAW pressure over 20 mm Hg usually produce little or no improvement in the CO, as reflected by flattening of the curve. *A,* Arrow reflects a shift to a higher ventricular function curve and stroke volume without a change in preload (this occurs with positive inotropic therapy). *B,* Arrow reflects a shift to a higher ventricular function curve and stroke volume at a lower preload level (this occurs with vasodilator therapy). *C,* Arrow reflects a shift to a lower preload and stroke volume while remaining on the same ventricular function curve (this occurs with diuretic therapy).

The fourth factor that affects myocardial oxygen demands is the *contractility* of the ventricle, that is, the degree of myocardial fiber shortening at any given preload and afterload. This factor is not directly monitored at the bedside because it requires simultaneous ventricular pressure and volume measurements. However, an evaluation of the contractile state of the ventricle can be obtained by calculating the work of the ventricle (stroke work) and using ventricular function curves. Fig. 14-3 illustrates various states of contractility as indicated by the amount of ventricular work performed at specific fiber lengths (preload).

Myocardial oxygen demands also can be markedly affected by pharmacologic interventions, such as vasodilators to decrease peripheral resistance, or by mechanical assistance to reduce afterload and improve LV function by diastolic counterpulsation.

Reduction of Infarct Size

Studies by Jennings and others have demonstrated the development of irreversible structural changes in cell mitochondria after 20 minutes of ischemia; however, it is known that the process of MI is a dynamic process that may progress over at least 24 hours. According to Cox and co-workers, the size of an ischemic zone may continue to increase for up to 18 hours. These data, plus the lack of a clear demarcation between infarcted and normal tissue, have promoted the concept of an ischemic or twilight zone of myocardium surrounding the central necrotic area of infarction. Presumably, the quantity of oxygen delivered to this area and the oxygen demands of an ischemic area (based on myocardial work requirements) determine the eventual outcome of the twilight area. With this phenomenon in mind, Maroko and Braunwald

Table 14-2. Methods of reducing myocardial ischemia

Desired effect	Method
↓ Myocardial oxygen demand	Treat tachycardia and/or dysrhythmia
	Treat hypertension
	Administer beta-adrenergic blockade
	Treat LV failure (decrease PAW pressure and LV size)
	Provide mechanical assist
↑ Myocardial oxygen delivery	Maintain normal Pao₂
	Maintain arterial diastolic pressure around 80 mm Hg
	Decrease PAW
	Maintain heart rate 50-60 beats/min
	Maintain normal hemoglobin
	Provide intraaortic balloon counterpulsation
	Provide thrombolytic therapy
	Perform coronary bypass surgery
	Perform acute angioplasty
↓ Cell injury	Use calcium antagonists
	Use hydrogen receptors
	Use oxygen free radicals

LV, Left ventricular; *PAW,* pulmonary artery wedge; *Pao₂,* arterial oxygen pressure.

systematically studied a number of interventions that might reduce myocardial injury and perhaps infarction. These studies have been limited by the lack of suitable methods for accurately determining the extent of infarction in patients. Serial enzyme curves, precordial ST mapping, and radioisotope techniques have been important but are not sufficiently quantitative for determining infarct size. Nevertheless, there is a great deal of physiologic experimental data indicating that pharmacologic and physiologic interventions probably can reduce infarct size.

Recent clinical studies have shown that early intravenous administration of beta blockers reduces ventricular dysrhythmias and may reduce infarction size after thrombolytic therapy. Table 14-2 lists factors or interventions that may decrease myocardial ischemia during AMI.

Acute Thrombolytic Therapy

Early studies documenting complete occlusion of the corresponding coronary artery in patients with AMI led to the concept of thrombolytic therapy, initially administered by the intracoronary route. Subsequently it has been shown in large clinical trials that intravenous administration of streptokinase, tissue-type plasminogen activator (t-PA) or anistreplase results in decreased mortality, particularly if it is provided in the first 4 to 6 hours after onset of symptoms. Other large clinical trials also have demonstrated reduced infarct size and improved LV function with early thrombolytic therapy. Early IV thrombolytic therapy results in lysis of the clot in 70% to 85% of patients, which manifests clinically by rapid resolution of chest pain and reduction of the ST elevation on ECG. LV function may recover more slowly from the ischemic insult. Thrombolytic therapy is contraindicated when decreased clotting ability might be dangerous to the patient. These new developments have revolutionized the management of the patient with AMI.

Most patients in whom coronary flow is reestablished by thrombolytic therapy demonstrate severe occlusive atherosclerotic lesions underlying the area of the thrombus. Thus these patients are at high risk for reocclusion and require continued anticoagulation therapy. Angioplasty at the time of acute thrombolytic therapy has been successful but carries some risk because of the anticoagulated state. Recent clinical studies have demonstrated that in patients who have received thrombolytic therapy it is better to wait 24 to 72 hours after thrombolytic therapy to perform the angioplasty procedure, which is indicated only if the patient continues to have chest pain or if chest pain recurs. The most serious complication of acute thrombolytic therapy is hemorrhage, including intracerebral and gastrointestinal bleeding. Fortunately, these events occur in only a small percentage of patients. Reocclusion may occur, necessitating repeat thrombolytic therapy or acute angioplasty.

Treatment of Associated Symptoms

The complexities of biomedical monitoring and the vigilance it requires may divert attention away from other symptoms associated with the MI. Pain and anxiety not only cause psychologic discomfort but can produce hemodynamic abnormalities that can jeopardize the patient's cardiovascular status.

Pain causes an increased sympathetic discharge, resulting in tachycardia and increased blood pressure. Because these factors increase myocardial oxygen requirements, immediate treatment is important. Severe pain also may precipitate a vasovagal reaction, resulting in marked sinus bradycardia and hypotension caused by excessive parasympathetic activity. In this case atropine, as well as a narcotic for pain relief, may be useful.

Similar hemodynamic responses occur with the situational anxiety of hospitalization; sedation is both effective and necessary in most patients.

COMPLICATIONS OF ACUTE MYOCARDIAL INFARCTION

Complications of AMI, which may occur at various stages, are associated with increased mortality. Treatment of complications is directed at returning cardiovascular function toward normal, either by pharmacologic or by physiologic means. In general, the patient with an AMI is considered to be at high risk for cardiac surgery, and aggressive medical treatment usually is used before surgical intervention. This section deals with the complications most commonly seen after an AMI.

Hypoxemia

Approximately 60% to 70% of patients suffering an MI develop transient LV dysfunction with elevation of the LVEDP. This elevation, in turn, increases pulmonary venous pressure, resulting in transudation of fluid from the pulmonary capillaries into the alveoli. The presence of fluid in the alveoli interferes with the transfer of oxygen at the alveolocapillary level and results in systemic hypoxemia that may not be evident clinically but is documented by arterial blood gas values. Because hypoxemia may contribute to cardiac dysrhythmias and further myocardial ischemia, oxygen is administered to return the Pao_2 to normal levels. Sufficient oxygen delivery usually can be achieved with a nasal cannula at low flow rates of 2 to 6 L/min. Repeated arterial blood gas measurements are necessary to document adequate oxygen administration. Abnormally high Pa_{O_2} levels may cause rises in systemic pressure and actually increase myocardial work.

Dysrhythmias

Treatment for dysrhythmic complications is discussed in the section on maintaining electrophysiologic stability (p. 345).

Thromboembolism

Pulmonary embolism, fostered by advanced age, inactivity, decreased cardiac output, and invasive cardiac catheters, continues to contribute to the mortality of patients in the coronary care unit. Anticoagulation should be used for the high-risk patient who has a history of thromboembolic disease, obesity, or congestive heart failure. Minidose heparin (5000 units administered subcutaneously every 12 hours) may be useful prophylactically in these situations, with few, if any, complications. Recurrent small pulmonary emboli should be suspected in the patient with repeated, unexplained episodes of tachypnea, tachycardia, dyspnea, cyanosis, or hypotension.

The rise in PA pressure with the occurrence of a pulmonary embolus causes a delay in the closure of the pulmonic valve, and there is fixed or wide splitting of the second sound. There may be an RV gallop. In severe cases there may be accompanying transient tricuspid insufficiency because of pulmonary hypertension. Recurrent small pulmonary emboli may precipitate pulmonary edema or recurring bouts of chest pain without roentgenographic evidence of an infarction. The occurrence of hemoptysis or a pleural friction rub, however, should be considered evidence of a pulmonary infarction. Hemodynamic monitoring can help establish the diagnosis of pulmonary embolus by demonstrating a high PA pressure in the presence of a normal or low PAW pressure.

Systemic emboli may occur from a thrombus on the endocardium in the area of infarction. Studies in which echocardiography was used have demonstrated mural thrombus in a high percentage of patients with anterior MI. Although the incidence of mural thrombi is high, the incidence of arterial emboli of clinical consequence is low, and it has not been established whether aggressive anticoagulation therapy in this patient group is useful in preventing morbidity and mortality. The use of echocardiography can identify the presence of an LV clot and assist in making a decision regarding anticoagulation. Anticoagulation and warfarin sodium (Coumadin) may be useful in reducing the risk of a systemic embolus, particularly in the patient with a protruding or mobile LV thrombus or with an anterior MI and congestive heart failure. Thrombolytic therapy may provide an additional approach to the patient with this complication.

Pericarditis

A pericardial friction rub can be heard in at least 10% to 20% of patients with an MI, particularly those with an anterior MI. The rub is usually transient, occurring on the second through the fifth day after the infarction. If the pain is severe, it may require analgesics or antiinflammatory drugs.

Ventricular Aneurysm

A ventricular aneurysm occurs in a later phase of an MI at any time from a few days to several weeks after the infarction. The diagnosis is difficult to establish by physical examination, although in midsystole and late systole there may be outward bulging when the precordium is palpated. It can be suspected in the patient with refractory heart failure, in the patient with an abnormally large cardiac silhouette or unusual shadow on a roentgenogram, and in the patient with paradoxic movement of the cardiac silhouette during fluoroscopic examination. A small group of patients have drug-resistant ventricular tachycardia associated with the aneurysm.

Surgical removal of the aneurysm is usually not performed during the first 6 to 12 weeks after AMI to allow time for cardiac function to stabilize. Earlier surgical intervention may be necessary, however, in the patient whose hemodynamic status is deteriorating.

Mitral Insufficiency

More than 50% of patients with an MI develop a transient systolic murmur at the apex, consistent with papillary muscle dysfunction. This complication usually occurs within the first few days after an AMI and is associated with a poorer prognosis. Varying degrees of mitral insufficiency may occur, depending on the extent of the infarction and ischemia of the papillary muscles and the LV loading conditions (both preload and afterload).

Hemodynamic features of mitral insufficiency classically include a dominant and elevated v wave in the PAW waveform. The timing of the v wave relative to the ECG T wave may reveal an earlier than normal appearance of the v wave as regurgitation occurs with initial myocardial fiber shortening. The presence of elevated PAW v waves

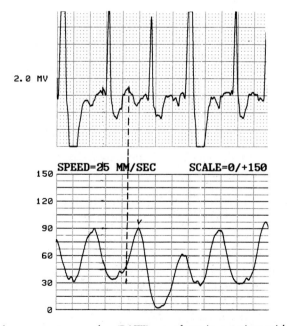

Fig. 14-4. This pulmonary artery wedge (PAW) waveform in a patient with atrial fibrillation (with aberrant beats) and mitral regurgitation remained in a permanent wedge position for 24 hours because it was mistakenly interpreted as a pulmonary artery (PA) waveform. This error is more likely to be made in the presence of atrial fibrillation with absent a waves on the PAW waveform and mitral regurgitation that produces early and elevated (90 mm Hg) v waves.

may be transient with ischemic episodes, or they may be persistent with LV failure or papillary muscle infarction or rupture (Fig. 14-4).

Vasodilator therapy during hemodynamic monitoring is an ideal treatment for these patients with a poorer prognosis because it not only decreases preload (LVEDP) but also decreases afterload. This reduction in afterload tends to promote forward cardiac output and minimize mitral regurgitation. An increase in forward flow decreases LV volume, which may improve function of the subvalvular apparatus of the mitral valve. When the condition is severe, counterpulsation may allow time before mitral valve replacement.

Occasionally an infarcted papillary muscle can rupture, resulting in flagrant mitral regurgitation. This complication is characterized clinically by the sudden onset of a loud holosystolic murmur and pulmonary edema that is resistant to drug treatment. Temporary management consists of afterload reduction with vasodilators and counterpulsation, but most patients require immediate mitral valve replacement after cardiac catheterization and coronary arteriography.

Patient Example

A 69-year-old woman was admitted to the emergency room complaining of several hours of severe chest pressure without associated nausea, vomiting, or shortness of breath. Past medical history included an anterior subendocardial MI 2 years previously. The patient was a smoker and was being treated for chronic hypertension. On admission her blood pressure (BP) was 120/70, heart rate was 64 beats/min, and respiratory rate was 18/min. Examination results were normal except for scant bilateral basilar rales and the presence of an S_4 heart sound.

The ECG obtained on the patient's admission showed no ST elevation but revealed ST depression in the anterolateral leads. The woman was admitted to the CCU where routine MI management was carried out, including administration of oxygen, heparin, nitroglycerin, and morphine. Serial enzyme values showed a creatine kinase (CK) of 430 with a CK-MB of 25%, along with a lactate dehydrogenase (LDH) of 291 approximately 36 hours after the patient's admission.

The patient's condition was stable for 2 days after admission when she suddenly complained of severe recurrent chest pressure, which was accompanied by marked dyspnea. BP was palpable at 80 mm Hg, heart rate was 106 beats/min, and respiratory rate was 28/min. She was cyanotic, cold, and clammy and slightly confused. Rales were present bilaterally to the apexes. A left parasternal thrill was felt, and a grade 5/6 systolic murmur was heard. The ECG revealed prominent ST depression in leads V_2 through V_4. On oxygen at 4 L/min, an arterial blood gas sample revealed Po_2 42 mm Hg, Pco_2 38 mm Hg, and pH 7.46. Dopamine infusion at 10 μg/kg/min was begun, a PA catheter was inserted, and the following hemodynamic data were obtained:

HR (beats/min)	108
BP systole/diastole (mm Hg)	86/58
PA systole/diastole (mm Hg)	82/50
PAW a/v/mean (mm Hg)	31/70/–
RA mean (mm Hg)	9
CO/CI (L/min; L/min/m²)	2.6/1.6
SVR (dynes/sec/cm^{-5})	1785
PVR (dynes/sec/cm^{-5})	615
Sao_2	0.81
Svo_2(PA)	0.47

Examination of the PAW pressure waveform reveals an extremely dominant and elevated *v* wave, resulting in a "ventricularized" appearance of the PAW (Fig. 14-5). The *v* wave is not only elevated; when correlated with the ECG, it can be seen to occur quite early, in timing with the T wave of the ECG. This early appearance almost obscures the *a* wave of the PAW waveform and indicates severe mitral regurgitation—in this case secondary to infarction of the papillary muscle. The elevated *v* wave also can be observed on the downslope of the PA waveform, giving an almost bifid appearance to PA systole (Fig. 14-6). The adverse effects of the very high pulmonary venous pressure are evident in the low arterial oxygen saturation. The cardiac output (CO) is severely depressed as blood regurgitates back into the left atrium rather than being ejected forward into the systemic circulation.

In an attempt to reduce afterload and promote forward flow, an infusion of dobutamine was begun while the patient was prepared for immediate insertion of an intraaortic balloon

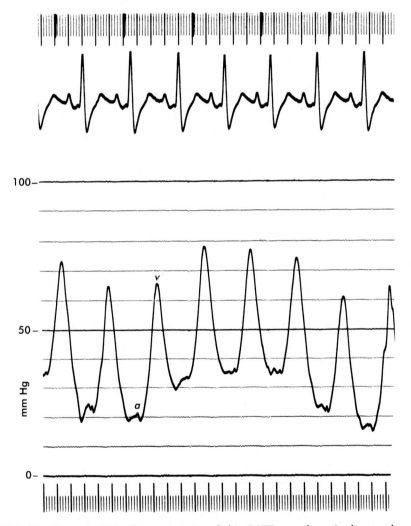

Fig. 14-5. The "ventricularized" appearance of this PAW waveform is due to the early, dominant, and elevated *v* wave of approximately 72 mm Hg produced by severe mitral regurgitation. The *a* wave of approximately 35 mm Hg is almost obscured in this PAW waveform.

From Daily EK, Schroeder JS: *Hemodynamic waveforms: Exercises in identification and analysis*, ed 2, St Louis, 1990, Mosby–Year Book.

pump (IABP) before cardiac catheterization and emergent surgery. The patient was discharged 13 days after mitral valve and coronary artery bypass graft surgery of the right and left anterior descending coronary arteries.

Right Ventricular Infarction

Identification of right ventricle infarction is important because the condition has a relatively good prognosis if managed properly. The cause is proximal occlusion of a dominant right coronary artery, resulting in extensive damage to the walls of both left and right ventricles and may include the intraventricular septum. This diagnosis

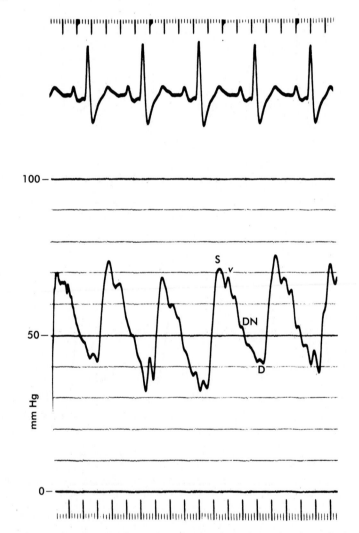

Fig. 14-6. The PA waveform in this patient displays a notch on the downslope that occurs shortly after peak systole and that corresponds in timing and value to the patient's PAW *v* wave (see Fig. 14-5). (*S*, Systole; *DN*, dicrotic notch; *D*, diastole.)

From Daily EK, Schroeder JS: *Hemodynamic waveforms: exercises in identification and analysis,* ed 2, St Louis, 1990, Mosby–Year Book.

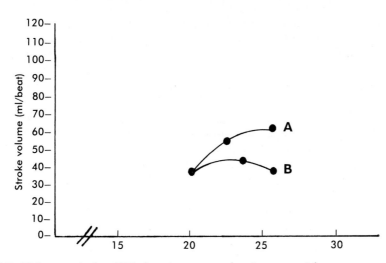

Fig. 14-7. Right ventricular (RV) function curves showing potential responses to volume loading in a patient with RV infarction and elevated right atrial (RA) pressure. *A* depicts an improvement in stroke volume (SV) after infusion, whereas *B* depicts no benefit from volume infusion. Ventricular function curves should be constructed to assess the individual patient's response to therapy.

is suspected when there is evidence of RV failure during an acute inferior infarction, and the condition can be diagnosed by the presence of ST-segment elevation in right side precordial leads V_2 through V_4. Clinical findings usually include distended neck veins in the absence of LV failure, with clear lungs and no S_3 gallop. Hypotension and varying degrees of heart block may be present. The marked venous distention can easily lure the physician into treatment with diuretics if RV infarction is not considered in the differential diagnosis. Diuresis decreases intravascular volume and ventricular filling and results in further hypotension and lowered cardiac output.

Hemodynamic monitoring is very useful in establishing the diagnosis of RV infarction by demonstrating a high CVP and RA pressure in the presence of a lower or normal PAW pressure.

Initial therapy is directed at volume loading to maintain adequate cardiac output. However, careful observation of the effects of volume loading on the stroke volume or cardiac output should be performed and individual ventricular function curves constructed (Fig. 14-7). RV volumetric measurements may be particularly helpful in the hemodynamic assessment of these patients (see Chapter 9). Close monitoring of the diastolic PA or PAW mean pressure is also necessary during fluid therapy in an effort to maintain adequate LV filling pressures without precipitating pulmonary edema. Inotropic support may be required to improve stroke volume and ejection fraction in some patients.

Patient Example

An 80-year-old man was transferred from the surgical ward with complaints of increasing chest tightness. He had undergone colonectomy for colon cancer 72 hours earlier. The ECG revealed ≥ 1 mm ST elevation in the inferior leads, as well as in leads V_{3R} and V_{4R}. The patient's neck veins were full, and jugular venous pressure was elevated. Lung fields were clear. A CVP line was present, which was exchanged for a right ventricular ejection fraction (RVEF) catheter positioned in the PA. The following hemodynamic and volumetric data were obtained:

Hemodynamic values

HR (beats/min)	72
BP systole/diastole (mm Hg)	102/72
PA systole/diastole (mm Hg)	21/12
PAW a/v/mean (mm Hg)	12/14/13
RA mean (mm Hg)	19
CO/CI (L/min; L/min/m^2)	2.7/1.7
SVR (dynes/sec/cm^{-5})	1840
PVR (dynes/sec/cm^{-5})	60
Sao_2	0.95
Svo_2(PA)	0.51

RV volumetric measurements

RVEF	0.28
RV stroke volume (ml/beat)	37
RV end-diastolic volume (ml)	132
RV end-systolic volume (ml)	95

The primary hemodynamic abnormalities consist of a severely depressed cardiac output and elevated RA pressure, with a normal PAW pressure or left heart filling pressure. The RA : PAW ratio is > 1, which is a common finding in RV infarction. Evaluation of the RA waveform reveals a dominant *a* wave, as well as a constrictive pattern of an exaggerated *y* descent (Fig. 14-8). It is difficult to appreciate the presence of Kussmaul's sign on such few beats in this tracing.

It would be tempting to administer a fluid challenge to this patient in an effort to increase left heart filling and, therefore, cardiac output. When the RV volumetric data are evaluated, however, it is clear that the patient's RV end-diastolic volume is already sufficient and that the primary deficit consists of reduced ejection as a result of RV infarction. Without improving RV contractility, increased volume would likely not increase CO but would further increase RV size, which, in turn, would decrease the LV size even more. On the basis of the volumetric data, the patient was begun on dobutamine infusion at 5 μg/kg/min. This therapy resulted in an improvement in the RVEF, with an increase in stroke volume and CO and a decrease in the RV end-systolic volume. Little change occurred in either the RA or PAW pressures. The patient recovered from his surgery, as well as his MI, and was discharged from the hospital 18 days later.

Cardiac Rupture

Acute cardiac rupture almost inevitably leads to sudden death and accounts for approximately 10% of hospital patient deaths caused by infarction. Physical examination and cardiovascular monitoring are not helpful in the prediction or care of this problem.

Ventricular Septal Defect (VSD)

Rupture of the ventricular septum is a well-known, albeit rare, complication that can occur with both anterior and inferior MIs, usually within 2 to 10 days after the infarction. This complication is characterized by the sudden onset of a palpable thrill and a loud pansystolic murmur at the lower left sternal border. Hemodynamic

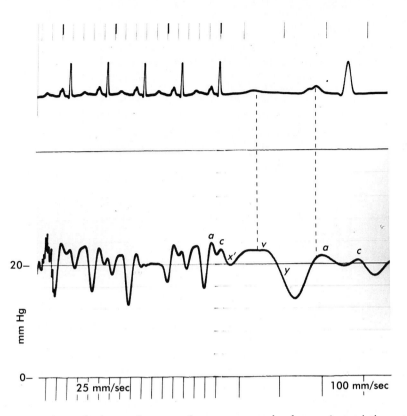

Fig. 14-8. This elevated RA waveform reveals an exaggerated *y* descent (constrictive pattern) commonly seen in patients with RV infarction. (Increasing the paper speed from 25 mm/sec to 100 mm/sec helps to identify the waveform components.) Kussmaul's sign, or minimal respiratory variation, is another common feature associated with the RA waveform in RV infarction.

From Daily EK, Schroeder JS: *Hemodynamic waveforms: exercises in identification and analysis,* ed 2, St Louis, 1990, Mosby–Year Book.

evidence of a VSD consists of a step-up (>10%) in the oxygen saturation of an RV or a PA blood sample compared with that of a superior vena cava (SVC) or RA blood sample. Depending on the size of the VSD, left-to-right shunting can cause pulmonary overcirculation, cardiac failure, and cardiogenic shock. Increased pulmonary blood flow via the shunt causes the thermodilution cardiac output measured in the PA to be high—despite obvious systemic hypoperfusion. In addition, the cardiac output curve demonstrates a secondary rise on the downslope of the curve as a result of early recirculation (Fig. 14-9). The increase in pulmonary blood flow also may cause the PA pressure to be somewhat elevated. An elevated and dominant *v* wave may be seen in the PAW waveform of patients with acute VSD. Its timing, however, is not early. Because early surgical intervention results in high patient mortality, treatment with afterload reduction (pharmacologically or mechanically) decreases the left-to-right shunting and allows time for initial healing of the infarcted area. In the patient who develops shock with drug-resistant heart failure, however, early surgical repair of the VSD may be required.

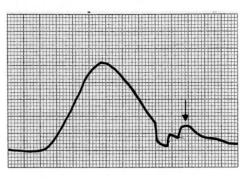

Fig. 14-9. Thermodilution cardiac output curve typical of a high flow rate. The arrow following the cessation of computer sampling marks the reappearance of thermal indicator as a result of a left-to-right shunt—ventricular septal defect (VSD).

Patient Example

A 55-year-old man with diabetes who had undergone above-the-knee amputation of the right leg 2 weeks previously was admitted complaining of substernal chest pain and shortness of breath for several hours. His blood pressure was 110/70, heart rate 80/min, and respiratory rate 20/min. Sparse bilateral basilar rales were present, and an S_3 was noted. No cardiac murmurs were present, and the neck veins were flat. The ECG showed ST elevation in the anterior leads. Because he was not a candidate for thrombolytic therapy, the patient was admitted to the CCU where an acute anterior MI was documented by ECG and subsequent enzyme elevations. Routine MI monitoring was carried out, in addition to administration of aspirin, oxygen, heparin, nitroglycerin, a beta blocker, and morphine.

On the second day of hospitalization the patient suddenly developed recurrent chest pain and severe dyspnea. His blood pressure fell to 70/50, and his heart rate rose to 112 beats/min. A loud systolic murmur and bilateral rales to the scapular angles were heard. A left parasternal thrill was palpated. Dopamine 5 μg/kg was started and a PA catheter inserted, revealing the following hemodynamic data:

HR (beats/min)	111
BP systole/diastole (mm Hg)	88/60
PA systole/diastole (mm Hg)	40/25
PAW a/v/mean (mm Hg)	19/30/24
RA mean (mm Hg)	12
CO/CI (L/min; L/min/m^2)	8.2/5.0
SVR (dynes/sec/cm^{-5})	566
PVR (dynes/sec/cm^{-5})	960
Sao_2	0.98
Svo_2 (PA)	0.84

The thermodilution CO determination is disproportionately high in view of the patient's hypotension. It does, however, represent an accurate determination of the flow of blood into the PA, which is increased as a result of the left-to-right shunt through a VSD. It does not reflect systemic flow, and it cannot be used to calculate the SVR (which is inaccurately low when the right-sided CO value is used in the calculation). A secondary rise on the downslope of the CO curve is another indication of recirculation secondary to the VSD (see Fig. 14-9).

Although the PAW v wave is dominant and elevated, a close assessment of its timing relative to the ECG T wave reveals normal timing of the v wave (Fig. 14-10).

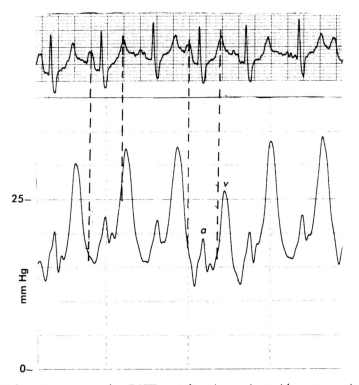

25—

mm Hg

0—

Fig. 14-10. Pulmonary artery wedge (PAW) waveform in a patient with acute ventricular septal defect (VSD) showing a dominant, elevated *v* wave (approximately 32 mm Hg) that occurs after the ECG T wave.

The oxygen saturation of the PA blood sample is abnormally elevated (84%). Obtaining a blood sample from the RA revealed an Sao$_2$ of 52%, providing the definitive diagnosis of VSD.

An IABP was rapidly inserted to reduce afterload and myocardial oxygen demands while improving forward flow. The patient was taken to the catheterization laboratory for coronary angiography, followed by surgical repair of the anteroapical septum and triple-vessel coronary artery bypass surgery. Although extensive pressor therapy was necessary postoperatively, the patient was discharged from the hospital 14 days after surgery.

Congestive Heart Failure

Congestive heart failure developing during AMI is closely related to the extent of LV infarction and generally implies a poorer prognosis. As indicated in Table 14-1, approximately 25% of patients with MI who do not receive thrombolytic therapy develop LV failure. Primary treatment for congestive heart failure is directed toward correction of systemic metabolic factors, such as acidosis, hypoxemia, and dysrhythmias, that may compromise cardiac output. Maintaining electrophysiologic stability and adequate coronary perfusion and reducing myocardial oxygen demands, as discussed previously, are also important.

The medical therapy for LV failure associated with an acute infarction is based on three hemodynamic objectives. The *first objective* is to maintain adequate arterial pressure to perfuse vital organs, particularly the heart. In some cases, this objective also may be accomplished by increasing cardiac output with afterload reduction. In more severe cases of LV failure, however, the patient may require peripheral vasoconstrictors to establish adequate perfusion pressure and to interrupt the vicious downward cycle that can occur once hypotension leads to myocardial ischemia and further LV dysfunction.

The *second objective* is to maintain adequate cardiac output and tissue perfusion to provide life-sustaining organ functions. This objective may be achieved by simply reducing afterload or, in more severe cases, by also administering positive inotropic agents to improve LV ejection.

Because elevation of LVEDP is the hallmark of LV failure, the *third objective* is to reduce the LVEDP (PAW pressure) if it is greater than 20 to 25 mm Hg. This treatment not only will relieve symptoms of dyspnea and improve arterial oxygenation but will decrease preload, reduce myocardial oxygen demands, and improve collateral coronary blood flow. Although diuretic therapy is the initial step toward achieving this objective, afterload reduction with use of a vasodilator has become increasingly recognized as valuable therapy and is discussed in Chapter 12.

Cardiogenic Shock

Cardiogenic shock develops in 8% to 10% of patients with an AMI. The primary physiologic hallmark of cardiogenic shock is inadequate perfusion and oxygen delivery to body tissues. Other accompanying changes include varying decreases in arterial pressure, cardiac output, and LV function. Clinical manifestations of cardiogenic shock may include hypotension, a cardiac index of less than 2.1 L/min/m^2, a urinary output of less than 20 ml/hr, tachycardia with a narrow pulse pressure, mental confusion, and decreased peripheral perfusion.

Pathology studies have demonstrated that patients who die during cardiogenic shock have infarcted at least 40% of their myocardium. Therefore cardiogenic shock reflects extensive myocardial necrosis, usually associated with severe triple-vessel occlusive coronary artery disease. As progressive cardiogenic shock and hypotension occur, coronary perfusion decreases, leading to development of other areas of focal necrosis and marked subendocardial ischemia throughout both ventricles. This progressive ischemia and infarction lead to further deterioration of ventricular function and death. A patient may have such extensive initial infarction because of occlusion of a major coronary artery (such as the proximal left anterior descending or left main coronary artery) that the patient dies rapidly of cardiogenic shock. Immediate reperfusion with early bypass surgery is now considered the treatment of choice for ongoing or impending cardiogenic shock, with resultant dramatic decreases in mortality of as much as 50%.

Physiologic concepts of medical treatment

Cardiogenic shock, as well as other forms of shock, causes multiple systemic abnormalities that must be identified and corrected to provide optimal chance for recovery. Most of these abnormalities are the result of decreased perfusion. Correction of factors that contribute to decreased tissue perfusion, as discussed earlier in this chapter, is important. Cardiac dysrhythmias, hypoxemia, and pain require prompt attention and treatment. In cardiogenic shock lactic acidosis occurs because of inadequate oxygen delivery to the tissues, which can lead to anaerobic metabolism and lactate production. Only partial compensation for acidosis can be achieved by hyperventilation and other buffer mechanisms. Use of sodium bicarbonate temporarily reverses the acidosis, promotes an optimal transmembrane potassium gradient, and improves the myocardial response to inotropic drugs.

Hemodynamic guidelines to therapy

Bedside hemodynamic monitoring during the administration of pharmacologic agents is essential to provide optimal hemodynamic function for the acutely infarcted heart when congestive heart failure or cardiogenic shock ensues. The initial goal of treatment is to provide adequate tissue perfusion to maintain the patient's life. Longer-term goals consist of providing temporary assistance to the left ventricle until spontaneous improvement in LV function occurs or stabilizing the critically ill patient in preparation for surgical therapy. Because of the marked variability in response to these potent therapeutic agents, it is mandatory that hemodynamic monitoring be initiated before using many of them.

Evaluation of the hemodynamic data also helps determine whether any factors other than pump failure are contributing to the cardiogenic shock. The development of a ruptured papillary muscle that causes severe mitral insufficiency or a ruptured ventricular septum can be diagnosed at the time of initiation of bedside hemodynamic monitoring, as discussed elsewhere in this chapter. Because both of these problems are amenable to aggressive afterload reduction and subsequent surgical therapy, the diagnosis can be critical.

Once hemodynamic monitoring has established baseline data, decisions about pharmacologic therapy are directed toward optimizing LV function at the lowest level of myocardial oxygen demands. These principles are similar to the treatment of LV failure, except that hypotension may be a more predominant part of this profile. Studies have shown that a coronary perfusion pressure below 80 mm Hg is directly related to coronary flow; collapse of the coronary artery occurs at approximately 40 mm Hg (Fig. 14-11). Thus every effort should be made to maintain coronary artery perfusion pressure at 60 to 80 mm Hg, even though this pressure may be at the expense of increasing myocardial oxygen demands. Table 12-4 lists a number of vasoactive agents and indicates the relationship between their effect on (1) improving contractility and (2) constricting peripheral arterioles to increase SVR. Because peripheral vasoconstriction and a high SVR usually are associated with cardiogenic shock, agents such as dopamine or dobutamine, that improve LV contractility and ejection fraction with minimal peripheral effects, are usually the initial drugs of choice. These agents shift the patient's ventricular function to a higher functional curve at the same level of preload (PAW) pressure (see Fig. 14-3). Thus adequate coronary perfusion pressure and cardiac output can be maintained temporarily while other potentially correctable problems are assessed.

The use of a positive inotropic agent should not substitute for providing optimal preload, or LV filling pressure, in the 15 to 22 mm Hg range. The patient in cardiogenic shock occasionally may have a low or normal PAW pressure in association with hypotension and a markedly reduced cardiac output. In this case treatment is aimed at increasing PAW pressure to the optimal range of 15 to 22 mm Hg by administration of IV fluid. As the diastolic volume and pressure in the left ventricle increase during IV fluid administration, stroke volume also will increase. If there is any possibility of a low PAW pressure, fluid loading as previously described should be initiated until the PAW pressure reaches approximately 25 mm Hg.

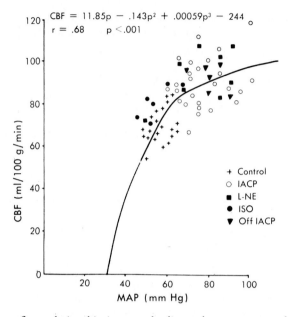

Fig. 14-11. Pressure-flow relationship in severely diseased coronary vascular bed. The graph demonstrates that L-norepinephrine *(L-NE)* and intraaortic counterpulsation *(IACP)* increase mean aortic pressure (MAP) and coronary blood flow (CBF). As MAP falls, CBF decreases; with a MAP of 30 or 40 mm Hg, the projected fall of CBF is to zero.

From Mueller H et al: *Trans NY Acad Sci,* Series II 34(4):309-333, 1972.

Once the patient's blood pressure is stabilized and optimal or high preload is determined, a trial of afterload reduction can be initiated to increase stroke volume at the same or lower preload. Use of nitroprusside in this situation requires extreme caution because of the accompanying hypotension in the patient with cardiogenic shock. As the afterload agent is increased, the stroke volume may improve sufficiently to prevent any fall in blood pressure and may allow a gradual tapering of the inotropic agent.

Mortality remains high in the patient with cardiogenic shock because of inadequate spontaneous improvement in the infarcted left ventricle to maintain sufficient cardiac output and blood pressure. Some of these patients are excellent candidates for intraaortic balloon pumping to further improve the relationship between LV work and output (see Chapter 11), especially if a definitive surgical procedure such as LV aneurysmectomy is planned.

REFERENCES

ACC/AHA Task Force report: Guidelines for the early management of patients with acute myocardial infarction, *J Am Coll Cardiol* 16:299, 1990.

Arven S, Boscha K: Prophylactic anticoagulation for left ventricular thrombi after acute myocardial infarction: a prospective randomized trial, *Am Heart J* 113:688-693, 1987.

Barden RM et al: Right ventricular infarction, *Cardiovasc Nurs* 19:7-10, 1983.

Bodai BI, Holcroft JW: Use of the pulmonary arterial catheter in the critically ill patient, *Heart Lung* 11:406-415, 1982.

Bolooki H et al: Clinical, surgical, and pathologic correlation in patients with acute myocardial infarction and pump failure, *Circulation* 44:1034-1042, 1971.

Chatterjee K: Pathogenesis of low output in right ventricular myocardial infarction, *Chest* 102:590S-595S, 1992.

Cox JL et al: The ischemic zone surrounding acute myocardial infarction: its morphology as detected by dehydrogenase staining, *Am Hrt J* 76:650, 1968.

Daily EK: Use of hemodynamics to differentiate pathophysiologic causes of cardiogenic shock, *Crit Care Nurs Clin North Am* 1:589-602, 1989.

Deepak V et al: A simplified concept of complete physiological monitoring of the critically ill patient, *Heart Lung* 10:75-82, 1981.

Forrester JS, Diamond GA, Swan HJC: Correlative classification of clinical and hemodynamic function after acute myocardial infarction, *Am J Cardiol* 39:137-145, 1977.

Forrester JS et al: Medical therapy of acute myocardial infarction by application of hemodynamic subsets. II. *N Engl J Med* 295:1404-1414, 1976.

Funk M: Diagnosis of right ventricular infarction with right precordial ECG leads, *Heart Lung* 15:562, 1986.

GISSI trial: long-term effects of intravenous thrombolysis in acute myocardial infarction—final report of the GISSI study, *Lancet* 2:871-874, 1987.

Goodman JS, Shah PK: How—and when—to suspect post-MI mechanical complications, *J Crit Illness* 5:681-692, 1990.

ISIS-2 (Second International Study of Infarct Survival Collaborative Group): Randomized trial of intravenous streptokinase, oral aspirin, both, or neither among 17,187 cases of suspected acute myocardial infarction:ISIS-2, *Lancet* 2:349, 1988.

Isner JM: Right ventricular myocardial infarction, *JAMA* 259:712-718, 1988.

Jennings RB: Early phase of myocardial ischemic injury and infarction, *Am J Cardiol* 24:753-765, 1969.

Kelly DT et al: Use of phentolamine in acute myocardial infarction associated with hypertension and left ventricular failure, *Circulation* 47:729-735, 1973.

Kennedy JW et al: Western Washington random-ized trial of intracoronary streptokinase in acute myocardial infarction, *N Engl J Med* 312:1477-1482, 1983.

Kent KM et al: Beneficial electrophysiologic effects of nitroglycerin during acute myocardial infarction, *Am J Cardiol* 33:513-516, 1974.

Lewis PS: Evaluation of the patient sustaining a right ventricular infarction and nursing implications, *Crit Care Nurse,* Jan-Feb: 50-54, 1983.

Loeb HS, Gunnar RM: Hemodynamic monitoring in a coronary care unit, *Heart Lung* 11:302-320, 1982.

Maroko PR, Braunwald E: Modification of myocardial infarction size after coronary occlusion, *Ann Intern Med* 79:720-723, 1973.

Mathewson HS: Pharmacologic regulation of hemodynamic variables, *J Cardiovasc Pulmonary Technology,* April-May: 33-49, 1982.

Mueller HS: Shock following acute myocardial infarction: assessment, pathophysiology, and therapy, *J Cardiovasc Pulmonary Technology,* June-July: 19-25, 1980.

Nishimura RA et al: Papillary muscle rupture complicating acute myocardial infarction: analysis of 17 patients, *Am J Cardiol* 51:373, 1983.

Parmley WW: The post-MI role of hemodynamic monitoring, *Hosp Pract* 17:169-175, 1982.

Pohjola-Sintonen and the MILLS study group: Ventricular septal and free wall rupture complicating acute myocardial infarction: experience in the Multicenter Investigation of Limitation of Infarct Size, *Am Heart J* 117:809-815, 1989.

Rahimtoola S: Treatment of pump failure in acute myocardial infarction, *JAMA* 245:2093-2096, 1981.

Shaver JA: Hemodynamic monitoring in the critically ill patient, *N Engl J Med* 308:277-279, 1983 (correspondence).

Smith B, Kennedy JW: Thrombolysis in the treatment of acute transmural myocardial infarction, *Ann Intern Med* 106:414, 1987.

Topol EJ: Tissue-type plasminogen activator in acute MI, *Cardiology,* April: 57-60, 1988.

Topol EJ et al: A randomized, multicenter trial of intravenous tissue plasminogen activator and emergency coronary angioplasty in acute myocardial infarction: results from the TIMI study group, *N Engl J Med* 317:518-588, 1987.

Verstraete M: New thrombolytic drugs in acute MI: theoretical and practical consideration, *Circulation* 76(suppl II):II-31, 1987.

Chapter 15

Hemodynamic Monitoring of the Patient on Mechanical Ventilation

Mechanical ventilatory support in critically ill patients is used (1) to improve oxygenation, (2) to treat alveolar hypoventilation, and (3) to reduce the work of breathing. Positive end-expiratory pressure (PEEP) frequently is applied to allow the reduction of the fractional concentration of oxygen in inspired gas (Fio_2) and to improve functional residual capacity and oxygen transport across the lungs. These interventions increase the intrathoracic pressure, improve lung compliance, and affect hemodynamic pressure measurements. However, their beneficial aspects can be offset by a deleterious reduction in cardiac output (CO) and oxygen delivery. The cardiovascular effects of positive-pressure mechanical ventilation relate directly to the increases in intrapleural pressure. This, in turn, is influenced by the particular mode of ventilation and the level of positive pressure applied. The addition of PEEP produces the most deleterious effects on the cardiovascular system and poses significant problems in the interpretation of hemodynamic waveforms and values. The degree of cardiovascular impairment associated with positive-pressure ventilation is determined by the patient's underlying cardiovascular and pulmonary function status. This discussion focuses on the changes in hemodynamics related to cardiovascular alterations as a result of positive-pressure ventilation.

PRELOAD

As intrathoracic pressure increases as a result of positive-pressure ventilation, the pressure gradient between the intrathoracic right atrium (RA) and the extrathoracic systemic veins is reduced, causing a decrease in venous return and, consequently, a decrease in right ventricular (RV) filling volume (preload). The deleterious effects of decreased venous return are more pronounced with large volume ventilations, the addition of PEEP, hypovolemia, or decreased venous tone.

At initiation of mechanical ventilation the left ventricular (LV) filling volume increases as the positive pressure forces blood out of the pulmonary capillaries through the pulmonary vasculature and into the left heart. This disparity soon subsides, however, as the reduced RV preload results in reduced stroke volume, which causes LV filling (preload) to be reduced similarly.

AFTERLOAD

As lung volume and alveolar pressure increase with mechanical ventilation, pulmonary vascular resistance (right heart afterload) becomes elevated. The degree of pulmonary vascular resistance increase is influenced by and proportional to the amount of airway pressure elevation. With significant elevations in RV afterload, the RV dilates and the intraventricular septum shifts, reducing LV filling capacity and volume and further decreasing LV compliance.

In contrast to the effects on right heart afterload, increased intrathoracic pressure of mechanical ventilation unloads the LV by increasing LV and aortic pressures relative to the extrathoracic aorta. This process may be highly beneficial to patients in congestive heart failure with high left heart afterload.

CARDIAC OUTPUT

The greatest disadvantage of positive-pressure mechanical ventilation, particularly PEEP, is its potential deleterious effect on CO. The decrease in venous return causes decreased RV filling and stroke volume and, hence, cardiac output. This is directly related to increases in intrapleural or airway pressure (Fig. 15-1) and is thought to be caused by the actual compressive effect of increased lung inflation that limits preload or cardiac filling. Increases in pulmonary vascular resistance (PVR), or right heart afterload, impose further limitation on ventricular output. Reductions in CO are most significant in the presence of underlying hypovolemia.

Inasmuch as tissue oxygenation depends not only on the oxygen saturation of blood but also on the blood flow, the effects of mechanical ventilation on CO must be carefully assessed:

$$\text{Oxygen delivery } (\dot{D}o_2) = CO \times \text{Arterial oxygen content } (Cao_2)$$

This formula for calculating oxygen transport shows the significance of both CO and the oxygen content in oxygen delivery or transport. If CO is severely depressed despite improvement in arterial oxygenation, it is possible to *reduce* rather than improve oxygen transport at the tissue level.

EXAMPLE: $\dot{D}o_2 = CO \times$ Arterial oxygen content (Hgb $\times$ Sao$_2$ $\times$ 1.34 ml/g Hgb $\times$ 10)

885 ml/min = 5 L $\times$ 177 (15 g $\times$ 0.88 $\times$ 1.34 ml/g Hgb $\times$ 10)

Normally, oxygen transport is greater than 1000 ml O$_2$/min. Despite the fact that

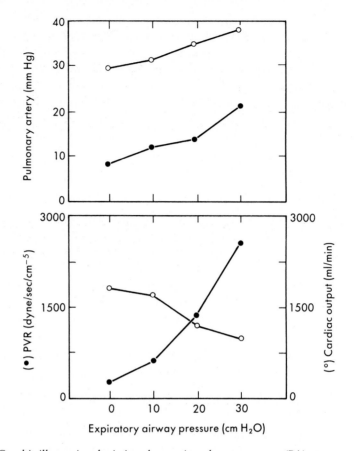

Fig. 15-1. Graphic illustration depicting changes in pulmonary artery (PA) pressure, pulmonary vascular resistance (PVR), and cardiac output (CO) with increased levels of positive end-expiratory pressure (PEEP). Note the marked increase in PVR with concomitant fall in CO as airway pressure is increased. The increase in PA pressure is much less dramatic because, although the PVR is high, the flow is low (P = F × R [pressure = flow × resistance]).

the CO in the preceding example is normal, oxygen delivery to the tissues is reduced because of hypoxemia (arterial saturation of 88%). Note the following example:

EXAMPLE: $\dot{D}o_2$ = CO × Arterial oxygen content

579 ml/min = 3 L × 193 (15 g × 0.96 × 1.34 ml/g Hgb × 10)

In this example a reduction in oxygen delivery to the tissues occurred secondary to reduced CO as a result of mechanical ventilation with PEEP despite improved oxygenation, as indicated by the increase in arterial saturation from 88% to 96%. This emphasizes the need to assess all the factors that contribute to oxygen supply rather than relying solely on the level of arterial oxygen saturation improvement.

HEMODYNAMIC PRESSURE MEASUREMENTS

Inasmuch as hemodynamic measurements obtained with mechanical ventilation are altered by the increases in intrapleural pressure, various attempts have been made to more accurately measure transmural hemodynamic pressures during mechanical ventilation. These have included (1) the use of esophageal balloons and pericardial cannulas to record intrathoracic pressures, which are then subtracted from the measured hemodynamic pressures to obtain effective or transmural pressures; (2) the discontinuance of mechanical ventilation of PEEP during the hemodynamic measurement; and (3) measurement of pressures at end-expiration as verified with transduced airway pressure. Discontinuing mechanical ventilation is generally not acceptable for several reasons. The sudden discontinuance of mechanical ventilation or PEEP can result in catastrophic hypoxemia and an immediate fall in functional residual capacity (FRC) and also can cause an initial sudden rise in venous return that does not reflect the true cardiovascular physiologic state of the patient. The use of esophageal balloons and intrapericardial cannulas to measure intrapleural pressures is fraught with a certain amount of vagaries and technical difficulties that preclude widespread clinical application.

Calculating transmural cardiac pressure by estimating intrapleural pressure and subtracting it from the measured cardiac pressure is performed in some centers. Mean intrapleural pressure relative to the atmosphere is normally about -5 cm H_2O or -3 mm Hg during spontaneous respirations. The true transmural intracardiac pressure, therefore, would be the measured pressure minus the intrapleural pressure.

EXAMPLE: Measured PAWm $-$ Pleural pressure $=$ Transmural PAWm pressure
$$8 \text{ mm Hg} - (-3 \text{ mm Hg}) = 11 \text{ mm Hg}$$

Because this difference is small and remains relatively constant during normal spontaneous breathing, it is not necessary to calculate the actual transmural hemodynamic pressures by subtracting -3 mm Hg from each pressure reading. However, as intrapleural pressures are increased to varying levels, the effect on measured hemodynamic pressures becomes more appreciable. The extent to which the intrapleural pressure is increased depends on the mode of ventilation. Control-mode ventilation (CMV) increases mean airway and intrapleural pressure 5 to 10 cm H_2O or 3 to 7 mm Hg. The factors that influence the extent to which CMV increases intrapleural pressure are (1) the inspiratory/expiratory ratio, (2) the peak airway pressure, (3) the airway resistance, and (4) the lung compliance.

PEEP therapy maintains the mean airway pressure positive during expiration. PEEP pressures < 10 cm H_2O have minimal effect on hemodynamic measurements, whereas levels > 10 cm H_2O directly affect hemodynamic measurements to varying degrees. Because the critical care patient whose condition warrants the use of mechanical ventilation with PEEP usually has lungs that are stiff and noncompliant, it is believed that only about 30% to 40% of the applied airway pressure is transmitted to the intrapleural space.

Positive-pressure mechanical ventilation not only causes varying changes in cardiovascular function; it also imposes significant artifact on measured hemodynamic waveforms and thus confounds interpretation of the patient's cardiovascular status. Reading all hemodynamic pressures at end-expiration helps reduce some of the respiratory artifact and provides some uniformity of measurement. End-expiration is associated with the least respiratory artifact and is least affected by intrapleural pressures, which should be close to baseline at this time. The respiratory effects of

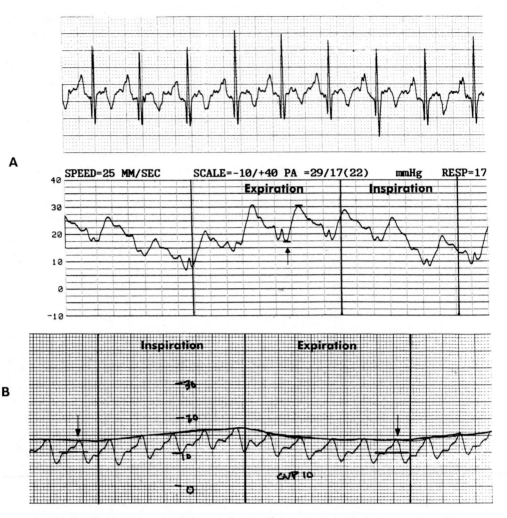

Fig. 15-2. A, Pulmonary artery *(PA)* waveform with spontaneous respiratory variation. Pressure read at end-expiration *(arrow* just before cyclic pressure decline) is 30/17 mm Hg. **B,** Central venous pressure (CVP) waveform with respiratory variation with mechanical ventilation. In this case, end-expiratory pressures are read just before the cyclic pressure rise *(arrow)* and average approximately 10 mm Hg.

positive-pressure ventilation on hemodynamic waveforms are directly opposite those associated with spontaneous respirations. Hemodynamic pressure waves rise during positive-pressure inspiration and fall during expiration. End-expiration can be identified on a graphic printout as the pressure wave just before the obvious cyclic rise (Fig. 15-2, *B*). This is facilitated in patients receiving a normal inspiratory to expiratory ratio inasmuch as the expiratory phase normally is about twice as long as the inspiratory phase. The timing is reversed in patients receiving inverse inspiratory to expiratory ratio. Measurement of airway pressures by means of a transducer connected to the ventilator tubing near the patient's endotracheal tube is a simple, accurate method of identifying the respiratory phases and the associated hemodynamic pressure changes (Fig. 15-3).

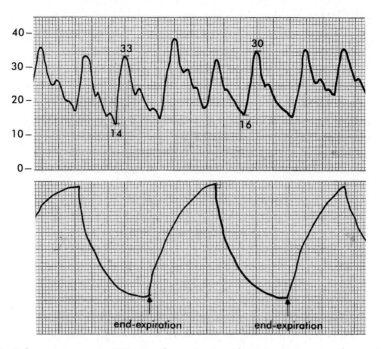

Fig. 15-3. Pulmonary artery (PA) waveform *(top)* with airway pressure *(bottom)* to aid in identification of end-expiration. PA pressure at end-expiration is approximately 31/15 mm Hg.

HEMODYNAMIC PRESSURES
Right Atrial Pressure

Measurement of the RA pressure relative to the atmosphere reveals an elevated RA pressure, reflecting the increase in intrathoracic pressure with mechanical ventilation. However, the actual RA transmural pressure (referenced to intrapleural pressure) usually is decreased as a result of the associated decrease in venous return. The degree to which venous return is impeded, and hence the amount the RA transmural pressure falls, depends primarily on the amount of increase in mean intrapleural or airway pressure. Because PEEP applies pressure at end-expiration (when airway pressure normally is at its lowest point), it greatly increases the mean airway and intrapleural pressure.

Pulmonary Artery Pressure

PA systolic, diastolic, and mean pressures are all usually elevated in patients receiving mechanical ventilation and PEEP. This is caused by the increase in PVR that occurs with increased airway pressure. Although venous return, stroke volume, and, therefore, CO fall as airway or intrapleural pressures are increased, the PVR increases dramatically (see Fig. 15-1). This increase in RV afterload, coupled with the decrease in RV preload or filling, may be responsible for the major physiologic effect of increased airway or intrapleural pressure.

Pulmonary Artery Wedge Pressure and/or Left Atrial Pressure

PAW and/or LA pressures measured in reference to the atmosphere usually are elevated in patients with increased intrapleural pressure. However, the transmural LA filling pressures (measured directly or indirectly through the PAW pressure) usually fall as airway or intrapleural pressures are increased, and venous return and, hence, diastolic filling volumes decrease.

The degree to which the measured PAW pressure actually reflects the left-sided filling pressure (LA) depends on the alveolar or airway pressure, the compliance of the lung, the location of the catheter tip, and the pulmonary venous or LA pressure. Transmission of increased airway pressure is markedly reduced when lungs become stiff and noncompliant as is the case in many patients receiving mechanical ventilation. However, it is possible for the measured PAW pressure to reflect alveolar pressure rather than pulmonary venous or LA pressure. This can occur if (1) the catheter tip is located in either zone 1 or 2 of the lung (Fig. 15-4), (2) alveolar pressures are increased to levels above the pulmonary intravascular pressure, or (3) the pulmonary venous or LA pressures are low. Fig. 15-4 illustrates the altered relationship between PAW and LA pressures and increased airway pressure with the catheter tip in two locations, above and below the LA. With the catheter tip in zone 1, the PAW reflects the increased alveolar pressure rather than the LA pressure. However, when the catheter tip is positioned in zone 3 (below the level of the LA), the PAW pressure reflects LA pressure until the airway pressure exceeds 10 cm H_2O.

Increasing airway pressure (with increased levels of PEEP) expands zones 1 and 2 and limits zone 3, which mandates positioning of the PA catheter tip in zone 3, below the level of the LA to achieve an accurate PAW pressure. This can be accomplished quite easily by positioning the patient in a lateral position, which automatically places the catheter tip below the LA level (*if* the patient is turned onto the side in which the catheter tip is located). Actual confirmation of catheter tip placement in zone 3 is achieved by a lateral chest x-ray radiograph, but this is not always possible. However, suspicion of the PAW as an inaccurate measurement of the patient's LA pressure should occur (1) when the PAW waveform lacks the normal components of an atrial waveform (*a* wave, *x* descent, *v* wave, *y* descent) and is associated with marked respiratory variations, (2) when the mean PAW pressure is higher than the pulmonary artery end-diastolic pressure (PAEDP), (3) when a blood sample obtained from the tip of an inflated catheter yields an oxygen saturation less than 95% (in patients who are not hypoxemic), and (4) when the change in PAW pressure during positive-pressure *inspiration* is much greater than the corresponding change in PA pressure. The last assessment was described recently by Teboul and colleagues as a useful and easily performed assessment to identify cases in which the PAW pressure measurements are not valid. This assessment is demonstrated in Fig. 15-5 in which the application of 20 cm H_2O PEEP is associated with an inspiratory pressure change of 15 mm Hg in the PAW pressure but only a 6 mm Hg change in the PA pressure. This pressure (p) change (Δ) ratio ($\Delta pPAW/\Delta pPA$), which should be close to 1, is more than twice normal and suggests that the PAW pressure likely is reflecting the alveolar pressure and not the LA pressure.

In patients with unilateral lung injury who receive PEEP therapy, the relationship between the PAW and LA pressures also may depend on location of the catheter in the injured or the normal lung. In these patients the PAW pressure may correlate more

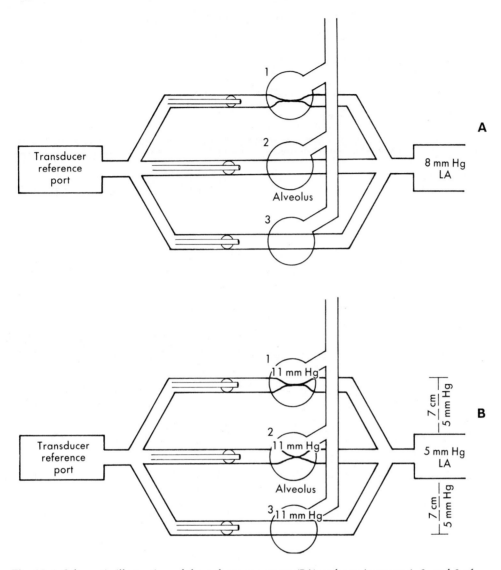

Fig. 15-4. Schematic illustration of the pulmonary artery (PA) catheter in zones *1, 2,* and *3* of pulmonary circulation. **A,** Represents pressures in these areas with normal, spontaneous respiration. **B,** Represents these pressures with positive end-expiratory pressure (PEEP) of 15 cm H_2O (11 mm Hg). Even in patients without increased airway pressure, the pulmonary artery wedge (PAW) pressure may not reflect left atrial *(LA)* pressure if the catheter tip is in zone 1, as in **A.** Increased airway pressure of 11 mm Hg results in collapse of the microvasculature when the catheter tip is located in either zone 1 or 2 and the LA pressure is low.

closely with the LA pressure when the catheter is in the injured lung rather than in the normal lung. This may occur because of alveolar flooding and localized atelectasis, which protects intraalveolar capillaries in the injured lung from the effects of increased airway pressure with PEEP. If the catheter tip is located in the normal lung, more accurate PAW pressure measurements also can be obtained by placing the patient in a lateral position with the "normal" lung down (Fig. 15-6). However, with

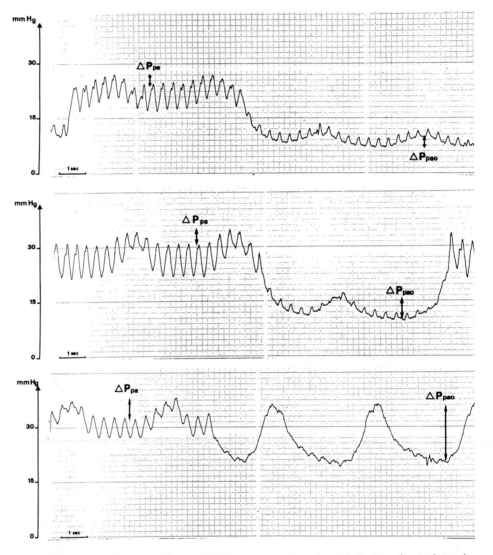

Fig. 15-5. Pulmonary artery (PA) and pulmonary artery wedge (PAW) waveforms from the same patient at the following different levels of end-expiratory pressure: zero end-expiratory pressure (ZEEP) *(top);* 15 cm H_2O *(middle);* and 20 cm H_2O *(bottom).* The amount of change (Δ) in PA pressure *(Ppa)* and PAW pressure *(Ppao)* from inspiration to expiration is denoted by the vertical lines and arrows. Note that at both ZEEP and 15 cm H_2O PEEP, the change in both pressures is similar (approximately 4 to 5 mm Hg). However, at 20 cm H_2O PEEP, the change in PAW pressure *(ΔPpa)* is about 15 mm Hg, whereas the change in PA pressure *(ΔPpa)* is only about 6 mm Hg. This greater change in PAW pressure suggests a shift to a non–zone III condition during balloon occlusion.

From Teboul JL et al: *J Crit Care* 7:22-29, 1992.

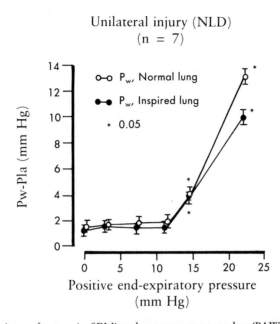

Unilateral injury (NLD)
(n = 7)

o—o Pw, Normal lung

●—● Pw, Inspired lung

* 0.05

Pw-Pla (mm Hg)

Positive end-expiratory pressure
(mm Hg)

Fig. 15-6. Comparison of mean (±SEM) pulmonary artery wedge (PAW) − left atrial (LA) pressure differences obtained from injured and normal lungs at various positive end-expiratory pressure (PEEP) levels in dogs with unilateral acid pneumonitis that were positioned with the normal lung in the dependent position *(NLD). Asterisk* denotes significant increase in PAW-LA difference that occurs at PEEP levels above 15 mm Hg.

From Hasan FM et al: *Am Rev Respir Dis* 131:246-250, 1985.

PEEP pressure above 15 mm Hg (11 cm H_2O), neither PAW nor LA pressure accurately reflects LV preload or filling.

Although the PAW pressure is used to reflect the LVEDP and volume, this relationship may be altered in patients with increased PVR. It has been noted that elevations in PVR cause the intraventricular septum to shift to the left, thereby decreasing LV end-diastolic volume. However, LVEDP may be elevated as a result of decreased compliance. This alteration in the pressure-volume relationship of the LV may overestimate the LV preload (as reflected by the PAW pressures) in the presence of reduced LV end-diastolic volume (Fig. 15-7).

Arterial Pressure

Peripheral arterial pressures remain unchanged or decrease with mechanical ventilation and PEEP. This is correlated with the decrease in CO that occurs with increasing levels of intrapleural pressure. The degree to which the arterial blood pressure falls depends on the amount of compensatory vasoconstriction that occurs with the decreased CO. The pulse pressure usually becomes narrower, reflecting decreased stroke volume. Exaggerated changes in the systolic arterial pressure in patients receiving mechanical ventilation are referred to as "reverse" or "positive pulsus paradoxus." A greater than 10 mm Hg change during mechanical exhalation, which is believed to indicate hypovolemia, can be eliminated with volume

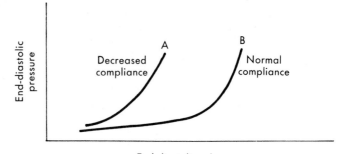

Fig. 15-7. Relationship between ventricular end-diastolic volume and end-diastolic pressure illustrating the effects of decreased compliance *(curve A)* on this relationship. With normal ventricular compliance *(curve B)*, relatively large increases in end-diastolic volume are accompanied up to a point by relatively small increases in end-diastolic pressure. In the noncompliant ventricle, small increases in end-diastolic volume are associated with marked increases in end-diastolic pressure.

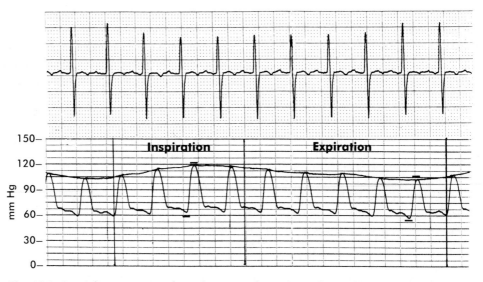

Fig. 15-8. Arterial pressure waveform during mechanical ventilation demonstrating reversed pulsus paradoxus with an inspiratory systolic pressure *rise* of approximately 17 mm Hg.

administration (Fig. 15-8). Figs. 15-9 and 15-10 depict various alterations in hemodynamic waveforms as a result of mechanical ventilation.

CLINICAL MANAGEMENT BASED ON HEMODYNAMIC PARAMETERS

The usefulness of monitoring hemodynamic parameters in patients receiving mechanical ventilation lies in its contribution to the formulation and titration of therapy. Because a favorable balance must be struck between the beneficial effects of improved oxygenation and the deleterious effects of decreased CO, hemodynamic

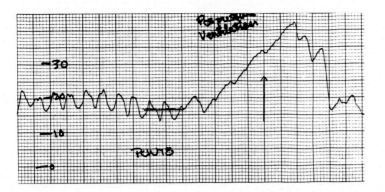

Fig. 15-9. Pulmonary artery wedge (PAW) waveform with mechanical ventilation demonstrating pressure artifact when the ventilator is triggered by a spontaneous breath (↑). Mean end-expiratory PAW pressure is approximately 16 mm Hg.

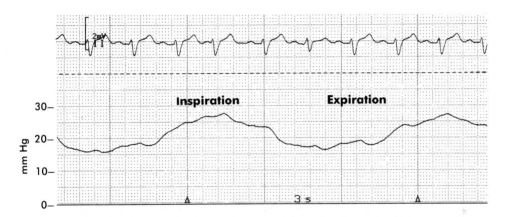

Fig. 15-10. This waveform obtained after balloon inflation in a patient receiving 20 cm H_2O positive end-expiratory pressure (PEEP) lacks the normal morphology of a pulmonary artery wedge (PAW) waveform and exhibits marked respiratory swings that suggest catheter tip location in zone 1 or 2. Such a pressure does not reflect the left atrial (LA) or left ventricular (LV) end-diastolic pressure.

monitoring provides essential information to attain this goal. The following are some of the more common therapeutic interventions employed to achieve this state of counterpoise.

Volume

With the drastic reductions in venous return and, hence, CO that can occur with increased intrathoracic pressure, it is frequently necessary to ameliorate these effects by administering volume to the patient even before mechanical ventilation is initiated. Hemodynamic signs of hypovolemia, decreased ventricular filling, and hypoperfusion include the following:

1. Low *transmural* CVP or RAm pressure
2. Low *transmural* PAWm or LAm pressure
3. Low CO

Clinical indications of decreased venous return and CO are flat neck veins, restlessness and confusion, reduced urine output, and cool, clammy skin. Volume infusion of a balanced electrolyte solution is often necessary to maintain transmural left heart filling pressures of 15 to 18 mm Hg in an attempt to optimize CO according to the Starling law. This can be graphically plotted as a ventricular function curve when CO measurements are made in addition to monitoring the transmural PAW pressure.

Positive Inotropic Agents

A low CO in patients receiving mechanical ventilation can result from causes other than decreased venous return and ventricular filling. Severe hypoxemia can result in myocardial ischemia even in the presence of normal coronary arteries. In addition, mechanical ventilation may compress the coronary arteries and reduce blood flow, resulting in LV dysfunction with reduced contractility and ejection fraction. Hemodynamic evidence of this condition includes the following:

1. Low CO
2. Normal or high *transmural* PAWm or LAm pressure

Because the transmural PAWm pressure is normal or high, further increases in volume would be inappropriate and could result in pulmonary congestion and increased interference with oxygenation. Positive inotropic agents such as dopamine, dobutamine, and epinephrine may be necessary to improve ventricular contractility and hence stroke volume.

Vasodilators

As CO falls with the use of mechanical ventilation, sympathetic stimulation causes reflex vasoconstriction to maintain an adequately perfusing blood pressure. This results in increased SVR, which serves to further reduce CO by increasing afterload. Vasodilating agents or afterload-reducing agents are often necessary to interrupt this vicious circle. Hemodynamic data that suggest the need for a vasodilator such as nitroprusside or nitroglycerin include the following:

1. Low CO
2. Normal or high *transmural* PAWm or LAm pressure
3. High SVR

Precise hemodynamic monitoring allows support of the cardiovascular system during mechanical ventilation with or without PEEP, thereby minimizing the negative effects on the cardiovascular system. Several interventions can be used to improve cardiac performance during mechanical ventilation. In addition, the use of intermittent mandatory ventilation (IMV) has been shown to be very useful in offsetting the negative effects of positive-pressure ventilation. IMV lowers the overall *mean* intrathoracic pressure by allowing normal negative inspiratory pressures to occur several times each minute. This improves venous return and CO even at higher levels of PEEP.

Patient Example

A 69-year-old man with cancer of the pancreas and signs and symptoms of pyloric obstruction underwent a vagotomy and gastrojejunostomy. His postoperative course was stormy, and the patient manifested acute postoperative respiratory distress that required Fio_2 greater than 60% and controlled ventilatory management. The patient's hemoglobin value was reduced to 12 g/dl (or 120 g/L). To maximize oxygen delivery and minimize dead space, PEEP therapy was added. A pulmonary artery and arterial catheter had been inserted before the operation in this high-risk surgical patient. The measured hemodynamic data in Table 15-1 were obtained just before and after the institution of mechanical ventilation with gradual increments of PEEP therapy.

The hemodynamic data in Table 15-1 reveal a CO value within normal range until a PEEP level of 15 cm H_2O is reached. The MAP, PAWm, and RAm pressures all fall within the normal range and are obtained at end-expiration while the patient is on mechanical ventilation. The *transmural* RAm and PAWm pressures were calculated after estimating the patient's intrapleural pressure with use of the following formula:

$$\text{Intrapleural pressure} = \text{Normal pleural pressure} + \text{CMV pressure} + 1/3\ \text{PEEP}$$

Table 15-2 reveals the estimated intrapleural pressure for each level of PEEP and the estimated transmural RA and PAW pressures when the intrapleural pressure is subtracted.

Table 15-1. Hemodynamic profile with *measured* hemodynamic pressures

Hemodynamic data	Positive end-expiratory pressure (PEEP levels)			
	0 cm H_2O	5 cm H_2O	10 cm H_2O	15 cm H_2O
Arterial saturation (%)	78	81	98	98
Arterial O_2 content (vol%)	12.5	13.0	15.8	15.8
CO (L/min)	4.8	4.9	4.3	3.7
MAP (mm Hg)	78	77	74	71
RAm (mm Hg)	3	5	6	5
PAWm (mm Hg)	11	10	12	13
Svo_2	51	52	59	50

CO, Cardiac output; *MAP,* mean arterial pressure; *RAm,* right atrial mean; *PAWm,* pulmonary artery wedge mean; Svo_2, venous oxygen saturation.

Table 15-2. Hemodynamic profile with *estimated* transmural hemodynamic pressures

Hemodynamic data	Positive end-expiratory pressure (PEEP levels)			
	0 cm H_2O	5 cm H_2O	10 cm H_2O	15 cm H_2O
Arterial saturation (%)	78	81	98	98
Svo_2 (%)	51	52	59	50
Arterial O_2 content (vol%)	12.5	13.0	15.8	15.8
CO (L/min)	4.8	4.9	4.3	3.7
MAP (mm Hg)	78	77	74	71
RAm measured and (transmural) (mm Hg)	3(6)	5(2)	6(2)	5(1)
PAWm measured and (transmural) (mm Hg)	11(14)	10(7)	12(8)	13(8)
Estimated intrapleural pressure (mm Hg)	−3	+3	+4	+5
Oxygen delivery (ml/min)	602	638	678	583

Svo_2, venous oxygen saturation; *CO,* cardiac output; *MAP,* mean arterial pressure; *RAm,* right atrial mean; *PAWm,* pulmonary artery wedge mean.

It also reveals the oxygen transport at each level of PEEP obtained from the following formula:

$$\text{Oxygen transport} = \text{CO} \times \text{Arterial oxygen content (Hgb} \times \text{Oxygen saturation} \times 1.34) \times 10$$

The data from Table 15-2 reveal an increase in arterial oxygenation from 78% to 81% at 5 cm H_2O PEEP. Inasmuch as the CO remained approximately the same, this change resulted in a desirable increase in oxygen delivery (from 602 to 638 ml/min), although it is still at a subnormal level particularly in this postoperative state. A look at the transmural RA and PAW mean pressures shows a decline in both filling pressures at 5 cm H_2O PEEP.

When PEEP is increased to 10 cm H_2O, there is a substantial increase in arterial oxygenation to 98%. Although the CO is reduced to 4.3 L/min, the proportionately larger increase in oxygen saturation results in improved oxygen transport to 678 ml/min. The transmural RA and PAW mean pressures remain low.

At 15 cm H_2O PEEP, the arterial oxygen saturation remains the same, but the CO is further reduced. The net result of this is a reduction in oxygen delivery despite improved arterial oxygenation. The transmural RA and PAW mean pressures remain low, reflecting reduced ventricular filling.

Thus in this patient it appears that a PEEP level of 10 cm H_2O is optimal in striking the balance between improved oxygenation and adequate cardiovascular function.

Subsequently, this patient's PEEP level was dropped to 10 cm H_2O and two units of whole blood were given to increase the patient's hemoglobin value and filling pressures and thus improve tissue oxygenation. This resulted in a hemoglobin level of 14 g/dl and the hemodynamic data found in Table 15-3.

The administration of blood resulted in several improvements. First, it increased the transmural filling pressures (RA and PAW), which resulted in improved CO according to the Starling law. Second, in increasing the hemoglobin to 14 g/dl, it increased oxygen transport to a normal level. Further increases in oxygen delivery to the tissues might be obtained by additional increases in CO, hemoglobin, or oxygen saturation of blood.

Table 15-3. Hemodynamic profile with measured and estimated transmural hemodynamic pressures following transfusion

Hemodynamic data	10 cm H_2O PEEP
Arterial saturation (%)	99
Arterial O_2 content (vol%)	18.6
CO (L/min)	5.1
Svo_2 (%)	72
MAP (mm Hg)	80
RAm, measured (transmural) (mm Hg)	9(5)
PAWm, measured (transmural) (mm Hg)	20(16)
Estimated intrapleural pressure (mm Hg)	+4
Oxygen delivery (ml/min)	947

PEEP, Positive end-expiratory pressure; CO, cardiac output; Svo_2, venous oxygen saturation; MAP, mean arterial pressure; RAm, right atrial mean; PAWm, pulmonary artery wedge mean.

This case illustrates the benefits of careful measurement and interpretation of hemodynamic parameters in a patient receiving mechanical ventilation with PEEP and its use in guiding and titrating therapy. It allows the selection of the appropriate intervention that will permit the best improvement in cardiovascular function and oxygenation.

REFERENCES

Agostoni E: Mechanics of the pleural space, *Physiol Rev* 52:57-128, 1972.

Bemis EC et al: Influence of right ventricular filling pressure on left ventricular pressure and dimension, *Circ Res* 34:498-504, 1974.

Benumof JL et al: Where pulmonary arterial catheters go: intrathoracic distribution, *Anesthesiology* 46:336-338, 1977.

Bradley TG et al: Cardiac output response to continuous positive airway pressure in congestive heart failure, *Am Rev Respir Dis* 145:377-382, 1992.

Cengiz M, Crapo RO, Gardner RM: The effect of ventilation on the accuracy of pulmonary artery and wedge pressure measurements, *Crit Care Med* 11:502-507, 1983.

DeGent GE, Greenbaum DM: Mechanical ventilatory support in circulatory shock, *Crit Care Clin* 9:377-393, 1993.

Ditchey RV, Costello D, Shebetai R: Effects of pressure and lung volume on left ventricular transmural pressure-volume relationships in humans, *Am Heart J* 106:46-51, 1983.

Gallagher TJ, Civetta JM, Kirby RR: Terminology update: optimal PEEP, *Crit Care Med* 6:323-326, 1978.

Guyton AC: *Textbook of medical physiology,* Philadelphia, 1981, WB Saunders Co.

Hasan FM et al: Influence of lung injury on pulmonary wedge-left atrial pressure correlation during positive end-expiratory pressure ventilation, *Am Rev Respir Dis* 131:246-250, 1985.

Hudson LD: Ventilatory management of patients with adult respiratory distress syndrome, *Semin Respir Med* 2(3):128-139, 1981.

Jardin F, Bourdarias JP: Influence of abnormal breathing conditions on right ventricular function, *Intensive Care Med* 17:129-135, 1991.

Klose R, Oswald PM: Effects of PEEP on pulmonary mechanics and oxygen transport in the late stages of acute pulmonary failure, *Intensive Care Med* 7:165-170, 1981.

Lozman J et al: Correlation of pulmonary wedge and left atrial pressures: a study in the patient receiving positive end-expiratory pressure ventilation, *Arch Surg* 109:270-277, 1974.

Mathru M et al: Hemodynamic response to changes in ventilatory patterns in patients with normal and poor left ventricular reserve, *Crit Care Med* 10:423-426, 1982.

Nelson LD, Houtchens BA, Westenskow DR: Oxygen consumption and optimal PEEP in acute respiratory failure, *Crit Care Med* 10:857-862, 1982.

Nelson LD, Snyder JV: Technical problems in data acquisition. In Snyder JV, Pinsky MR, editors: *Oxygen transport in the critically ill,* Chicago, 1987, Mosby–Year Book.

Patel HK, Yang KL: Transmission of PEEP to pleural pressure during mechanical ventilation, *Chest* 102:93S, 1992.

Philip C: Think transmural, *Crit Care Nurse* 2(2):36-43, 1982.

Pinsky MR: The hemodynamic effects of artificial ventilation. In Snyder JV, Pinsky MR, editors: *Oxygen transport in the critically ill,* Chicago, 1987, Mosby–Year Book.

Teboul JL et al: A comparison of pulmonary occlusion pressure and left ventricular end-diastolic pressure during mechanical ventilation with PEEP in patients with severe ARDS, *Anesthesiology* 70:261-266, 1989.

Teboul JL et al: A bedside index assessing the reliability of pulmonary artery occlusion pressure measurements during mechanical ventilation with positive end-expiratory pressure, *J Crit Care* 7:22-29, 1992.

Chapter 16

Hemodynamic Monitoring of the Postoperative Cardiac Surgery Patient

Pat O. Daily

The outcome for a patient undergoing cardiac surgery is determined by many factors. Three essential considerations are the patient's preoperative left ventricular function, the performance of the operation in an expedient, technically excellent manner, and the provision of optimum conditions for postoperative recovery. Preoperative left ventricular dysfunction predisposes the patient to the likelihood of low postoperative cardiac output and left ventricular failure. This problem should be anticipated, and the patient should be monitored vigilantly. Although a technically excellent operation may minimize postoperative problems, inadequate postoperative care may nullify that advantage and serve to increase morbidity and mortality.

The goals of optimum postoperative care are (1) to recognize, monitor, and assess all essential parameters, (2) to anticipate potential hemodynamic or pulmonary instability for a given condition or situation, (3) to detect deviations from acceptable ranges, and (4) to intervene appropriately to reestablish optimum function.

Postoperative monitoring is the basis for appropriate postoperative management. Effective monitoring requires not only specific monitoring techniques but also the knowledge of particular deviations that may occur. The techniques of hemodynamic monitoring that are employed after cardiac surgery are discussed in Chapters 5, 6, 7, 8, and 10. This chapter emphasizes specific problems detected during monitoring of the patient after cardiac surgery.

Maintenance of a balance between myocardial oxygen supply and demand is imperative in the postoperative setting during which the myocardium is particularly vulnerable to ischemia. Fig. 16-1 schematically illustrates the determinants of myocardial oxygen consumption ($M\dot{V}O_2$), namely preload, afterload, and contractility, as well as those of myocardial oxygen supply ($M\dot{D}O_2$). Thus, it is apparent that hemodynamic monitoring of the determinants of both myocardial oxygen supply and demand is vital to assessment and management of the patient's condition after cardiac surgery.

A major objective after cardiac surgery is the restoration of hemodynamic and ventilatory independence from supportive assistance while ensuring adequate tissue perfusion and gas exchange. Thus maintenance and monitoring of both cardiovascular and pulmonary parameters are equally essential. Incorporation of data from clinical assessment, as well as hemodynamic monitoring, pulmonary function, and clinical laboratory studies, provides the most accurate postoperative management.

Many immediate outcomes or postoperative problems can be anticipated on the basis of the patient's preoperative status. A patient with a low cardiac index, elevated left-sided pressures, and/or an ejection fraction of less than 50% preoperatively is more likely to have problems with left ventricular dysfunction after surgery. There should be few surprises in the postoperative period if the clinician knows the patient's preoperative cardiac status.

A patient with single-vessel coronary artery disease and no previous infarction or episodes of cardiac failure most likely will experience no significant postoperative complications. However, the patient with multiple coronary artery lesions, previous infarction, and decreased ejection fraction tends to have a slower recovery and may need pharmacologic support of cardiac output.

The patient with valvular heart disease and a hypertrophied ventricle, as might be seen with preoperative aortic stenosis, is prone to hyperdynamic states postoperatively in which the generation of excessive cardiac output and hypertension might cause problems. Such a state markedly increases the demand for oxygen. Inotropic support is certainly not indicated for the patient whose ventricle is hypertrophied and generating cardiac outputs of more than 8 L/min. Instead, afterload reduction is appropriate to decrease systemic vascular resistance (SVR) and thereby reduce hypertension, left ventricular work requirements, and myocardial oxygen consumption. Care must be taken to monitor the *pulse pressure* of the patient who is receiving vasodilator therapy rather than to rely entirely on the mean arterial pressure (MAP). A blood pressure of 175/45 mm Hg produces a MAP of 88 mm Hg that at first glance seems acceptable. However, this represents a pulse pressure of 130 mm Hg and an increased work requirement to support the high systolic pressure. At the same time, diastolic perfusion pressure is quite low and may be inadequate for coronary perfusion to meet energy requirements of a hypertrophied ventricle. In contradistinction, a blood pressure of 135/68 mm Hg represents a pulse pressure of 67 mm Hg and an MAP of 90 mm Hg. Although the mean pressure is essentially the same as in the previous example, the systolic work requirement is appreciably lower and diastolic perfusion pressure is enhanced. This manipulation of blood pressure can be achieved with appropriate use of vasodilator therapy and careful monitoring of arterial blood pressure.

Volume requirements for this patient also must be considered in view of the hypertrophic state. A hypertrophied ventricle is stiff and less compliant. Large, sudden increases in volume may cause marked elevation of pulmonary venous pressure that

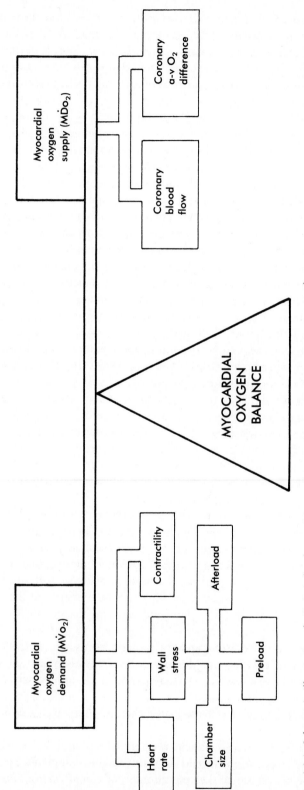
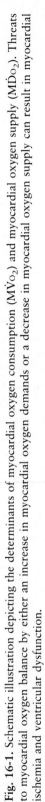

Fig. 16-1. Schematic illustration depicting the determinants of myocardial oxygen consumption ($M\dot{V}o_2$) and myocardial oxygen supply ($M\dot{D}o_2$). Threats to myocardial oxygen balance by either an increase in myocardial oxygen demands or a decrease in myocardial oxygen supply can result in myocardial ischemia and ventricular dysfunction.

may result in pulmonary edema. In the noncompliant ventricle, small changes in left ventricular volume result in larger changes in left ventricular end-diastolic pressure (LVEDP) and left atrial (LA) or pulmonary artery wedge (PAW) pressure. These measured values may overestimate left ventricular diastolic volume in a patient with a hypertrophied ventricle. Protecting the left ventricle from excessive oxygen demands is the key feature in the postoperative care of the patient with pure ventricular hypertrophy.

Diseases of valvular insufficiency with chronic volume overload result in dilation of the ventricular chamber. Although concomitant ventricular hypertrophy also may occur, the dilation completely alters the hemodynamic profile. This patient is more prone to postoperative low cardiac output states and hypotension. Even after surgical correction of the valve, the patient may require increased left ventricular volumes. Preload monitoring by means of LA or PAW pressure or pulmonary artery end-diastolic pressure (PAEDP) is useful in this situation to assess volume requirements and responses in cardiac output and SVR.

In some patients with pulmonary disease—arterial or parenchymal—the PAW or PAEDP may not accurately reflect LA pressure. Consequently, an LA line may be placed intraoperatively to allow postoperative monitoring of the LA pressure. In contrast to the patient with hypertrophy, the patient with ventricular dilation demonstrates smaller increases in LA and PAW pressures with larger increases in volume. These pressures therefore may underestimate left ventricular diastolic volume. The optimum filling pressure for this patient should be determined by monitoring LA or PAW pressure response to volume therapy and measuring cardiac output to determine which filling pressure range produces optimum cardiac output according to the ventricular function curve. Actual plotting of the individual patient's ventricular function curve is very helpful in assessing optimum preload levels.

In low cardiac output states, particular attention must be given to SVR. Because MAP is a function of both cardiac output and SVR, MAP alone may not reflect the adequacy of cardiac output. If cardiac output begins to fall, SVR most likely will increase to maintain blood pressure. Monitoring MAP alone may not illustrate early hemodynamic changes in the patient. The key features in the care of this patient are to determine and maintain adequate filling pressure and to assess the need for pharmacologic support of cardiac output with positive inotropic and/or afterload-reduction therapy.

EFFECTS OF ANESTHESIA AND SURGERY

Proper interpretation of postoperative monitoring data also requires knowledge of the effects of cardiac surgery and anesthesia on the cardiovascular and pulmonary systems. Myocardial depression occurs during the intraoperative phase and may extend into the postoperative period. Although there are multiple causes of myocardial depression, periods of intraoperative myocardial ischemia are most common.

Induction of anesthesia can be a particularly vulnerable time for the patient with cardiac disease. The physiologic stress of intubation can potentially cause a rapid release of catecholamines, with resultant hypertension and tachycardia. Such an episode might precipitate significant ischemia and even infarction in the patient with coronary artery disease. This alone is a major reason for maintaining patients on a regimen of prescribed beta-blocking or calcium blocking agents until the time of surgery. This same catecholamine response can result in serious falls in cardiac output in patients with minimal cardiac reserve. Another contributing factor in such a patient is relative hypovolemia caused by chronic diuretic therapy and fluid restriction preoperatively. Resulting hypotension can again produce serious myocardial ischemia. To avoid such complications the anesthesiologist will take care to ensure that patients receive adequate hydration and sedation before induction of anesthesia.

The optimum time for placement of monitoring lines is before induction of anesthesia. If the high-risk patient can be identified, it is desirable to have baseline hemodynamic parameters available, so that problems can be detected early and treated before the development of significant hypotension or hypertension that might result in ischemia. Monitoring is initiated with the placement of ECG leads, a central venous sheath, an arterial pressure catheter, and in some patients a pulmonary artery (PA) catheter. In some instances a direct LA pressure catheter may be inserted during surgery in lieu of, or in addition to, the PA catheter. The use of this catheter requires extreme care to prevent air or clot embolization in the arterial system. To avoid this potentially lethal complication, the LA catheter is always aspirated before it is flushed or connected to the infusion line. It also should be clearly marked so that it is never used for withdrawal of blood samples or administration of any fluid or medication. Insertion of a urinary catheter before surgery is desirable because it allows continuous intraoperative and postoperative monitoring of urinary output. This continuous monitoring permits indirect assessment of cardiac output and renal function and precludes bladder distention.

Many anesthetic agents result in cardiac depression; however, with appropriate selection of the type of anesthetic agent and method of administration, this effect can be minimized. One approach is to administer large IV doses of fentanyl or newer synthetic narcotics with diazepam or midazolam. This method minimizes cardiac depression but causes respiratory depression, which may last several hours postoperatively, necessitating support with a ventilator and careful monitoring of oxygenation.

Another major cause of myocardial depression is the myocardial ischemia that is produced by cross-clamping of the ascending aorta to allow valve replacement or other intracardiac repairs. Aortic cross-clamping excludes perfusion to the coronary arteries, resulting in myocardial ischemia and ventricular dysfunction. Significant protection is afforded by myocardial hypothermia, coronary perfusion, and cardioplegia, but this protection is not complete. When the aorta is not cross-clamped, long periods of induced ventricular fibrillation during surgery may result in subendocardial ischemia and ventricular dysfunction. In addition to depressing myocardial function and contractility, ischemia may aggravate or cause dysrhythmias.

Whole-body hypothermia (30° to 32° C) is used during cardiopulmonary bypass to reduce body metabolism and oxygen demand. Although the patient is rewarmed to 37° C before cardiopulmonary bypass is discontinued, this reduction in temperature causes vasoconstriction and increased SVR, which may extend into the postoperative period. More recently, cardiopulmonary bypass is conducted at normothermia with continuous retrograde warm cardioplegia. The efficacy of this method has not been clearly established. As rewarming occurs, vasoconstriction decreases and the vascular space increases, resulting in relative hypovolemia and hypotension. Because this hypotension is caused by hypovolemia, it can be recognized hemodynamically by a low central venous pressure (CVP) or PAW pressure and appropriately managed by blood or fluid replacement.

If cardiopulmonary bypass is prolonged, widespread systemic effects may occur. Microemboli, consisting of blood-cellular elements, fat aggregates, and protein breakdown products, may form in the pump and embolize to the lungs, heart, brain, and kidneys. Embolization and occlusion of the capillary beds of these organs result in decreased perfusion, which may lead to focal necrosis. The production of anaphylatoxins C3a and C5a may be significant. With modern cardiopulmonary bypass techniques and improved oxygenators and filters, however, this problem has been minimized. Prolonged cardiopulmonary bypass, with extended periods of low perfusion pressure, increases the risk of tissue ischemia and the incidence of coagulation abnormalities. Other sources of myocardial ischemia during surgery include inadequate analgesia, which causes catecholamine release, prolonged hypotension, prolonged hypertension, which causes dysrhythmias, and hypoxemia.

At the conclusion of cardiopulmonary bypass, two mediastinal tubes are inserted to prevent accumulation of blood and to monitor blood loss. One tube is positioned anterior to the heart in the midline, and another right-angle chest tube is positioned from the superior aspect of the diaphragm to the posterior pericardium. If the right or left pleural space was opened during the surgical procedure, a chest tube also is inserted at this time.

The orotracheal or nasotracheal airway established for the anesthetic is left in place in practically all patients. This provides for assisted ventilation in the early postoperative period when respiratory depression from anesthesia may be present. A safer, smoother transition from anesthesia and surgery can be achieved when sedation can be maintained during the rewarming phase, a period of great potential hemodynamic instability.

TRANSFER TO INTENSIVE CARE UNIT

A critical period in the patient's postoperative course occurs during the transfer from the operating room to the intensive care unit (ICU). Serious dysrhythmias, volume changes, and blood pressure changes can occur during this relatively short time. The goal is to optimize conditions for a smooth transition from the operating room to the ICU. ICU personnel should know what to expect and be prepared to minimize inefficiency that is inherent in the confusion upon the patient's arrival. One method of facilitating a smooth transfer is by means of communication with the operating room team. The box on p. 388 illustrates a written report format that can be sent by the anesthesiologist as the patient's chest is being closed. This is generally about 45 minutes to 1 hour before arrival. The report is brief but outlines the monitoring and pharmacologic support to be expected. Also included are approximate ventilator settings, so that time is not wasted preparing the ventilator for the patient after arrival in the ICU. Any problems that developed during surgery also can be outlined. This allows extra time to set up additional monitoring systems and to

Sample postoperative ICU advance information sheet

Patient name_____

Age_____Preoperative weight_____

Diagnosis_____

Other health problems_____

Surgical procedure_____

Operative problems_____

(Check or complete the following)

A. RESPIRATORY (Please notify Inhalation Therapy)

1. Ventilator requested?_____ Type?_____
   Anticipated tidal volume?_____ PEEP?_____ cm H_2O
2. T-piece system requested (no ventilator needed)?_____
3. Patient will be extubated?_____
4. Humidified mask oxygen?_____

B. MONITORING

1. Arterial catheter?_____ Location_____
2. CVP catheter?_____ Location_____
3. PA catheter?_____ Location_____
4. LA catheter?_____

C. INTRAVENOUS INFUSIONS PRESENTLY IN USE

Dopamine_____ Epinephrine_____ Nitroglycerin_____

Dobutamine_____ Calcium chloride_____ Lidocaine_____

Isoproterenol_____ Nitroprusside_____

Others_____

D. PLEASE PREPARE A FRESH INFUSION OF_____

_____ Standard _____ Double _____ Other

E. SPECIAL INFORMATION

1. Left ventricular device in use
   _____Intraaortic balloon
   _____Other
2. Request cardiac outputs early postoperatively_____
3. Miscellaneous_____

   _____

F. LABORATORY STUDIES DRAWN IN O.R. AND TIME DRAWN

Coagulation panel_____ Potassium_____

Hematocrit, platelets_____ Enzymes_____

Blood gases_____ Other_____

Estimated time of arrival in ICU _____ AM _____ PM

_____

PEEP, Positive end-expiratory pressure; *CVP*, central venous pressure; *PA*, pulmonary artery; *LA*, left atrial.

secure extra staff members if necessary. A quick "on-the-way" call from the operating room personnel just before the patient's departure also ensures optimum readiness to admit the patient to the ICU.

When the patient is connected to the monitoring equipment in the ICU, priorities should be established to minimize problems and confusion. One approach follows:

1. Connect the ECG monitoring leads for immediate monitoring of the heart rate and detection of dysrhythmias or cardiac arrest. During this time, blood pressure may be monitored by a portable electronic monitor from the operating room to the surgical ICU.

2. Connect the ventilator to the patient's airway. Adequate ventilation can be checked by watching the patient's chest move during respiration. Air movement into both lungs must be confirmed by auscultation of both the right and left sides of the chest. Because serious errors may occur when reliance is placed solely on spirometer tidal volume measurements, adequacy of ventilation is accurately determined by arterial oxygen saturation measurements. To avoid hypoxia, ventilation is initiated with 80% oxygen; the percentage of oxygen is then decreased as guided by Pao_2 determinations.

3. Connect the pulse oximeter sensor to the oximeter.

4. Connect venous and PA pressure lines to their appropriate transducers, IV infusion systems, and oximeter, if appropriate. At this time, after noting mean arterial pressure, clarify volume and drug infusion rates, as well as hemodynamic parameters desired by the physician. This is also a good time to quickly note the amount of drainage in the chest tube drainage system.

5. Connect the arterial pressure line to its appropriate transducer and IV infusion systems.

6. Milk or strip the chest tubes, record the amount of drainage, and connect them to the vacuum source if suction is to be applied.

7. Measure and empty urine drainage from the operating room and begin hourly urine output monitoring.

8. Insert a nasogastric tube to prevent abdominal distention from positive-pressure ventilation.

9. Connect the bladder temperature probe.

10. Clarify with the attending physician expectations, potential problems, and unique features for the care of the patient.

11. Continue rewarming measures such as the use of warm blankets or blood warmers if the patient is still hypothermic.

12. Once the patient is hemodynamically stable and ventilation is adequate, obtain a chest x-ray film with portable equipment. This film serves several purposes: it establishes a baseline from which to compare subsequent changes in mediastinal or cardiac size; it rules out pneumothorax; and it identifies the location of the endotracheal tube, nasogastric tube, and intracardiac monitoring catheters. It is particularly important to ensure that the endotracheal tube is positioned neither near the larynx nor in the right or left bronchus. The optimum location of the endotracheal tube tip is 1 to 2 cm above the carina. The examination also serves to monitor changes in pulmonary vascularity, which can reflect abnormalities in cardiac function and fluid balance. At this time, also obtain blood samples for

arterial blood gases, serum potassium, hematocrit, and coagulation studies, if warranted.

13. Obtain a 12-lead ECG to serve as a baseline from which to interpret any changes.

EARLY POSTOPERATIVE MONITORING
Assessment of Cardiac Output

Inasmuch as low cardiac output is the most common immediate postoperative problem, it is crucial to carefully assess and measure cardiac output. The thermodilution technique of cardiac output measurement is most commonly used in the critical care setting (see the discussion in Chapter 8). A minimum of 12° difference between the injectate and the core temperature is necessary to reliably measure ensuing temperature differences.

If serial thermodilution cardiac outputs are not measured postoperatively, arterial pressure monitoring may be used as the hemodynamic parameter that reflects cardiac output. Systemic hypotension always suggests the possibility of a low cardiac output and inadequate tissue perfusion. Metabolic acidosis, as detected by arterial blood gas values, may be caused by tissue hypoperfusion. Additional, less direct evaluation of tissue perfusion may be obtained by monitoring changes in the peripheral circulation. Peripheral perfusion can be assumed to be adequate if extremities are warm and have rapid capillary filling and full peripheral pulses (radial, dorsalis pedis, and posterior tibial). A urinary output greater than 40 ml/hr also usually indicates an adequate cardiac output.

Although low cardiac output in the postoperative setting may be caused by preoperative or perioperative factors, hypovolemia, decreased myocardial contractility, and cardiac tamponade are the three most likely causes of postoperative low cardiac output and hypotension. However, assessment of intravascular volume and vascular resistance during rewarming is also crucial and plays a major role in providing early hemodynamic stabilization. Alterations in cardiac output postoperatively must be assessed and interpreted with regard to the determinants of cardiac output, namely preload, afterload, and contractility (see Table 16-1).

Preload, the ventricular filling volume (or pressure), is clinically assessed by the RA, LA, or PAW pressure. Decreases in filling volume, or hypovolemia, in the postoperative setting may occur as a result of actual blood loss or as a result of fluid shifts from the vascular space to the interstitial spaces. The use of mannitol during cardiopulmonary bypass also increases diuresis after bypass, which can further reduce vascular volume. However, the most common cause of decreased filling, or hypovolemia, postoperatively relates to the increase in vascular space that occurs as the patient rewarms after induced hypothermia. As the peripheral vessels begin to dilate with temperature rise, the vascular space and thus the requirements for additional volume increase. This requirement should be anticipated and appropriate vasodilators and volume administered to establish adequate circulation volume before this occurrence.

Careful monitoring and maintenance of optimum ventricular filling pressures allow time to recognize and treat developing hypovolemia before serious hypotension occurs. For this reason, MAP should always be evaluated along with the CVP or PAW/LA pressure and heart rate response. It is initially possible for the MAP to remain relatively unchanged because of SVR changes in spite of decreases in intravascular volume. An increase in heart rate with a downward trend in filling pressures should alert the clinician to the possibility of developing hypovolemia, even though MAP has not dropped markedly. Right- and left-sided filling pressures that are both low (less than 8 and 12 mm Hg, respectively) provide confirmation of hypovolemia. Changes in right-sided pressures appear later than left-sided changes because of the more compliant nature of the venous system.

Another less common cause of relative hypovolemia resulting from changes in the vascular space is an allergic reaction. An antigen-antibody response from drug or transfusion reactions can result in decreased SVR caused by histamine release. The resultant hypotension is caused by insufficient volume to fill the increased vascular space. The change in preload requirement will result in decreased CVP and LA or PAW pressure. Temporary support of blood pressure can be achieved with vasopres-

Table 16-1. Evaluation of inadequate cardiac output

Findings	Causes	Correction
BP or MAP ↓ Right- and left-sided filling pressures ↓ Urine output ↓ Peripheral circulation ↓	Hypovolemia	Volume expansion
BP or MAP ↓ Right- and left-sided filling pressure ↓ Peripheral circulation adequate Urine output adequate	↓ Peripheral vascular resistance Allergic response	Volume expansion Alpha-adrenergic drugs (e.g., methoxamine)
BP or MAP ↓ CVP/RA ↓ and left-sided filling pressure ↑ Peripheral circulation ↓ Urine output ↓	Left-sided heart failure LA thrombus Intraoperative myocardial infarction Valve malfunction	Inotropic agents; afterload reduction Surgical correction Inotropic agents; diuretics; afterload reduction Surgical correction
BP or MAP ↓ CVP/RA ↑ and left-sided filling pressure ↓ Urine output ↓ Peripheral circulation ↓	Right-sided heart failure Pulmonary embolism Valve malfunction	Inotropic agents; Heparin; vasopressors; possibly surgery Surgical correction
BP or MAP ↓ Right- and left-sided filling pressure ↑ Urine output ↓ Peripheral circulation ↓	Cardiac failure Cardiac tamponade	Inotropic agents; diuretics Surgical correction
Dysrhythmias	Hypoxemia Hypokalemia Hypocalcemia Hypomagnesemia Drug-induced Surgical trauma Other (idiopathic)	Maintenance of adequate Pao_2 Potassium replacement Calcium replacement Magnesium replacement Withholding of further medication Additional measures (pharmacologic treatment, electroversion)

BP, Blood pressure; *MAP*, mean arterial pressure; *CVP*, central venous pressure; *RA*, right atrial; *LA*, left atrial; *Pao₂*, arterial oxygen pressure.

sors until the causative factor is removed or treated and vascular volume has been restored.

The fluid replacement of choice varies from institution to institution. There is a trend in most centers to maintain patients in a state of normovolemic hemodilution (anemia). Minimal blood replacement decreases the risk of virus transmission and conserves valuable blood products. Maintenance of the hematocrit value at 25% to 30% is acceptable for most patients. Transfusion of blood for hematocrits below this level is indicated. This, of course, would not apply to any patient with serious bleeding. Iron therapy can be initiated in the postoperative period to aid in the restoration of a normal hematocrit value. For individuals with significant left ventricular dysfunction, a lower hematocrit level may not be indicated. Lower oxygen-carrying capacity will necessitate an increase in heart rate or cardiac output to maintain adequate oxygen delivery to tissues. This extra demand might outweigh the benefits of normovolemic anemia. Care also must be taken to monitor such a patient for dysrhythmias that could be hypoxic in origin. Volume replacement for most patients will most likely be either crystalloid (normal saline), colloid (albumin), hetastarch, or a combination of these.

Decreased afterload or resistance may occur postoperatively as a result of anaphylaxis (a reaction to blood, protamine, or drug allergy) or sepsis.

Ventricular contractility, another determinant of cardiac output, frequently is depressed immediately after cardiac surgery as a result of the effects of anesthesia and hypothermia, as well as ventricular ischemia. Calculated stroke work indexes of the left and right ventricles are used as a reflection of their contractile state (see Table 16-1).

Afterload, in the clinical setting, is reflected by the resistance to ventricular ejection (SVR for the left side, pulmonary vascular resistance [PVR] for the right side) (see Table 16-1). Because afterload is inversely related to cardiac output, it is important to monitor and effectively manipulate this hemodynamic parameter to improve flow. Increased afterload that manifests by elevated SVR is a common postoperative occurrence as a result of hypothermia, increased circulating catecholamines, and surgical stimulation. High afterload may exist despite normal arterial blood pressures if cardiac output is reduced (pressure = flow × resistance). Therefore, calculation of the SVR is clinically necessary to evaluate afterload of the left side of the heart.

Patient Example 1

A 50-year-old man underwent an uncomplicated aortic valve replacement. On arrival in the ICU, he was still well sedated (not yet able to be aroused) and hypothermic. A PA catheter inserted before induction remained in place. Initial vital signs demonstrated elevated MAP and SVR. Immediately after his arrival, nitroprusside therapy was begun to control hypertension. Over the next 2 hours, right- and left-sided filling pressures gradually decreased as heart rate increased. Cardiac index also fell despite reductions in SVR. After 2 hours, the patient's temperature had risen to 36° C. Vasodilation had occurred from both rewarming and nitroprusside therapy, creating a state of relative hypovolemia. Hemodynamic stability was achieved in this patient with adequate fluid administration.

During hypothermia, SVR can be quite elevated, and this greatly increases the oxygen demand of the heart. This is a period in which patients also are prone to

Patient example 1

	Arrival	30 min	1 hr	90 min	2 hr	3 hr
HR (beats/min)	92	90	94	100	110	80
MAP (mm Hg)	110	100	90	85	70	85
PAW (mm Hg)	8	8	7	5	4	8
CVP (mm Hg)	10	10	10	8	7	10
CI (L/min/m^2)	3.4	—	3.2	—	2.8	4.0
SVR (dynes/sec /cm^{-5})	2000	—	1600	—	1100	1100
Temperature (° C)	34	34	35	35	36	36
Rx	—	0.5 µg/kg/min nitroprusside	1 µg/kg/min nitroprusside	1.5 µg/kg/min nitroprusside	1 µg/kg/min nitroprusside; volume therapy	1 µg/kg/min nitroprusside; 400 ml saline; 250 ml albumin

hypertension. Excessive pressure elevation places stress on new suture lines, increasing the risk of potential tears in the suture lines, with resultant hemorrhage. Vasodilators are used to treat hypertension by reducing vascular resistance and to enhance peripheral perfusion. When vasodilator therapy is begun, great care must be taken to watch for changes in preload requirements. The rewarming process almost always requires additional fluid administration.

If the right- and left-sided filling pressures rise after fluid replacement but hypotension and low cardiac output persist, *myocardial failure* with decreased contractility must be considered. In this case positive inotropic agents may be required to improve cardiac output and blood pressure. Cases of severe myocardial depression may necessitate a combination of positive inotropic agents and vasodilators to optimize cardiac output. In this instance it is essential to use serial cardiac output determinations with calculation of SVR to maintain the proper balance of inotropic agents and vasodilators for maximal cardiac output.

Patient Example 2

A 47-year-old woman underwent uncomplicated mitral valve replacement for recurrent mitral stenosis. After surgery, she remained in a state of low CO even with the administration of IV dopamine. Four hours postoperatively, the patient's cardiac index was 1.45 L/min/m^2 and the SVR was 2350 dynes/sec/cm^{-5}. The addition of IV nitroprusside with concomitant volume therapy resulted in a significant increase in cardiac index to 2.21 L/min/m^2 and a decrease in SVR to 1370 dynes/sec/cm^{-5} (Fig. 16-2).

Left ventricular failure is recognized by decreasing peripheral perfusion, which usually is seen in the form of decreased pulses, capillary refill, skin temperature, and urine output. Forward flow of blood is impaired by depressed contractility. As blood flow backs up in the pulmonary vasculature, rales will be evident when breath sounds are assessed. A rise in SVR is predictable as a result of an attempt to maintain blood pressure. The resulting increase in afterload further compromises cardiac performance. The left ventricle's inability to handle volume also will be reflected by an increase in left-sided filling pressures (mean LA or PAW pressure).

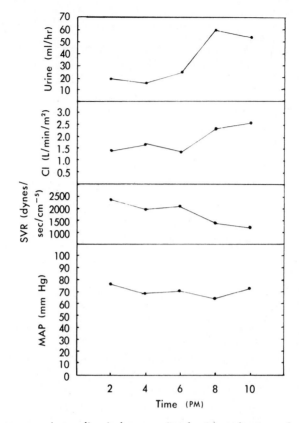

Fig. 16-2. Improvement in cardiac index associated with reduction of systemic vascular resistance in response to intravenous nitroprusside therapy. The slight decrease in mean arterial pressure suggests that the reduction of excessive systemic vascular resistance is responsible for the increase in cardiac index. (*MAP*, Mean arterial pressure; *SVR*, systemic vascular resistance; *CI*, cardiac index.)

Ventricular contractility may be excessive in the later postoperative period. This is more commonly seen in patients with preexisting ventricular hypertrophy (such as in aortic stenosis, idiopathic hypertrophic subaortic stenosis, or systemic hypertension), as well as in conjunction with the administration of positive inotropic agents. Increased contractility markedly increases myocardial oxygen consumption and causes systemic hypertension, which endangers suture lines and grafts and can cause hemorrhage. Reductions in contractility, if necessary, can be achieved with the use of beta-blocking agents or calcium channel blockers that possess negative inotropic effects.

The persistence of inadequate cardiac output after correction of hypovolemia may be caused by *cardiac tamponade*. This complication also manifests as a markedly elevated venous pressure and low arterial pressure. The diastolic pressures of both the right and the left sides of the heart tend to equilibrate because of the constriction of the heart by the accumulation of blood in the pericardial space. There also may be a characteristic pattern to the RA or RV pressure (see Chapter 6). An excessive output of blood through the chest tubes (>300 ml/hr) before the development of systemic hypotension may suggest impending cardiac tamponade. Although a paradoxical pulse (fall in systolic pressure >10 mm Hg during inspiration) is usually present in cardiac tamponade, the use of a positive pressure ventilator obscures these signs. Their absence therefore does not rule out the complication of cardiac tamponade. Significant mediastinal widening, as determined by serial chest radiographs provides strong evidence that cardiac tamponade may be responsible for a low cardiac output. Bedside echocardiography, direct or transesophageal, may be useful to detect significant fluid or clot collection around the heart and to evaluate right and left ventricular contractility. Surgical removal of the clotted blood is the definitive management of cardiac tamponade. However, fluid replacement to ensure adequate filling (despite already high filling pressures) and administration of inotropic agents to optimize cardiac contractility are important adjuncts in preparing the patient for reoperation.

Patient Example 3

A 60-year-old woman underwent distal right coronary endarterectomy with saphenous vein bypass grafts from the aorta to the distal right, left anterior descending, and circumflex coronary arteries because of preinfarction angina resulting from coronary artery disease. Postoperative hypotension slowly developed and persisted even though the filling pressures (CVP and PAW) increased to 15 mm Hg after blood replacement (Fig. 16-3). Her extremities remained cool. Comparison of the chest x-ray film taken immediately postoperatively (Fig. 16-4, *A*) with that taken 5 hours postoperatively (Fig. 16-4, *B*) revealed marked mediastinal widening. Cardiac tamponade was suspected, and reoperation was immediately performed. At surgery blood clots surrounding the heart were removed, and bleeding was controlled. After this surgery, arterial pressure and tissue perfusion returned to normal without the use of vasopressors.

Abnormal heart rates and rhythms may cause decreases in cardiac output (CO = HR × SV). Very slow heart rates, which can be seen postoperatively as a result of excessive hypothermia, can reduce cardiac output despite relatively normal stroke volumes. Augmentation of the heart rate by use of the implanted atrial or ventricular pacing wires or by pharmacologic means may be necessary to augment cardiac output. Tachycardias frequently occur postoperatively in the presence of hypovolemia. Excessive heart rates (> 120 beats/min) may reduce cardiac output and coronary filling time, as well as increase myocardial oxygen consumption. If the heart rate remains rapid after adequate volume restoration, pharmacologic intervention with calcium channel blockers or beta blockers may be necessary to reduce the rate and improve the oxygen supply and demand balance.

The immediate detection and accurate diagnosis of *dysrhythmias* are important because of the potentially adverse effect of dysrhythmias on cardiac output caused by impaired diastolic filling time. Ventricular extrasystoles may indicate myocardial irritability and the increased probability of more serious dysrhythmias to follow. Hypoxemia, hypokalemia, and cardiovascular drugs are frequent causes of postoperative dysrhythmias. These contributory causes should be carefully looked for and treated when dysrhythmias are present. In the absence of specific etiologic factors, antidysrhythmic treatment or cardioversion, or both, are used.

Other causes of low cardiac output postoperatively include inadequate prosthetic valvular function or residual RV or LV outflow obstruction. Abnormal valve sounds during auscultation of the heart may indicate prosthetic valvular malfunction, but right- or left-sided heart catheterization with angiography must be performed to confirm the diagnosis. LA thrombus formation is a rare and extremely serious

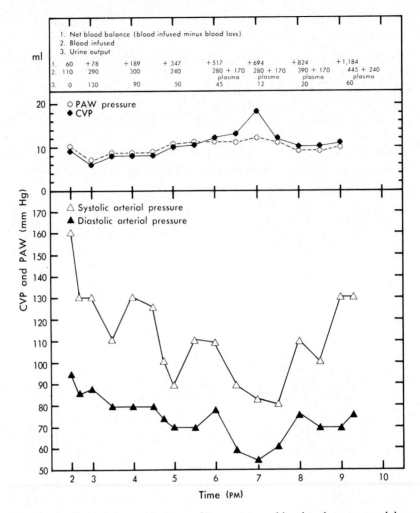

Fig. 16-3. Changes in vital signs with time and in response to blood replacement and dopamine. Although the central venous pressure *(CVP)* and the pulmonary artery wedge *(PAW)* pressure rise during fluid replacement, the arterial pressure falls until the blood balance is significantly increased and dopamine is added. At the time of the patient's return to surgery, the blood replacement is 1184 ml more than the measured loss, and the patient is given an additional 750 ml of plasma. The fluid replacement, along with the dopamine, results in an arterial pressure of 130/70 mm Hg.

complication, causing low cardiac output. It most often occurs after mitral valve replacement in association with atrial fibrillation. Unrecognized coronary artery disease or intraoperative myocardial infarction also may cause low cardiac output and hypotension. Serial monitoring of cardiac enzymes and ECGs assists in the diagnosis.

CARDIOVASCULAR EFFECTS ASSOCIATED WITH RESPIRATION

Inasmuch as tissue perfusion and gas exchange are essential for cellular metabolism, monitoring of pulmonary function and oxygenation is an essential adjunct to monitoring the cardiovascular system. For example, inadequate ventilation results in carbon dioxide retention and hypoxemia. If this inadequate ventilation

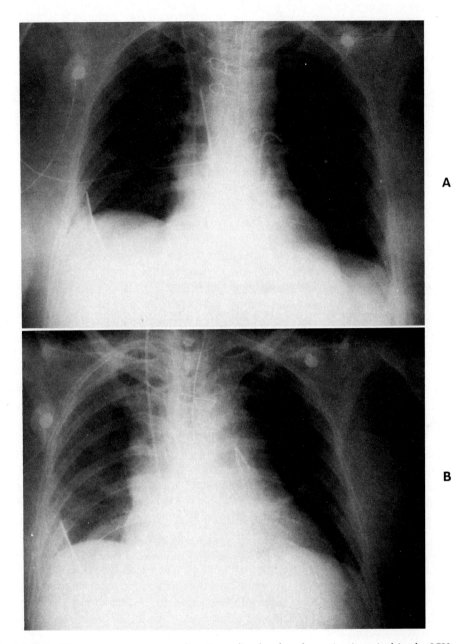

Fig. 16-4. A, Chest reoentgenogram taken immediately after the patient's arrival in the ICU. The mediastinum is not widened, and there is no apparent fluid collection in the pleural spaces. The chest tubes in the right pleural space and in the mediastinal space are apparent. Swan-Ganz catheter is visualized in the left pulmonary artery. A nasogastric tube is present in the esophagus and stomach. **B,** Chest roentgenogram taken 4½ hours later. There is considerable mediastinal widening, consistent with cardiac tamponade.

persists, respiratory and metabolic acidosis in conjunction with hypoxemia will depress cardiac function. This negative inotropic effect is aggravated by a depressed response to inotropic agents because of acidosis and hypoxia, and the result is progressive cardiac failure.

Continuous measurement of mixed venous oxygen saturation ($S\bar{v}o_2$) is very helpful in assessing the adequacy of cardiac output and oxygen delivery to the tissues (see the discussion in Chapter 10). Declines in $S\bar{v}o_2$ to 60% or less indicate a decrease in oxygen supply or an increase in oxygen demand and frequently precede any other hemodynamic change. Assessment of the components of oxygen delivery (cardiac output, hemoglobin, and arterial oxygen saturation) should be made whenever the $S\bar{v}o_2$ falls 5% to 10%. $S\bar{v}o_2$ has been shown to be a sensitive indicator of postoperative overall or global tissue oxygenation.

After cardiac surgery the primary concerns regarding respiration are the work of breathing, gas exchange, and maintenance of acid-base balance. A normal, resting person requires 2% to 5% of the basal energy for respiratory function, whereas this requirement markedly increases postoperatively. Several factors responsible for the increased work of postoperative ventilation are the following:

1. A decrease in chest wall compliance resulting from thoracotomy and pain-induced muscle spasm
2. A decrease in lung compliance resulting from a reduction in pulmonary surfactants (left-sided heart failure of any cause results in pulmonary venous congestion, further reducing lung compliance; chronic preoperative pulmonary edema also will render the lungs less compliant in the postoperative period)
3. Increased production and retention of airway secretions resulting in elevated airway resistance
4. Postoperative shivering causing decreased chest wall compliance

To decrease the work of breathing after surgery, all patients receive mechanical ventilatory assistance. Experience has shown that this practice also reduces the incidence of dysrhythmias and cardiac arrest. Assisted ventilation with use of an endotracheal tube is maintained for 48 to 72 hours after surgery. Low-pressure, high-volume cuffs on contemporary endotracheal tubes allow maintenance of intubation for periods of up to 1 week without damaging effects to the trachea.

Ventilatory assistance by means of a closed airway requires careful control and monitoring of ventilation and oxygenation, including respiratory rate (with or without triggering by the patient), tidal volume, and percentage of inspired oxygen. Minute-to-minute adequacy of ventilation is estimated by observing the degree of excursion of the patient's chest wall during ventilation. Auscultation of the lungs for bilateral inspiratory sounds affords additional evidence of ventilation adequacy. Spirometer measurement alone should not be relied on to ensure ventilation is adequate. Apnea alarms and equipment to continuously monitor end-tidal carbon dioxide and flow rates facilitate further monitoring of respiratory function in the critically ill patient.

During ventilator assistance, continuous monitoring of arterial oxygen saturation (Sao_2) is used to determine the adequacy of ventilation (Table 16-2). Adjustments in ventilatory management frequently are necessary to maintain Sao_2 at 95% or more. Frequent blood gas analyses also are necessary to assess carbon dioxide production and pH.

Ideally, the minute volume of ventilation is adjusted by varying the respiratory rate, tidal volume, and dead space to obtain a $Paco_2$ of 40 mm Hg. In practice, maintaining the $Paco_2$ at exactly 40 mm Hg requires inordinate time and attention. Therefore it is easier to slightly hyperventilate the patient to maintain a $Paco_2$ in the 30- to 40-mm Hg range. This slight respiratory alkalosis has minimal impact on the cardiovascular system.

Oxygen administration is determined by Sao_2 and Pao_2 assessment. In general, the fractional inspired oxygen concentration (Fio_2) is increased to whatever level is necessary to maintain an Sao_2 above 95% and a Pao_2 in the normal range of 90 to 100 mm Hg. An Fio_2 greater than 60% for more than 3 to 4 hours has been associated with oxygen toxicity; however, inasmuch as the harmful effect of hypoxemia may surpass the potential of adverse effects from oxygen toxicity, the Fio_2 is increased to whatever level is necessary to maintain a Pao_2 above 50 mm Hg. A higher Pao_2 may be required if there is anemia, increased oxygen demand caused by fever, or a low cardiac output. Repeated assessment of pH from arterial blood gas analyses is essential for complete cardiorespiratory monitoring.

Table 16-2. Evaluation of arterial blood gases

Findings	Cause	Correction	
		Mechanical ventilation	Extubation
$Paco_2$ ↑ Sao_2 or Pao_2 ↓ or NL	Inadequate ventilation Rewarming with shivering	↑ Tidal volume ↑ Respiratory rate ↓ Dead space	↓ Sedation Respirator
pH ↓ or NL	↑ Secretions	Aspiration of secretions	Coughing, deep breathing Nasotracheal suctioning
	Pneumothorax Bronchospasm Respirator malfunction	Chest tube Bronchodilator Correction of respirator	Chest tube Bronchodilator
Sao_2 or Pao_2 ↓ $Paco_2$ ↓ or NL pH NL	Pulmonary A-V shunting Pulmonary edema	↑ Fio_2 Inotropic agents PEEP Diuretics Correction of underlying cause	↑ Fio_2 via mask or cannulas Inotropic agents, diuretics Possibly ventilator with PEEP Correction of underlying cause
	Cardiac failure Atelectasis	See Table 16-1 Pulmonary physiotherapy Bronchoscopy, if severe and intractable	See Table 16-1 Coughing, deep breathing Physiotherapy Possibly bronchoscopy
Sao_2 or Pao_2 ↑ or NL $Paco_2$ ↓ pH ↑ or NL	Pain, anxiety causing hyperventilation	Decrease in minute volume Addition of dead space	Sedation
	Metabolic alkalosis	Replacement of electrolytes, fluid	Replacement of electrolytes, fluids

Paco₂, Arterial carbon dioxide pressure; *Sao₂*, arterial oxygen saturation; *Pao₂*, arterial oxygen pressure; *NL*, normal; *A-V*, arteriovenous; *Fio₂*, fractional inspired oxygen concentration; *PEEP*, positive end-expiratory pressure.

POSTOPERATIVE MONITORING AFTER 24 TO 48 HOURS

In most patients, vital signs stabilize within the first 24 hours after surgery. Drainage from the chest tube stops, and blood replacement no longer is necessary. Ventilatory support usually is not required, and removal of the endotracheal airway is well tolerated. Oxygen can be delivered by mask or nasal cannula, if required. At this point, arterial, PA, and/or LA pressure lines are removed. Usually, a CVP line is left in place for up to 48 hours postoperatively to permit blood sampling and drug administration. ECG monitoring is continued for the duration of the period in the ICU and is continued for 1 or 2 days by use of telemetry.

Tables 16-3 and 16-4 present some guidelines regarding this type and frequency of postoperative monitoring.

As the patient's condition stabilizes and improves, monitoring consists of less frequent recording of temperature, respiratory rate, pulse, and blood pressure by cuff measurement. Daily measurement of intake and output and patient's weight is

Table 16-3. Monitoring guidelines for the postoperative patient

Monitored parameters	Postoperative period			
	1-24 hr	24-72 hr (with pharmacologic support)	24-72 hr (without pharmacologic support)	72-120 hr
NONINVASIVE				
ECG	Continuous	Continuous	Continuous	Daily and prn
Blood pressure	—	q 1-2h	q 2-4h	q 4h
Respiratory rate	q 15-20 min	q 1-2h	q 2-4h	q 4h
Temperature	q 15-20 min	q 1-2h	q 4h	q 4h
Peripheral circulation	q 15-20 min	q 1-2h	q 2-4h	q 4h
Intake and output	q 1h	q 1-2h	q 8h	q 8h
Chest x-ray film	Immediately and prn	Daily and prn	Daily and prn	Daily and prn
INVASIVE				
CVP/RA pressure	q 15-20 min	q 1-2h	q 2-4h	prn
Arterial pressure	q 15-20 min	q 1-2h	q 2-4h	prn
LA pressure	q 15-20 min	q 1-2h	q 2-4h	prn
Chest tube drainage	q 15-20 min	prn	prn	prn

CVP, Central venous pressure; RA, right atrial; LA, left atrial.

Table 16-4. Postoperative laboratory analysis guidelines

Laboratory analysis	Postoperative period (hr)		
	1-24	24-72	72-120
Arterial blood gas	Immediately and q 4h	prn	prn
Chemistry panel	q 8h	Daily and prn	Daily and prn
Hematocrit	Immediately and q 4h	Daily	Daily
Potassium	Immediately and q 4h	Daily and prn	Daily and prn

continued. Assessment of circulatory adequacy, including vital signs, observation, and examination, is performed as deemed necessary by the patient's condition and the amount of pharmacologic support. Routine laboratory tests consist of complete blood cell count (CBC), serum electrolyte values, arterial blood gas analyses, blood urea nitrogen (BUN) and creatinine determinations, ECG, and chest x-ray studies. In most cases daily determinations suffice, but more frequent assessments are made when indicated. During this later postoperative period, the more important monitoring goals include detection of hypotension, respiratory distress, and dysrhythmias. Even more important is the capability to immediately detect and respond to unexpected cardiac arrest. Telemetry ECG monitoring for several days is an essential aspect of early cardiac arrest detection and treatment.

MONITORING FOR OTHER POSTOPERATIVE COMPLICATIONS

Some of the more common postoperative problems have already been discussed. Others occur frequently enough to be looked for in each patient's postoperative course.

Hemorrhage

Excessive bleeding after cardiac surgery, which necessitates reoperation, occurs in approximately 1% to 5% of patients. Thus the CVP or PA pressure, as well as the arterial pressure, should be closely monitored. External blood loss is monitored every 15 minutes by measuring chest tube drainage. Clotting of the chest tube may occur, so that measured blood loss may be less than the actual loss. For this reason assessment of the blood loss must be correlated with the arterial pressure, ventricular filling pressures, and chest x-ray films. The definition of excessive blood loss is somewhat arbitrary. An accepted figure for total average blood loss is 400 ml/m² body surface average. General guidelines for reoperation for hemorrhage are bleeding in excess of 300 to 400 ml/hr for the first 2 hours, 250 ml/hr from 3 to 6 hours, and more than 200 ml/hr for the next 4 hours. Excessive bleeding also may be related to a coagulopathy and should be confirmed by clotting studies.

Embolization

Systemic arterial emboli during or after cardiac surgery are infrequent but may occur any time. The most usual source is from a thrombus on prosthetic cardiac valves. Other sources are from a clot on suture lines on the left side of the heart, LA thrombi, calcium from the aortic or mitral valve, or thrombus from a left ventricular aneurysm. A rare cause is tumor embolization occurring at the time of surgery for removal of an LA myxoma or other left-sided cardiac tumor. To detect embolization, the most important systems to monitor are the central nervous system (mental status), kidneys (renal function), mesenteric arteries (acute abdominal pain), and peripheral arteries (loss of distal pulse). Central nervous system effects are extremely diverse, ranging from slight changes in cerebration to coma or hemiparalysis. Pulmonary embolization may cause respiratory distress. Although an abnormally low Pao_2 may suggest pulmonary embolism, more commonly the Pao_2 is not significantly decreased. A suspicion of pulmonary embolism based on the presence of tachycardia, tachypnea, and patient agitation and apprehension should be confirmed by a pulmonary ventilation-perfusion scan and, if indicated, a pulmonary arteriogram. If the embolus is large, a fall in cardiac output and hypotension may occur.

Renal Failure

Postoperative renal failure is associated most commonly with preexisting renal disease and long periods of cardiopulmonary bypass with low flow rates, or prolonged low cardiac output after surgery. Current trends toward more liberal fluid administration in the postoperative period have decreased the incidence of postoperative renal failure. Maintenance of adequate intravascular volume and cardiac output are paramount in the prevention of renal failure. Renal failure must be recognized as early as possible to prevent fluid and electrolyte overload. Inadequate renal function is evident by a decrease in urine sodium and decreased creatinine clearance. A patient at risk or who appears to be developing acute renal failure will benefit from early assessment of these studies. Creatinine clearance will decrease long before marked elevations in serum creatinine occur, thus providing an early, more specific indicator of renal function. Monitoring hourly urine output in conjunction with frequent serial potassium and BUN or creatinine determinations will provide other valuable information regarding renal function.

Central Nervous System Complications

Postoperative complications involving the central nervous system are frequent and require diligent monitoring of the patient's motor or sensory abilities and mental status. Diffuse cerebral dysfunction most frequently occurs in the older patient after a period of hypotension, either intraoperatively or postoperatively. Air or particulate material embolization also may cause these changes. More focal central nervous system abnormalities usually result from emboli or from hypotension in association with occlusive disease of the carotid, vertebral, or intracranial arteries.

Postoperative delirium or psychosis is another central nervous system complication. Its exact cause remains undetermined, but diffuse microembolization of the intracranial arteries during cardiopulmonary bypass, as well as deep hypothermia and circulatory arrest, may be factors. Other possibilities include deprivation of sleep and sense of time during intensive postoperative care. The diagnosis is established by recognition of the inability to concentrate, hallucinations, and paranoid or delusional psychotic behavior. To a great degree it can be prevented by affording adequate opportunities for the patient to sleep, allowing the patient access to both a clock and calendar, and assisting in orienting the patient to time. Most patients are aware of their hallucinations, which is a source of tremendous anxiety to them. These patients require a significant amount of reassurance that they are not "losing their minds" and that the hallucinations will pass. It also might be helpful to discuss the effects that narcotics might have in contributing to their condition. This will help reinforce the fact that the situation is only temporary. If psychotic behavior does occur, it almost always disappears before or shortly after discharge from the hospital.

Cardiac Arrest

One of the most important goals of monitoring after cardiac surgery is the immediate detection of cardiac arrest. Only by immediate detection and resuscitation can the patient's life be spared and the central nervous system's function be optimally preserved. The primary mode of detection of cardiac arrest is continuous ECG monitoring and arterial pressure monitoring. Caution must be used in placing total reliance on electronic monitoring for detection, because dislodgment of the ECG leads may result in an oscilloscopic pattern closely resembling asystole or ventricular fibrillation. Before resuscitation (and especially before defibrillation) is begun, absence of effective cardiac activity should be confirmed by palpation of the brachial or femoral arteries. Palpation of the carotid arteries may interfere with cerebral circulation or stimulate the carotid sinus nerves and should be avoided. Without continuous electronic monitoring, cardiac arrest is recognized by a sudden loss of consciousness and loss of brachial and femoral artery pulses. Even though cardiac activity may be present or detected by observation of the chest wall or stethoscopic examination of the heart, resuscitation measures should be instituted if the brachial and femoral pulses are absent or inadequate.

REFERENCES

Bodai BI, Holcroft JW: Use of the pulmonary arterial catheter in the critically ill patient, *Heart Lung* 11:406-416, 1982.

Connors JP, Avioli LV: An update on cardiac surgery, *Heart Lung* 10:323-328, 1981.

Cosgrove A et al: Blood conservation in cardiac surgery, *Cardiovasc Clin* 12:165, 1981.

Fernando H et al: Late cardiac tamponade following open heart surgery: detection by echocardiography, *Ann Thorac Surg* 24:174-177, 1977.

Futral J: Postoperative management and complications of coronary artery surgery, *Heart Lung* 3:477-486, 1977.

Harken D: Postoperative care following heart-valve surgery, *Heart Lung* 3:839, 1974.

Kirklin JM, Barrat-Boyes BG: *Cardiac surgery,* New York, 1993, Churchill Livingstone.

McCauley KM, Brest AN, McGoon DC: *McGoon's cardiac surgery: an interprofessional approach to patient care,* Philadelphia, 1985, FA Davis.

Norback CR, Tinker JH: Hypothermia after cardiopulmonary bypass in man, *Anesthesiology* 53:277-280, 1980.

Palmer PN: Advanced hemodynamic assessment, *Dimens Crit Care Nurs* 1:139-144, 1982.

Ream AK, Fogdall RP: *Acute cardiovascular management: anesthesia and intensive care,* Philadelphia, 1982, JB Lippincott.

Reddy PS: Hemodynamics of cardiac tamponade in man. In Reddy PS, Leon DF, Shaver JA, editors: *Pericardial disease,* New York, 1982, Raven Press.

Seifert PC: Protection of the myocardium during cardiac surgery, *Heart Lung* 12:135-142, 1983.

Sladen RN: Management of the adult cardiac patient in the intensive care unit. In Ream AK, Fogdall RP, editors: *Acute cardiovascular management: anesthesia and intensive care,* Philadelphia, 1982, JB Lippincott.

Thurer RL, Hauer JM: Autotransfusion and blood conservation, *Curr Probl Surg* 19:97-156, 1982.

Viljoen JF: Anesthesia and monitoring techniques for open heart surgery in the adult, *Surg Clin North Am* 55:1217-1228, 1975.

Weeks KR et al: Bedside hemodynamic monitoring: its value in the diagnosis of tamponade complicating cardiac surgery, *J Thorac Cardiovasc Surg* 68:847-856, 1974.

Wilson RS et al: The oxygen cost of breathing following anesthesia and cardiac surgery, *Anesthesiology* 39:387-393, 1973.

Woods SL, editor: *Cardiovascular critical care nursing,* New York, 1983, Churchill Livingstone.

Young LC: Coronary artery surgery: commonplace yet complicated, *Crit Care Nurse* 1:15-24, 1981.

Chapter 17

Hemodynamic Monitoring During Critical Care Transport

Ronald Pearl

During the past 20 years, technologic advances in neonatal, pediatric, and adult intensive care have resulted in the development of increasingly sophisticated critical care transport systems. Whether the transport occurs by air or ground, it poses one of the most challenging environments in which to provide optimal patient care. The goal during critical care transport is to provide a level of care equal to that available in the ICU. The availability of this level of care during transport is a crucial factor in the development of regionalized medical programs, such as trauma, perinatal, and pediatric critical care.

The goals and operations of medical transport programs throughout the world vary greatly. Although most programs are hospital-based, some are operated by privately owned companies. Team selection varies, but most programs use some combination of physicians, nurses, respiratory therapists, and paramedics. The mode of transportation may be ambulance, helicopter, airplane, or a combination of vehicles. Transports usually are initiated by physician-to-physician referral, utilizing communication centers to coordinate the transport process.

The principles of critical care transport are based on the characteristics of and interaction among three components within the transport environment (Fig. 17-1). The people in the environment, including team members, patients, and vehicle operators, are dependent on both the equipment and transport vehicle for optimum

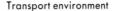

Transport environment

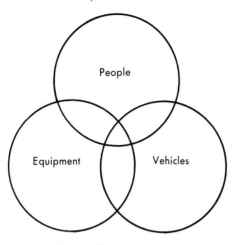

Ambient air/barometric pressure

Fig. 17-1. The transport environment.

patient outcome. Conversely, the vehicle and equipment are only as efficient as the individuals operating them. The physical laws that exist in the aeromedical transport environment influence all of the entities within that environment. Dalton's law describes the characteristics of ambient air at altitude, and Boyle's law states the effects of barometric pressure on volume. Understanding the role of these factors in the transport environment is required to optimize the efficiency, safety, and quality of patient care.

The appropriateness of an individual patient for critical care transport is a function of both the diagnosis and the underlying pathophysiology. Critically ill patients who require transport may have cardiovascular disease (dysrhythmias, myocardial infarction, congestive heart failure, aortic aneurysm), respiratory disease (pneumonia, adult respiratory distress syndrome, respiratory failure, pulmonary embolism), renal disease, neurologic disease, trauma, and all types of shock. The decision to transport a patient is based on the patient's clinical status and hemodynamic stability, as well as the anticipated stability during transport. This chapter discusses some of the elements in the transport environment that are encountered in the intensive care setting. Important aspects of aviation physiology pertinent to air transport, as well as characteristics that set air and ground transport apart, are included. The various monitoring techniques applied to the transport environment are reviewed in the final section of this chapter.

TRANSPORT ENVIRONMENT
Aviation Physiology

To appreciate the effects of the transport environment on both the patient and the team, the physiologic effects of altitude must be understood. Two physical laws govern these phenomena. The first law, Boyle's law, states that the volume of a gas is inversely proportional to its pressure when the temperature remains constant. Thus, as altitude increases and atmospheric pressure decreases, the volume of air will expand. The effects of increasing altitude on volume of gas follow*:

Altitude (ft)	Atmospheric pressure (mm Hg)	Expansion factor
Sea level	760	1.0
5000	633	1.2
10,000	523	1.5
18,000	380	2.0

Boyle's Law is the basis for dysbarisms in transport. Dysbarisms, or pressure-induced changes in the body, result from an increase or decrease in ambient barometric pressure. Body structures that contain partially or completely trapped gas—that is, the lungs, gastrointestinal tract, middle ear, and sinuses—are at risk for compromise. At a cabin altitude of 8000 feet, a 30% gas expansion occurs. A small undetected pneumothorax at sea level can result in respiratory distress at altitude. The expansion of trapped gas in the gastrointestinal tract may result in abdominal distention, causing respiratory failure, stress on suture lines, pain, and rupture. Aerotitis media results from the effects of the pressure differences on the middle ear. During ascent, air in the middle ear expands and is vented through the eustachian tube

*From Ferrara A, Harin A: *Emergency transfer of the high-risk neonate,* St Louis, 1980, Mosby–Year Book.

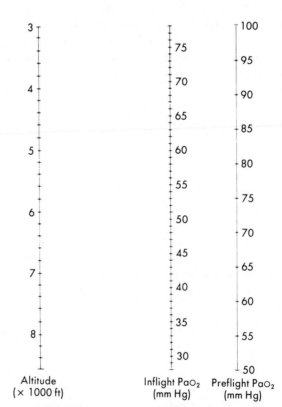

Fig. 17-2. Nomogram for predicting in-flight arterial oxygen tension from cabin altitude and preflight arterial oxygen tension.

From Henry JN, Krenis LJ, Cutting RT: *Surg Gynecol Obstet* 136:49-53, 1973.

into the throat. During descent, the air in the middle ear contracts. If pressure cannot be equalized by venting air through the eustachian tube, pain and trauma to the middle ear may result. Similarly, barosinusitis results from the inability of the sinuses to adjust to ambient pressure differences and can cause severe discomfort if pressures are not equalized.

The second gas law that affects aviation physiology is Dalton's law. Dalton's law states that the total pressure of a mixture of gases is equal to the sum of the partial pressures of each gas in the mixture. Thus the partial pressure of an individual gas is the product of the total pressure of the mixture and the fractional concentration of the individual gas. For example, oxygen always contributes 21% of the partial pressure in air. However, when the total pressure of the mixture changes, as with altitude, so will the partial pressure of a gas. For instance, at sea level atmospheric pressure is 760 mm Hg, so that the partial pressure of oxygen (P_{O_2}) is 760 mm Hg $\times$ 0.21 = 160 mm Hg. At an altitude of 8000 feet, the atmospheric pressure decreases to 565 mm Hg. However, the proportion of oxygen in the air remains constant, so that the P_{O_2} decreases to 565 mm Hg $\times$ 0.21 = 119 mm Hg (Fig. 17-2).

Adequate arterial oxygenation is a major concern for both patients and crew during air medical transport. Arterial oxygen pressure (Pa_{O_2}) depends on both the partial pressure of oxygen in the alveoli (PA_{O_2}) and the gradient between alveolar and arterial oxygen tension ($P(A-a)_{O_2}$. Pa_{O_2} is lower than the P_{O_2} in the inspired gas for two reasons. First, alveolar gas is fully saturated with water vapor (47 mm Hg at 37° C), which reduces the partial pressures of all the other gases. Second, and more important, oxygen is continually being removed from the alveolar gas and replaced by carbon dioxide. The respiratory quotient is the ratio of oxygen utilization to carbon dioxide production. Under most circumstances the ratio is approximately 0.8. The alveolar gas equation allows estimation of the P_{O_2} in the alveolar gas as follows:

$$PA_{O_2} = (FI_{O_2}) \times (BP - 47) - (PA_{CO_2}/0.8)$$

where:

BP = Barometric pressure

PA_{CO_2} = Alveolar carbon dioxide tension

FI_{O_2} = Fractional inspired oxygen concentration

PA_{O_2} = Alveolar oxygen tension

Thus, in a normal person breathing room air at sea level, the alveolar P_{O_2} is $0.21 \times (760 - 47) - 40/0.8 = 100$ mm Hg. The normal gradient between alveolar P_{O_2} and arterial P_{O_2} is approximately 5 to 10 mm Hg, so that a normal Pa_{O_2} is 90 to 95 mm Hg. In a normal person breathing air at an altitude of 8000 feet (barometric pressure of 565 mm Hg), the alveolar P_{O_2} is 65 mm Hg, so that the arterial P_{O_2} will be 55 to 60 mm Hg. In a person with any type of respiratory embarrassment, the Pa_{O_2} would be further reduced. To avoid or minimize these problems in aeromedical transports, two prophylactic measures are practiced. First, supplemental oxygen is given at a percentage necessary to maintain an acceptable Pa_{O_2} (Fig. 17-3). Second, in fixed-wing aircraft the cabin is pressurized to near sea level when possible.

Critical Differences in the Transport Environment

Within the transport environment, a level of care similar to that of the ICU must be available. However, the transport environment has certain characteristics

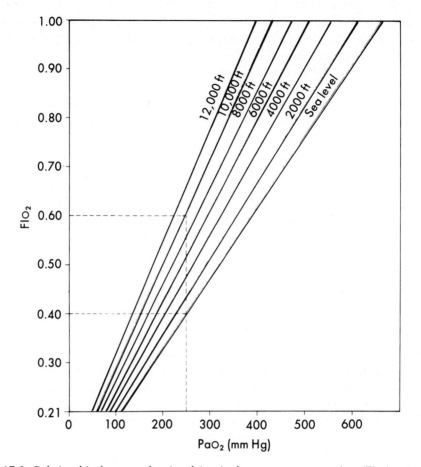

Fig. 17-3. Relationship between fractional inspired oxygen concentration (Fio_2), pressure altitude, and arterial oxygen pressure (Pao_2). This graph shows that if an Fio_2 of 0.4 is required to maintain a Pao_2 of 250 mm Hg at sea level, then an Fio_2 of 0.6 will be required at an altitude of 9000 ft to maintain the same Pao_2.

From Ferrara A, Harin A: *Emergency transfer of the high-risk neonate,* St Louis, 1980, Mosby–Year Book.

that are different from the usual intensive care setting. These characteristics must be initially recognized, thoroughly understood, and incorporated into the plan of care.

Gravitational forces and turbulence

When an aircraft changes speed (as in landing and taking off) or turns, the body experiences a gravitational force. Turbulence is experienced when there are rapid changes in wind speed and direction, either horizontally or vertically. Both of these factors have implications for patient care and team comfort, with safety being a top priority. People or equipment that are not secured quickly become projectiles when an increased gravitational force or turbulence is encountered. For this reason, all passengers are always secured to their seat or stretcher, and all equipment is secured or stored in accordance with Federal Aviation Administration (FAA) regulations.

An effect of the gravitational force is a transient blood-fluid redistribution. For instance, during aircraft takeoff, the acceleration force would be from the front to back of the plane. If the patient were lying supine, with the head to the rear of the cabin, a transient increase in venous return could occur from redistribution of blood from the legs. This phenomenon would be desirable in a patient with hypovolemic shock but contraindicated in a person with congestive heart failure, increased intracranial pressure, or an eye injury. During landing, the effects would be the reverse: the deceleration force would be from back to front. Although the practical application of this phenomenon has not been investigated, it bears consideration in aeromedical transport.

Turbulence is probably most annoying for the transport team. Turbulence may make delivery of patient care more difficult and can produce symptoms of motion sickness. Motion sickness, caused from vestibular stimulation, often results when the horizon becomes unstable or when a person sits facing backwards or sideways. Symptoms include headache, nausea, vomiting, diaphoresis, and pallor. The steps that can be taken to minimize symptoms include (1) restriction of head movement, (2) visual fixation on a stationary object, (3) loosening of restrictive clothing, (4) good ventilation, and (5) medication. Generally, prophylactic oral or transdermal medication (e.g., scopolamine) should be administered 30 to 60 minutes before flight. Once motion sickness has occurred, oral medication will be ineffective and may itself precipitate vomiting.

Vibration

Mechanical vibration is experienced to varying degrees in both ground and air ambulances. The biologic effects of mechanical vibration have been investigated primarily in military personnel. Such effects as changes in arterial blood pressure, altered respiratory function, and decreases in body temperature, with changes in peripheral nerve conduction time, have been documented. Probably more applicable to the transport team are the symptoms of headache, motion sickness, and general fatigue. Vibration also can cause monitor artifacts, making ECG and hemodynamic interpretation difficult.

Noise

The effects of noise in ICUs have been well documented. However, the noise in the transport environment has a different impact. The decibel level in ICUs has been recorded between 60 and 70 dB, whereas the decibel level in an aircraft is between 85 and 110 dB (a decibel difference is equal to a factor of two). High decibel noise over a span of time can create such symptoms as general physical discomfort, headache, and fatigue. In time, without proper protection, detectable hearing loss may occur. The use of ear plugs is encouraged if transport is by airplane or by ground ambulance when sirens may be used. Helicopter transport personnel wear either headsets or helmets to protect their hearing and to facilitate communication among team members.

The high noise level also affects patient care. As the noise level increases, conversation becomes difficult and communication is impeded. Monitor beepers and alarms are of little value because they generally are too soft to hear. In addition, blood pressure, breath sounds, and heart sounds cannot be auscultated inasmuch as the transmission from a standard stethoscope is inadequate. Alternative methods of assessment include visual inspection, monitors with digital displays, and invasive monitoring when necessary.

Space and lighting considerations

The interiors of air and ground ambulances are configured in many different ways, but they all have one characteristic in common, that is, limited space. A conventional configuration is that of having the stretcher on one side of the vehicle, a bench or seats to accommodate three persons opposite the stretcher, and a single seat at the head of the patient. There is often minimal space between the patient and the crew. Essential supplies usually are maintained in carry-on packs. Many transport vehicles are designed to store supplies and equipment securely and within reach of the care giver.

Direct lighting sources are available in the patient care areas of most transport vehicles. These sources are augmented indirectly by sunlight from the cabin windows. High-intensity spot lighting also is available on many carriers. Because patient assessment becomes more difficult at night as visual acuity decreases, it is advisable to bring a portable external light source such as a flashlight to aid visual acuity.

Electrical power and oxygen supply

In planning the care of a patient during transport, it must be remembered that the unlimited power sources in the hospital are replaced by limited and exhaustible resources during transport.

Some type of electrical power is a necessity for most types of monitoring equipment. An inverter system should be installed in the transport vehicle. The inverter converts electrical power from the vehicle's power source to power that is usable by the transport equipment. A common inverter provides 110 V of AC power at 60 Hz.

In the transfer of patients from hospital to vehicle or from vehicle to vehicle, it is imperative to have a continuous source of power. Currently, most transport equipment utilizes nickel cadmium, gel cell, or 9-V batteries. This battery power allows for continuous monitoring during entrance to and exit from the transport vehicle or during any time when electrical power is not available. Product guides generally describe battery life as averaging from 2 to 20 hours of continuous use, depending on the specific piece of equipment. The longevity of an individual battery, however, can never be absolutely confirmed before each transport. It is necessary therefore to take alternative power sources, including extra battery packs and power cords to attach to the vehicle's inverter.

Most patients who are transported require oxygen therapy, whether by nasal prongs, mask, ventilator, or bag-valve-mask ventilation. Because the patient is moved from place to place, a portable oxygen source is imperative. A standard E cylinder with regulator and flowmeter is small, easy to move, and adequate in volume. Equally efficient is the Linde Walker liquid oxygen system, which is lightweight and holds approximately 1000 liters of oxygen. Frequently, a larger, nonportable oxygen system, such as an H or M tank, can be permanently installed in the transport vehicle. This option is highly desirable for long transports or when high gas consumption is anticipated.

To ensure that an adequate amount of oxygen is taken on transport, it is essential to calculate the amount of oxygen to be used *before departure*. The equation for calculating the amount of time a cylinder will last is as follows:

$$\text{Duration (minutes)} = \frac{\text{Gauge pressure (psi)} \times \text{Gauge factor}}{\text{Liter flow per minute}}$$

The gauge pressure, indicated in pounds per square inch (psi) on the gauge dial, represents the pressure of the compressed gas in the cylinder. As the volume of gas in the cylinder decreases, so does the pressure. Therefore the number of minutes that oxygen will flow until the tank is empty is equal to the gauge pressure multiplied by the gauge factor divided by the liter flow per minute. Standard tank sizes with corresponding gauge factors follow:

Common tank sizes	Capacity (liters)	Gauge factors
E	670	0.28
M	3470	1.57
H and K	6900	3.14

EXAMPLE: If an E cylinder has a gauge pressure reading of 1800 psi and a 6 L/min liter flow is needed, the cylinder would last 84 minutes.

$$\text{Duration} = \frac{\text{Gauge pressure (psi)} \times \text{Gauge factor}}{\text{Liter flow}}$$

$$84 \text{ min} = \frac{1800 \text{ psi} \times 0.28}{6 \text{ L/min}}$$

In calculating the amount of oxygen to be taken on a transport vehicle, it is important to consider certain variables: (1) the patient's condition may be more critical than reported and hence require more oxygen; (2) the patient will require more oxygen at altitude than on the ground; (3) the patient's condition may deteriorate during transport and require more oxygen; (4) there may be unexpected travel delays necessitating a longer use of oxygen; and (5) equipment may fail, causing an unnecessary loss of gas. To avoid the potential problems associated with these variables, it is advisable to carry twice the amount of oxygen anticipated. In all cases a bag-valve-mask should be carried in the event of a total oxygen supply depletion.

TECHNIQUES IN MONITORING
Effects of Altitude on Equipment

The physical laws present in the transport environment affect not only the patient and the team but also the equipment used. Boyle's law is of the most concern. Briefly restated, as altitude increases and barometric pressure decreases, the volume of a gas will expand. This law has a direct impact on any equipment with trapped air space, including Foley catheter balloons, endotracheal tube cuffs, air splints, pulmonary artery (PA) catheter balloons, IV bottles, and pneumatic trousers.

Intravenous solutions in plastic bags rather than glass bottles are suggested for use on transport for several reasons. First, the flow rate of IV solutions in either glass or plastic alters considerably because of the pressure changes during aircraft ascent or descent. However, the effects on the flow rate are considerably greater with glass containers. Second, glass bottles break easily during turbulence or movement. Finally, glass bottles are difficult to pack and require more space in supply boxes.

Special precautions also are necessary for other equipment with air-filled spaces. Circulation in the extremities should be checked frequently in patients with pneumatic trousers or air splints in place. Consideration should be given to deflating Foley catheter balloons on reaching altitude and reinflating on landing.

Endotracheal tube cuffs pose a special problem. Because cuff expansion at altitude can cause tracheal mucosal damage, a slight cuff deflation is advisable on ascent. During descent, however, an endotracheal tube leak may result that is inaudible because of background noise. Endotracheal tubes with high–residual volume cuffs and those with foam cuffs partially overcome these concerns.

PA catheter balloons require the injection of approximately 1 to 1.5 cc of air for placement in the wedge position. If the balloon remains inflated during ascent to 10,000 feet, this amount of air will expand 1.5 times, or from 1.5 to 2.25 cc, possibly causing balloon rupture and PA damage or rupture. Therefore it is important that the balloon of the catheter be completely deflated and the PA waveform be continuously monitored during ascent.

Criteria for Selecting Transport Equipment

The criteria for evaluating the applicability of equipment for the transport environment are different from those used in the ICU. Equipment must be capable of functioning in the rugged and unpredictable environment of transport. All transport equipment must be able to withstand severe mechanical, thermal, and electrical stresses, constant vibration, and changes in atmospheric pressure.

Four general guidelines can be used in evaluating equipment for critical care transport. The first guideline is that the equipment must be portable because it is both moved from vehicle to vehicle and carried alongside the patient. A dependable battery is crucial for continuous, uninterrupted monitoring when AC power is unavailable or impractical. The second criterion is that the equipment be of reasonable size and weight. Ease of movement remains important, and allowance for the limited space within the transport vehicle also is considered. The third guideline ensures that transport equipment has full intensive care monitoring capability. To provide continuous critical care services between institutions, intensive care standards must be maintained. Provision should be made for direct arterial pressure, PA pressure, and central venous pressure monitoring, as well as for multiple drug infusions. Finally, transport equipment must be reliable and durable. Optimum care and safety of the patient depend on equipment that functions during all the events encountered during transport. In addition, equipment must be durable enough to withstand the knocks and jolts that are inevitable during transport. Proper equipment is vital to the effective transport of any patient. Team members must have confidence in its reliability, a thorough knowledge of its operation, and an understanding of its limitations.

Equipment Options
Cardiac monitor

As alluded to earlier, the cardiac monitor used during transport must provide the level of hemodynamic monitoring necessitated by the patient's medical condition. A number of multiple function transport systems are now available that allow the clinician to monitor arterial, PA, and venous pressures, as well as the ECG (Fig. 17-4). The oscilloscope and digital numbers must be easily read and impervious to vibration and movement that can cause annoying artifacts. Calibration and zeroing of the channels must be uncomplicated and quick. Finally, the battery must be reliable, have at least 2 hours of power, and require a minimal amount of recharging time once depleted.

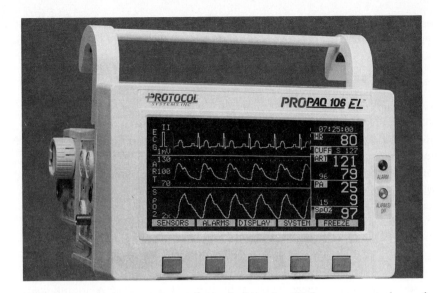

Fig. 17-4 A typical transport monitor allows display of multiple pressures and waveforms. (*ECG,* Electrocardiogram; *ART,* arterial; *Sp*o_2, pulse oximetry; *PA,* pulmonary artery.)

Noninvasive blood pressure monitoring

Multiple-channel monitors often can accommodate other functions, including noninvasive blood pressure monitoring. Single-function units reproduce the patient's systolic and diastolic blood pressure, as well as pulse rate, by means of digital display. The noninvasive blood pressure monitor is useful for observing trends in the hemodynamic status but for the critically ill patient should serve as an adjunct to arterial and PA monitoring. It is important to note that this type of noninvasive measurement may be more susceptible to vibration from the aircraft or ambulance and occasionally displays erroneous readings. Noninvasive blood pressures also may be taken by use of Doppler amplification or by palpation of the distal upper extremity artery with a sphygmomanometer and cuff.

Pulse oximetry

Perhaps no other physiologic system is affected by the transport environment as acutely as the respiratory system. Pulse oximetry allows for continuous monitoring of respiratory stability by rapidly and noninvasively measuring the patient's arterial oxygen saturation. The use of oximetry thus enables the team to recognize hypoxia and assess the effectiveness of oxygen therapy. The oximeter may be part of a multiple-function monitor or may be a battery-powered self-contained unit. The pulse oximeter most often provides a digital display of the patient's arterial oxygen saturation level and heart rate.

Capnometry

End-tidal carbon dioxide (CO_2) monitoring is being used increasingly in the transport environment to assess the placement of the endotracheal tube and monitor the adequacy of ventilation. Capnometry is a noninvasive mode of monitoring that measures the partial pressure of end-tidal CO_2. Some monitors can calculate the amount of CO_2 in the patient's expired air and provide a digital display and waveform. Other CO_2 devices use a color detector that indicates CO_2 concentrations.

Defibrillator

Consistent with critical care standards, the ability to deliver electrical countershock should be available for all transported patients. In addition, a defibrillator with an oscilloscope can be used in place of the cardiac monitor when pressure monitoring is not necessary, thus decreasing the amount of equipment that is taken. The defibrillator should be simple to operate, require a minimal number of steps to energize the paddles, and have a strip recorder to document ECG tracings. The batteries must be easily interchangeable, easily stored, and of sufficient capacity to deliver 20 to 30 countershocks at maximal joules if necessary.

Defibrillation is accomplished routinely in the air and ground transport environments and employs the standard countershock precautions. Defibrillation precautions in transport include following advanced cardiac life support defibrillation standards for selecting energy levels, appropriate paddle placement, and cautionary measures in countershock delivery.

Semonin-Holleran et al. discuss the use of integrated monitoring systems that allow a defibrillator to be attached to an existing monitor. These augmented systems use special pads that provide hands-off defibrillation, as well as external pacing and cardiac monitoring. These advances are particularly well-suited for the transport setting, inasmuch as they provide a measure of safety in the close proximity of the patient care area.

Cardiac output computer

If the patient's condition warrants the presence of a PA catheter, cardiac output measurement is valuable in evaluating the patient's hemodynamic status before transport. Cardiac output values usually are obtained at the referring facility, as well as on arrival at the receiving hospital. However, some output computers are small enough to be carried during transport and are particularly useful when the transit time will extend over several hours.

The technique involved in measuring cardiac output by the thermodilution method is described elsewhere in this text. The technique used during transport is similar to that used in the ICUs. Cardiac output measurements should not be taken during periods of turbulence or excessive vibration.

Intraaortic balloon pump

Critical care transport has evolved to a level at which the patient who requires intraaortic balloon counterpulsation may safely and efficiently be transferred from one hospital to another. This type of transport is becoming increasingly more common as patients with acute cardiac decompensation are being moved to tertiary centers for cardiovascular treatment modalities unavailable in the smaller hospitals.

The counterpulsation system for transport generally involves four units: the pump console, the monitor, the drive gas for the pump, and the battery pack. The components are either secured to the floor of the transport carrier with belts or to a frame configured with a locking mechanism. Balloon pumps designed specifically for transport generally are smaller, lighter-weight units that can be moved simultaneously with the patient with relative ease.

It is imperative that the transport vehicle have an electrical inverter in place to serve as the primary power source for the balloon pump. Different pump models have different amperage requirements and place varying demands on the carrier's electrical system. It is vital that the capability of the electrical inverter and the power requirements of the balloon pump be evaluated before the use of the system during an actual patient transport. Auxiliary power sources, including battery pack and ancillary drive gas cylinders, should be available in the event the inverter cannot function properly.

The effects of altitude on balloon counterpulsation have been evaluated in a limited number of studies. Kramer and Snow observed that although the distensibility of an elastic balloon may be affected by altitude, the atmospheric pressure changes most probably would not affect the function or size of a nonelastic intraaortic balloon. It is important, however, to note that as altitude increases, there may be potential for volume expansion in the enclosed gas system. The capability of pneumatic systems varies by product, but it generally is advisable to complete precautionary filling cycles on ascent and descent, as well as incrementally, until pressurization has been achieved or, in the case of rotor wing aircraft, flight altitude has been reached.

If the patient is to be transported by air, it is important to notify the pilot as to the planned departure so that the reconfiguration of the aircraft can take place. This rearrangement of the patient care area accommodates the increased equipment and personnel. It is further necessary to allot adequate time so that the pilot can complete the necessary weight and balance calculations and confirm that all equipment has been adequately secured.

Coordination of multiple resources is required to ensure that this type of transport is successfully completed. In addition to equipment requirements, additional personnel such as balloon pump specialists are included on the medical team. In the close confines of transport, it is essential that the team members understand their respective patient care responsibilities and how to function in the moving environment. Support staff personnel should be available to assist in providing safe entrance and egress from all transport vehicles. Because of the complexities of transporting patients who require the use of the balloon pump, serious consideration should be given to utilizing only those teams experienced in the use of such therapies in transport.

Intravenous lines and infusion pumps

The critically ill patient who is transported often has in place a number of intravenous lines for fluid and drug administration. When the patient is moved or when the IV fluid must be hung a short distance above the patient, as in an aircraft or ambulance, the infusion rate may vary.

When accurate or limited infusions are indicated, a pumping device should be employed. As with other transport equipment, infusion pumps should be lightweight and portable. Battery power usually depends on the rate of flow as well as the duration of use. It is advisable to have a power cord available to use with the carrier's electrical inverter should the battery power be insufficient or malfunction.

The pump's visual display should be easily readable and the infusion settings uncomplicated and quickly alterable. Visual alarms should be augmented by the standard audio alarm. Ideally these pumps should inform the care giver of the reason for the alarm (e.g., a digital display indicating that there is "air in the line"). Many of the new transport pumps have this feature available.

There now are multichannel infusion pumps that can accommodate two to three individual infusions. These new pumps are valuable in transport because they eliminate the need to carry several infusion devices. Most infusion devices have specific tubing requirements. However, the infusion cartridge or tubing may be adaptable to standard microdrip or macrodrip chamber tubing, thus minimizing the time necessary to transfer multiple IV lines before transport.

Syringe pumps are most commonly used for neonatal and pediatric transports, but they also may be used for the adult patient who requires a drug infusion that is given in small doses—in which the increments must be closely observed. Syringe pumps often accommodate several sizes of syringes and require only the attachment of standard extension tubing.

A pressure bag frequently is used for lines through which fluid must be given rapidly. It is applied to the IV bag in the same fashion as in the ICU. However, caution should be taken in using the device in the air transport environment. Because the pressure bag is an air-filled container, it is subject to the effects of altitude previously discussed in this chapter. As the aircraft ascends, the volume of air in the pressure bag will increase, which may result in the fluids infusing faster than anticipated or the infusion bag emptying completely. Because it is often difficult to ascertain the fluid level of the enclosed IV bag, these effects may go unnoticed and create untoward effects for the patient. In the case of the trauma patient who receives large amounts of fluid through large-bore catheters, such cautionary notes may be of less significance.

Pulmonary artery and arterial lines

Comprehensive monitoring during transport frequently requires the use of a PA catheter and an arterial catheter. The methods, techniques, and problems associated with using these catheters have been thoroughly discussed elsewhere in this book; these facts certainly apply during transport. Disposable pressure tubing and transducers have made it possible to provide invasive monitoring systems that are similar to those used in the ICU. In the transport setting it is necessary to keep such monitoring systems relatively uncomplicated because of limited space and increased movement of the patient during transfer between vehicles.

The PA and arterial catheters must be well-secured to avoid accidental dislodging during frequent movement or turbulence. As in the ICU the infusions to these lines should be continuous to ensure catheter patency. Continuous infusion may be provided by use of a moderately inflated pressure bag or an infusion pump. The infusion pump is used most often in pediatric patients whose infusion rates must be minimal and accurate. Finally, the transducer-reference port must be kept at right atrial (RA) level for accurate measurement. Taping the transducer-reference port to the patient's side is one method of securing it during transport.

Patient Care

Preparation for transport begins at the time of the referral of the patient. The first issue to be addressed is whether or not the patient should be transported. The answer is obtained by a consultation between the referring and receiving physicians and the transport team responsible for the patient's care. The variables involved include the following: (1) the severity and acuteness of the patient's illness, (2) whether the patient's condition can be stabilized before transport, (3) the modes of transport and the types of transport carriers available, (4) the anticipated interhospital transport time, and (5) the capability of the available transport team. The physiologic factors relating to air and surface transport discussed earlier in this chapter need to be considered as well. Compensation for the effects of transport on the patient can be achieved, provided the transport program personnel are aware of specific problems and can manage them properly.

The patient should be under the care of the transport team during the entire transport process. Transfer of patient care responsibilities under other circumstances—for example, at an airport after deplaning—is strongly discouraged. Continuity of patient care may be jeopardized in such circumstances in which the transfer of a patient is not accomplished in the hospital environment. Except in the most unusual circumstances, the patient's condition can be stabilized with the therapies provided in the referring hospital. Usually, major new therapies do not have to be initiated during the transport. Patients suffering from cardiogenic shock and/or severe and unstable respiratory insufficiency will not tolerate movement well.

Patient stabilization before transport may include the following: (1) the treatment of shock with the administration of blood and other replacement parenteral solutions and the use of cardioactive agents, (2) the treatment of respiratory insufficiency with the initiation of endotracheal intubation and assisted ventilation, and (3) the insertion of indwelling arterial, venous, and PA catheters.

Serious consideration should be given to inserting an endotracheal tube before transport in patients who (1) are in borderline respiratory insufficiency requiring oxygen by mask or prongs or (2) have a compromised cardiac output resulting from increased work of breathing. With the endotracheal tube in place, assisted ventilation can be controlled more easily. Insertion of an endotracheal tube in a moving environment with limited working space is fraught with problems.

The multifactor respiratory influences of oxygenation, ventilation, and the work of breathing on the cardiovascular and neurologic systems mandate that patients who require assisted ventilation be carefully assessed before transport. Because the transport team frequently has to change the ventilator settings during their initial management of the patient in the referring hospital, patients with severe respiratory insufficiency, central nervous system disease, or an unstable cardiovascular system may require further stabilization measures before transport.

The same considerations taken into account for an endotracheal tube also apply to the insertion of central venous, PA, and arterial lines. These lines should be inserted before leaving the referring hospital whenever there is anticipated need. Dependable and secure means of providing IV fluids and monitoring the cardiovascular system are essential during transport. It is essential that flow through these lines be free enough to withstand the frequent changes in gravity that occur in the transport environment as a result of movement of the patient in and out of ambulance carriers and through hospitals. A continuous infusion system ensures the patency of the lines. In addition, all lines must be securely taped at the insertion site and at the connection points to prevent dislodgment or disconnection. These lines experience a greater amount of tension than most. Accurate labeling of IV bags and IV tubing close to the patient decreases confusion in the limited space.

It is essential that critically ill patients be observed closely for signs of clinical change (specifically deterioration) from the moment the actual transport begins to the time the patient's care is transferred to another team within a hospital facility. The clinical changes of particular concern relate to the cardiovascular and pulmonary systems. Patients in shock can become hypotensive when moved. Cardiac arrest is not uncommon under such circumstances if the shock state has not been carefully evaluated and reversed before movement. Continuous monitoring of the ECG and direct arterial pressure is essential in such patients. Measurement of the CVP and/or PA pressure also is important.

Respiratory insufficiency can easily be accentuated during transport by (1) inadvertent changes in assisted ventilation, (2) changes in the ambient oxygen concentration that are not compensated for, (3) catastrophic changes such as endobronchial intubation or pneumothorax, or (4) gravitational factors and factors associated with surface and airplane movement. Because of the dynamic state of their pathophysiologic condition, patients with respiratory insufficiency are prone to changes in their clinical state even if transport is not under way.

Patient assessment in the transport environment, although somewhat different from that in the ICU, is not impossible. A thorough baseline clinical assessment and reliable monitoring techniques are essential. The patient's clinical status may be evaluated noninvasively by assessing the pulse rate, blood pressure, capillary refill, mentation, urinary output, and skin temperature. Although the noise level precludes the use of auscultation, meaningful data can be obtained by palpation and visualization. For example, inasmuch as breath sounds cannot be heard, increased respiratory effort is assessed by visualizing the respiratory muscles and feeling chest expansion. Recognizing the limitations of the environment and planning for them decrease many potential problems.

Placement of the patient, the transport team, and the equipment in the transport vehicle must allow for the appropriate care of the patient. It is useless to take a full complement of team members if they all cannot participate in patient care during transport. Potential clinical problems must be anticipated before loading the vehicle. For example, a patient with recurrent ventricular tachycardia would certainly require a defibrillator and antidysrhythmic drugs in close proximity. Likewise, the team member most proficient at airway management would sit at the head of a patient with respiratory insufficiency. Oxygen, suction, and ventilatory support would be readily available.

The impact of transport on the patient's disease state should not be underestimated. The rigors of the transport environment can easily threaten the status of a patient with a tenuous clinical condition. With adequate preparation at the referring hospital and careful monitoring and attention to patient care during transport, the necessary level and quality of patient care can be delivered.

REFERENCES

Alfaro R: Pneumatic anti-shock trousers: when and how to use them, *Dimens Crit Care Nurs* 1:9, 1982.

Armstrong HG: *Principles and practices of aviation medicine*, Baltimore, 1979, Williams & Wilkins.

Barger J: Strategic aeromedical evacuation: the

inaugural flight, *Aviat Space Environ Med* 57:613-616, 1986.

Birnbaum ML: Prehospital and interhospital transport of adults. In Shoemaker WC et al editors: *Textbook of critical care,* Philadelphia, 1989, WB Saunders.

Bureau of Medicine and Surgery: *United States naval flight surgeon's manual,* ed 2, Washington, DC, 1978, US Government Printing Office.

Clark JG et al: Initial cardiovascular response to low-frequency whole body vibration in humans and animals, *Aerosp Med* 38:464-467, 1967.

Darga AF, Kline EM: Cardiovascular emergencies. In Lee G, editor: *Flight nursing: principles and practice,* St Louis, 1991, Mosby–Year Book.

Dhenin G: *Aviation medicine: health and clinical aspects,* London, 1978, Tri-Med, Ltd.

Dhenin G: *Aviation medicine: physiology and human factors,* London, 1978, Tri-Med, Ltd.

Egan DF: *Fundamentals of respiratory therapy,* ed 3, St Louis, 1977, Mosby–Year Book.

Ehrenwerth J, Sorbo S, Hackel A: Transport of critically ill adults, *Crit Care Med* 14:543-547, 1986.

Ernsting J: Prevention of hypoxia: acceptable compromises, *Aviat Space Environ Med* 49: 495-502, 1978.

Floyd WN, Brodersen AB, Goodno JG: Effect of whole body vibration on peripheral nerve conduction time in the rhesus monkey, *Aerosp Med* 44:281-285, 1973.

Hackel A, editor: Critical care transport, *Int Anesthiol Clin* 25(2), 1987.

Hansen PJ: Air transport of the man who needs everything, *Aviat Space Environ Med* 51:725-728, 1980.

Hart HW: The conveyance of patients to and from the hospital, 1720-1850, *Med History* 22:397-407, 1978.

Henry JN, Krenis LJ, Cutting RT: Hypoxemia during aeromedical evacuation, *Surg Gynecol Obstet* 136:49-53, 1973.

Hoffman JR: External counterpressure and the MAST suit: current and future roles, *Ann Emerg Med* 9:419-421, 1980.

Icenogle TB et al: Long distance transport of cardiac patients in extremis: the mobile intensive care

(MOBI) concept, *Aviat Space Environ Med* 59:571-574, 1988.

Johnson A: Treatise on aeromedical evacuation: I. Administration and some medical considerations, *Aviat Space Environ Med* 48:546-549, 1977.

Johnson A: Treatise on aeromedical evacuation: II. Some surgical considerations, *Aviat Space Environ Med* 48:550-554, 1977.

Kramer RP, Snow NJ: Technical considerations for transporting patients by air ambulance with intra-aortic balloon pumps, *J Extracorporeal Technol* 18:145-150, 1986.

McNeil EL: *Airborne care of the ill and injured,* New York, 1983, Springer-Verlag.

McSwain N: Pneumatic trousers and the management of shock, *J Trauma* 17:719-724, 1977.

Noise, hearing damage, and fatigue in general aviation pilots, AC No. 91-35, Washington, DC, 1972, Department of Transportation, Federal Aviation Administration.

Oxer HF: Carriage by air of the seriously ill, *Med J Aust* 64:537-540, 1977.

Parsons CJ, Bobechko WP: Aeromedical transport: its hidden problems, *Can Med Assoc J* 126: 237-243, 1982.

Poulton RJ, Kisicki P: Physiologic monitoring during civilian air medical transport, *Aviat Space Environ Med* 58:367-369, 1987.

Semonin-Holleran RS, Rouse M: Biomedical technology: using it during patient transport, *J Air Med Transport* 10:7-12, 1991.

Shenai JP: Sound levels for neonates in transit, *J Pediatrics* 90:811-812, 1977.

Shenai JP, Johnson GE, Varney RV: Mechanical vibration in neonatal transport, *Pediatrics* 68: 55-57, 1981.

Spearman C, Sheldon R: *Egan's fundamentals of respiratory therapy,* ed 4, St Louis, 1977, Mosby–Year Book.

Stoner DL, Cooke JP: Intratracheal cuffs and aeromedical evacuation, *Anesthesiology* 41:302-306, 1974.

United States Naval Flight Surgeon's Manual, ed 2, The Bureau of Medicine and Surgery, 1978.

West JB: *Respiratory physiology: the essentials,* ed 2, Baltimore, 1979, Williams & Wilkins.

Appendix A

Abbreviations

AMI	Acute myocardial infarction	LV dp/dt	Rate of left ventricular pressure rise (mm Hg/sec)
Ao	Aorta		
Ao dp/dt	Rate of aortic pressure rise (mm Hg/sec)	LVEDP	Left ventricular end-diastolic pressure
AV	Atrioventricular	LVSWI	Left ventricular stroke work index
a-v	Arteriovenous		
a-v Do_2	Arteriovenous oxygen difference	MAP	Mean arterial pressure
		$M\dot{D}o_2$	Myocardial oxygen supply
Cao_2	Oxygen content in arterial blood	MI	Myocardial infarction
		$M\dot{V}o_2$	Myocardial oxygen consumption
CI	Cardiac index		
CO	Cardiac output	O_2ER	Oxygen extraction ratio
CPAP	Continuous positive airway pressure	PA	Pulmonary artery
		$P(A - a)o_2$	Alveolar-arterial oxygen pressure difference
Cvo_2	Oxygen content in venous blood	$Paco_2$	Partial pressure of carbon dioxide in arterial blood
CVP	Central venous pressure		
$\dot{D}o_2$	Oxygen delivery per minute	PAd	Pulmonary artery diastolic
$\dot{D}o_{2\ crit}$	Critical level of oxygen delivery per minute	PAEDP	Pulmonary artery end-diastolic pressure
EF	Ejection fraction	PAo_2	Partial pressure of oxygen in alveolus
FA	Femoral artery		
Fio_2	Fractional inspired oxygen concentration	Pao_2	Partial pressure of oxygen in arterial blood
HR	Heart rate	PAW	Pulmonary artery wedge
IABP	Intraaortic balloon pump	Pco_2	Carbon dioxide pressure
IVC	Inferior vena cava	PDA	Patent ductus arteriosus
LA	Left atrium/atrial	PEEP	Positive end-expiratory pressure
LLSB	Lower left sternal border		
LV	Left ventricle/vetricular		

PMI	Point of maximal impulse (of left ventricle on precordium)	RVSWI	Right ventricular stroke work index
P_{O_2}	Oxygen pressure	Sa_{O_2}	Oxygen saturation of hemoglobin in arterial blood
PVC	Premature ventricular contraction	SEP	Systolic ejection period (sec/min)
Pv_{O_2}	Partial pressure of venous oxygen	SV	Stroke volume
PVR	Pulmonary vascular resistance	SVC	Superior vena cava
RA	Right atrium/atrial	Sv_{O_2}	Oxygen saturation of hemoglobin in venous blood
RV	Right ventricle/ventricular	$S\bar{v}_{O_2}$	Mixed venous (PA) oxygen saturation
RVEDP	Right ventricular end-diastolic pressure	SVR	Systemic vascular resistance
RVEDV	Right ventricular end-diastolic volume	$TcPa_{O_2}$	Transcutaneous partial pressure of oxygen in arterial blood
RVEF	Right ventricular ejection fraction	$\dot{V}_{O_2}$	Oxygen consumption per minute
RVESV	Right ventricular end-systolic volume		

Dot over a letter indicates per unit of time.

Appendix B

Normal Resting Values

Site	Pressure range	Oxygen saturation (%)
Superior vena cava (a/v/m)	<8/<8/2 to 6	60-75
Right atrium (a/v/m)	<8/<8/2 to 6	60-75
Right ventricle (sys/dias/end-dias)	15 to 30/0 to 5/2 to 6	60-75
Pulmonary artery (sys/dias/m)	15 to 30/10 to 15/10 to 20	60-75
Pulmonary artery wedge (a/v/m)	<12 to 15/<12 to 15/4 to 12	99
Left atrium (a/v/m)	<12 to 15/<12 to 15/4 to 12	95-99
Left ventricle (sys/dias/end-dias)	100 to 140/0 to 5/5 to 12	95-99
Aorta (sys/dias/m)	100 to 140/60 to 80/70 to 100	95-99

Measurement	Units	Range
Cardiac output	L/min	4-8
Cardiac index	L/min/m^2	2.5-4
Stroke volume	ml/beat	60-130
Stroke index	ml/beat/m^2	35-70
Oxygen consumption	ml/min	200-300
	ml/min/m^2	120-130
Oxygen delivery	ml/min	750-1000
Oxygen extraction ratio	%	22-32
Arteriovenous oxygen difference	vol %	3-5.5
Pa_{O_2}	mm Hg	95-100
Pv_{O_2}	mm Hg	40
Pa_{CO_2}	mm Hg	38-42
Plasma HCO_3	mEq/L	23-25
pH	—	7.38-7.42
Pulmonary vascular resistance	units	<2
	dynes/sec/cm^{-5}	30-180
Systemic vascular resistance	units	15-20
	dynes/sec/cm^{-5}	900-1400
Ca_{O_2}	vol%	18-20
Cv_{O_2}	vol%	14-16
Ejection fraction (left heart)	%	58-75
(right heart)	%	40-55
Sa_{O_2}	%	95-100
Sv_{O_2}	%	60-75

a, a wave; v, v wave; m, mean pressure; *sys*, systolic; *dias*, diastolic; *end-dias*, end-diastolic.

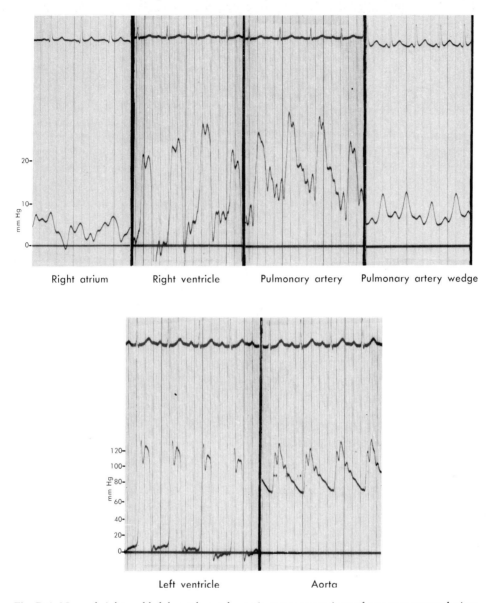

Fig. B-1. Normal right and left heart hemodynamic pressure tracings of a person at rest during spontaneous respiration.

Appendix C
Dubois Body Surface Charts

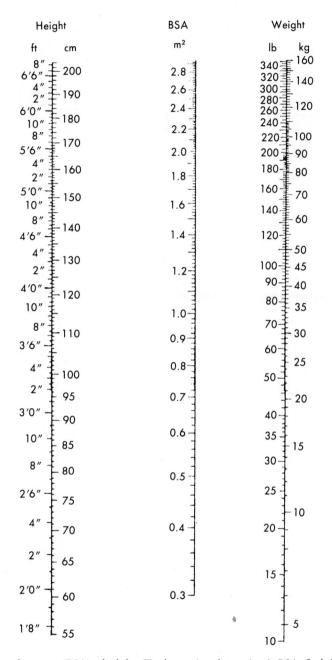

Fig. C-1. Body surface area (BSA) of adults. To determine the patient's BSA, find the patient's height in either feet or centimeters in the left column and the patient's weight in pounds or kilograms in the right column. Connect these two points with a ruler. The BSA is indicated at the point where the ruler crosses the middle column.

From DuBois EF: *Basal metabolism in health and disease*, ed 3, Philadelphia, 1936, Lea & Febiger.

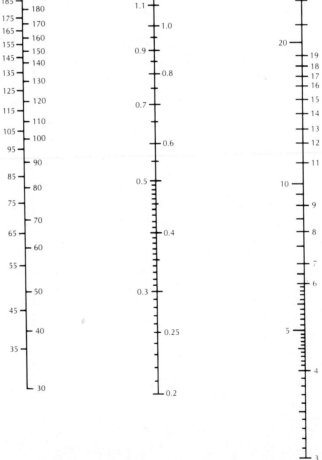

Fig. C-2. Nomogram to determine body surface area (BSA) in children.

Redrawn from Cole CH, editor: *The Harriet Lane handbook*, Chicago, 1984, Mosby–Year Book; based on data from Gelian EA, George SL: *Cancer Chemother Rep* 54:225, 1970.

Appendix D

Nursing Diagnoses and Patient Care Plans for Patients Undergoing Hemodynamic Monitoring

NURSING DIAGNOSIS: 1. Decreased Cardiac Output

Goals	Nursing intervention(s)	Rationale
Patient will demonstrate optimal hemodynamic function: CI 2.5-4 L/min/m^2 PAEDP/PAWm or LAm 10-20 mm Hg RAm 4-8 mm Hg MAP 70-80 mm Hg HR 50-100 beats per min without ectopy SVR 900-1400 dynes/sec/cm^{-5} PVR <180 dynes/sec/cm^{-5} Normal arterial blood gases Normal hemoglobin level Urinary output ≥40 ml/hr Svo$_2$ 60%-77% Oxygen delivery to tissues ≥1000 ml/min	Monitor preload (RA and PAEDP, PAW, or LAm) and administer appropriate fluids and medications as ordered.	Optimize preload to ↑ systolic ejection according to Starling's Law.
	Measure CO and CI and calculate SVR and PVR. Administer appropriate medications as ordered. Plot ventricular function curves.	High afterload → ↓ CO
	Calculate LVSWI and RVSWI. Administer appropriate medications as ordered.	High LVSWI or RVSWI → ↑ heart work and MV̇o$_2$.
	Monitor ECG for rate, rhythm, and ectopy, and determine patient's hemodynamic response to changes in rate or rhythm. Treat according to protocol. Implement emergency measures as necessary.	Very fast heart rates may ↓ ventricular filling and, thus, SV. Very slow heart rates (< 50) may → inadequate CO (CO = HR × SV). Dysrhythmias reduce CO.
	Physically assess patient (vital signs, heart and lung sounds, skin color and temperature, fluid balance, mentation, and jugular vein distention), and report any significant changes.	Baseline heart and lung sounds necessary to determine onset of changes associated with cardiac abnormality; ↓ mentation or ↑ restlessness may be early indication of ↓ CO.
	Measure arterial blood gases and Hgb levels and report significant changes. Administer appropriate therapy as ordered.	Optimize O$_2$ delivery by maintaining CO, Sao$_2$ and Hgb at normal levels.
	Measure hourly urine output and report if <30 ml/hr.	To assess renal perfusion and function and prevent dysfunction resulting from ischemia.
	Measure Svo$_2$ and report reductions of 10% for 2-3 min or if <60%.	Decrease in Svo$_2$ indicates decreased tissue perfusion. Svo$_2$ < 60% associated with poor prognosis.
	Reduce patient's activity and stress.	Reduced activity and stress will decrease O$_2$ demands.
	Relaxation techniques	

NURSING DIAGNOSIS: 2. Altered Peripheral Tissue Perfusion Related to Compromised Circulation Associated with Invasive Monitoring

Goals	Nursing intervention(s)	Rationale

Patient will demonstrate:
  Optimal skin integrity
  Normal skin color and temperature
  Equal arterial pulses in all extremities
	Assess catheter insertion site daily; cleanse site, apply iodophor ointment and new sterile dressing.
	Assess skin color, temperature and sensitivity in area around catheter insertion site. Report any significant changes.
		Inflammation at catheter insertion site associated with infection and/or thrombophlebitis.
		Alteration in tissue perfusion may result in ↑ in skin temperature below catheter site. An ↑ in skin temperature with pain or tenderness is associated with thrombosis or thrombophlebitis.

	Palpate and compare pulses in each extremity. Report any changes.	A ↓ or loss in arterial pulsations distal to catheter insertion site is associated with arterial insufficiency caused by thrombus formation.
	Assess characterized extremity for evidence of edema by measuring opposite extremity at the same anatomic location.	Edema is characteristic manifestation of ↓ tissue perfusion caused by venous interference.

NURSING DIAGNOSIS: 3. Potential for Infection Related to Invasive Monitoring

Patient will be free of infection as demonstrated by:
  Normal temperature
  Normal WBC
  Negative cultures of blood or catheter tip
	Check patient's temperature every 4 hr and as needed, and report any significant changes.
	Change catheter and catheter site every 4 days.
	
	Change IV fluid, tubing, stopcocks, and transducer every 48-72 hr.
	Inspect and cleanse catheter insertion site every day, and apply iodophor ointment and clean sterile dressing.
	Do not use IV solution containing glucose.
		Increase in patient's temperature associated with infectious process.
		
		Risk of infection increases with duration of catheter placement >5 days.
		Static fluid potential source for bacterial growth.
		
		Skin and old blood are potential sources for infection. Iodophor ointment reduces bacterial growth.
		Glucose solutions promote growth of bacteria.

NURSING DIAGNOSIS: 3. Potential for Infection Related to Invasive Monitoring—cont'd

Goals	Nursing intervention(s)	Rationale
	Place sterile dead-ender caps on all stopcocks.	Open stopcock port allows bacteria to enter.
	Use aseptic technique when withdrawing from or flushing the catheter.	Prevent contamination of open system.
	Use closed system blood withdrawal device.	Minimize opening of system and collection of old blood.
	Carefully remove all traces of blood from stopcock ports after obtaining blood sample from catheter.	Old blood promotes growth of bacteria.
	Use sterile plastic catheter sleeve over PA catheter.	Maintain external portion of catheter sterile to permit catheter advancement, if necessary.
	Use closed system for CO injectate.	Minimize opening of system.
	Use catheters with antimicrobial coating.	

NURSING DIAGNOSIS: 4. Potential for Injury Related to (A) Hemorrhage, (B) Thromboemboli, (C) Venous Air Embolism, (D) Pulmonary Infarction or Hemorrhage, or (E) Cardiac Dysrhythmias or Conduction Disturbances

Goals	Nursing intervention(s)	Rationale
A. Patient will remain without hemorrhage	Keep all catheter connecting sites visible, and observe frequently for possible hemorrhage.	Major blood loss can occur without notice from stopcocks or loose connections that are hidden beneath dressings or bed linens.
	Tighten all catheter connecting sites and stopcocks every 4 hr and as needed.	Plastic connections become loose over time and leakage can occur.
	Restrain patient, if necessary.	A restless or confused patient may pull catheter out, or connecting tubing apart.

NURSING DIAGNOSIS: 4. Potential for Injury Related to (A) Hemorrhage, (B) Thromboemboli, (C) Venous Air Embolism, (D) Pulmonary Infarction or Hemorrhage, or (E) Cardiac Dysrhythmias or Conduction Disturbances—cont'd

Goals	Nursing intervention(s)	Rationale
	After removal of arterial catheter, apply firm pressure to insertion site for 10 min before checking and applying pressure dressing.	Allow clot to form at insertion site to seal vessel opening.
	Discontinue systemic heparinization several hours before catheter or sheath removal.	
B. Patient will remain without thrombus as evidenced by: Patent catheter Unimpeded infusion or flush Undamped waveform with adequate dynamic response	Use heparinized IV solution with continuous flush device to continuously infuse all catheter ports and sideport of sheath, if used.	Continuous forward flow and use of heparin is associated with ↓ thrombus formation at catheter top or around catheter in sheath.
	Always aspirate and discard before gently flushing any catheter. If unable to aspirate, do not flush catheter. Periodically aspirate and manually flush catheter or activate flush device (every 4-6 hr).	Remove any fibrin or clot from within or at tip of catheter to prevent injection of clot material. Forward movement of heparinized fluid prevents clot formation.
	Do not fast flush arterial catheter longer than 2 sec; manually flush arterial catheter by gently tapping plunger of flush syringe with no more than 2-4 ml fluid.	Vigorous flushing of arterial catheter with large amounts of fluid can result in cerebral embolization.
	Maintain 300 mm Hg pressure on infusion bag.	300 mg Hg ± required to maintain forward flow of heparinized solution via flush device.
	Remove all traces of blood from catheter, tubing, and stopcocks after withdrawing blood; flush completely.	Residual blood in catheter, tubing, or stopcock can form small clots that can occlude catheter or be injected into patient.

NURSING DIAGNOSIS: 4. Potential for Injury Related to (A) Hemorrhage, (B) Thromboemboli, (C) Venous Air Embolism, (D) Pulmonary Infarction or Hemorrhage, or (E) Cardiac Dysrhythmias or Conduction Disturbances — cont'd

Goals	Nursing intervention(s)	Rationale
C. Patient will remain without venous air embolism	Tighten all catheter connecting sites and stop-cocks every 4 hr and as needed; check frequently.	Plastic connections become loose over time permitting intake of air into system.
	Place dead-ender caps on all stopcock ports.	Open or vented ports permit intake of air.
	Keep all connections or possible openings into system below level of heart.	Air intake more likely to occur through loose connection or open port when patient is in an upright position and takes a deep breath.
	Remove all air from IV solution bag.	Air in bag and solution can enter tubing and catheter.
	Have patient hum or suspend respirations when vascular system is open and near or above heart level.	Air intake through open port occurs during inspiration.
	After removal of venous catheter that was in place for a long period of time, apply petrolatum and occlusive dressing to insertion site.	Air intake can occur through the open tract formed by long-dwelling catheter, especially in thin person with little subcutaneous tissue.
D. Patient will be free of pulmonary infarction or hemorrhage as evidence by: Normal respirations No hemoptysis Normal ABG values Normal chest film	Continuously monitor PA wave form at distal tip of PA catheter.	Forward migration of catheter into a wedged position will be evidenced by PAW waveform.
	Inflate balloon to wedge catheter briefly (<20 sec).	Minimize cessation in blood flow to reduce risk of pulmonary ischemia or infarction.
	Leave balloon of PA catheter deflated with stopcock open and syringe removed.	Open stopcock with syringe off permits passive deflation should any air remain in balloon.
	Monitor PAEDP instead of PAW (if close relationship).	Reduce risks caused by inflation of balloon and cessation of blood flow in branch of PA.

NURSING DIAGNOSIS: 4. Potential for Injury Related to (A) Hemorrhage, (B) Thromboemboli, (C) Venous Air Embolism, (D) Pulmonary Infarction or Hemorrhage, or (E) Cardiac Dysrhythmias or Conduction Disturbances—cont'd

Goals	Nursing intervention(s)	Rationale
	Check location of catheter tip after insertion and as needed by PA chest film.	Catheter tip can migrate forward with blood flow into a wedge position (particularly during first 24 hr).
	Continuously observe waveform during *slow* balloon inflation; stop inflation at first appearance of PAW waveform. Do not inflate 7-Fr catheter with more than 1.5 cc air.	Overinflation of balloon can cause rupture of vessel.
	Do not inflate balloon with air if resistance is met.	Catheter may be in a small branch of the PA and already mechanically wedged, or balloon may already be inflated.
E. Patient will remain free of life-threatening dysrhythmias or conduction disturbances	Continuously monitor waveform from distal port of catheter.	Appearance of RV waveform indicates catheter tip is in RV and could cause ventricular dysrhythmias.
	Monitor daily chest film.	Check for coiling of catheters in RV or RA, which could cause dysrhythmias.
	If RV waveform appears, quickly inflate balloon of catheter.	Catheter tip in RV can produce ventricular dysrhythmias; with balloon inflation, catheter tip will be covered and should float to PA.
	To remove catheter, deflate balloon actively and completely with syringe and quickly remove catheter.	Rapid removal of catheter with fully deflated balloon should result in few, if any, dysrhythmias.
	Follow emergency protocols for occurrence of life-threatening dysrhythmias.	

NURSING DIAGNOSIS: 5. Anxiety Related to Fear of Technologic Equipment and Procedures Associated with Hemodynamic Monitoring

Goals	Nursing intervention(s)	Rationale
Patient will: Verbalize feelings Demonstrate a relaxed manner Verbalize familiarity with hemodynamic monitoring procedures and equipment	Assess ability and readiness to learn the following, when appropriate: Reasons for hemodynamic monitoring Function and purpose of hemodynamic monitoring equipment Explanation of procedures related to hemodynamic monitoring.	Readiness to learn facilitates meaningful learning and retention of knowledge. Knowing rationale and purpose of hemodynamic monitoring reduces anxiety.
	Instruct patient in relaxation techniques.	Use of energy-release techniques helps reduce anxiety.
	Listen attentively, encourage verbalization, and provide a caring touch.	Reassures patient that he or she is not alone.

NURSING DIAGNOSIS: 6. Sleep Pattern Disturbance Related to Invasive Monitoring Procedures

Patient will have undisturbed sleep	Do not awaken or reposition patient to obtain hemodynamic parameters.	Hemodynamic measurements may be obtained with patient in supine, right or left lateral positions, or 45-degree semi-Fowler's position as long as air-reference stopcock is adjusted to mid-RA level and transducer is rezeroed.
	Instruct in relaxation techniques.	Energy-release techniques help relax patient and aid in sleep.
	Provide quiet, dimly lit environment.	Quiet, dark environment is more conducive to sleep.

Glossary

afterload Tension developed by the ventricle during systole. The arterial systolic pressure best reflects this parameter.

autoregulation Local control of blood flow by the blood vessels not mediated by neural activity.

Bowditch's law An increase in heart rate resulting in an increase in the contractile tension developed.

cardiac reserve Ability of the cardiac muscle to increase its cardiac output under stress (normally 300% to 400% over resting values).

carotid body (chemoreceptor) Cells adjacent to the carotid sinus that regulate respiration by responding to changes in Pa_{O_2}, Pa_{CO_2}, and pH.

carotid sinus (baroreceptors) Pressure or stretch receptors at the carotid bifurcation that maintain blood pressure through reflex mechanisms.

central venous pressure Pressure in the superior vena cava.

central venous return Venous blood flowing into the right atrium.

chronotropic Relating to the heart rate.

contractility Force of contraction when preload and afterload are held constant.

counterpulsation Action of circulatory assist pumping device synchronized counter to the normal action of the heart.

damping Diminished amplitude of pressure waves.

diastolic augmentation Increase in arterial diastolic pressure produced by counterpulsation of a circulatory assist device. This increase results in increased retrograde blood flow into the aortic root and coronary arteries.

diastolic filling pressure Pressure in the ventricle during diastole (filling period).

dp/dt Rate of pressure rise per unit of time. Another index of contractility but difficult to measure at the bedside.

ejection fraction Proportion of blood ejected from the ventricle per beat compared with end-diastolic volume.

Frank-Starling law The response to an increase in ventricular volume is an increase in myocardial fiber length, resulting in an increase in tension developed. This increase in tension results in an increase in the contractile force of the next beat and an increased stroke volume.

inotropic Relating to the force of a muscle contraction.

Kussmaul's sign Paradoxic rise in venous pressure and neck vein distention during inspiration; occurs in constrictive diseases.

La Place relation Tension of a wall of a sphere directly related to the pressure inside the cavity and to its radius; the tension is inversely related to the wall thickness.

mean pressure Time-averaged pressure, sometimes indicated by a dash over the value.

oxygen consumption Amount of oxygen in milliliters per minute used by the body to maintain aerobic metabolism.

preload Initial stretch of the myocardial fiber at end-diastole. The ventricular end-diastolic pressure and volume reflect this parameter.

pulmonary vascular resistance Resistance to forward blood flow through the lungs.

pulsus alternans Alternating strong and weak pulses caused by alterations in stroke volume.

pulsus bisferiens Double-peaked pulse associated with hypertrophic cardiomyopathy or aortic regurgitation.

pulsus paradoxus Decrease of more than 10 mm Hg in systolic blood pressure during spontaneous inspiration.

pulsus parvus Small pulse with low pulse pressure.

stroke volume Amount of blood ejected by the ventricle per heartbeat.

systemic vascular resistance Resistance to arterial blood flow.

systolic ejection period Time spent in systole per minute.

transducer Device that converts one type of energy into another.

Index